DIABETES AND HYPERTENSION: LIFESTYLE DISEASES-NEW RESEARCH FINDINGS

Edited by

Tanya Singh

ALLIED
HEALTH
PRESS

Diabetes and Hypertension: Lifestyle Diseases-New Research Findings

Editor: **Tanya Singh**

Allied Health Press
4164 Lakeshore Road
Burlington ON L7L 1A4
Canada
www.alliedhealthpress.com
Email: orders@arclereducation.com

ISBN: 978-1-77956-763-5

ABOUT THE EDITOR

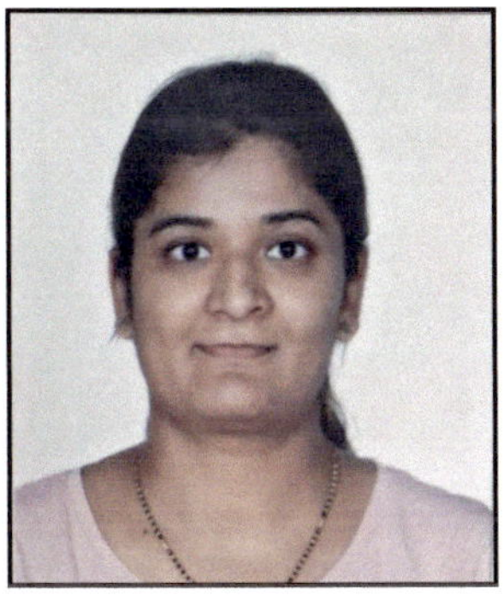

Tanya Singh is a biologist with a strong foundation in molecular biology, genetics, and mitochondrial research. She holds a Master of Science degree in Medical Biotechnology from the Postgraduate Institute of Medical Education and Research (PGIMER), Chandigarh, and has worked as a Scientific Assistant at the Tata Institute of Fundamental Research (TIFR), Hyderabad. During her time at TIFR, Tanya contributed to cutting-edge research in cellular and molecular biology, with a particular focus on mitochondrial function and genetic regulation. Her work reflects a deep commitment to scientific inquiry and a passion for exploring the mechanisms that govern life at its most fundamental level.

Brief Table of Contents

Detailed Table of Contents

CHAPTER 3

LIST OF FIGURES

LIST OF TABLES

PREFACE

The world is faced the COVID-19 pandemic that affected lives in multiple dimensions, with new viruses and conditions emerging each year. Apart from the physical, emotional, and financial damage wreaked, of prime importance is care for non-communicable diseases such as diabetes and hypertension.

> *"Man may be the captain of his fate, but he is also the victim of his blood sugar."*
> *—Wilfrid G. Oakley; Transactions of the Medical Society of London (1962), 78:16*

According to the WHO Fact Sheet, diabetes was the direct cause of 1.6 million deaths in 2021 and 47% of all these happened before the age of 70 years. Other challenges of diabetes are that the symptoms may appear suddenly and a major challenge is medication adherence.

Hypertension is estimated to affect 1.13 billion people across the globe with two-thirds in low/middle-income countries. The only way we can know if we have hypertension is by getting it measured by a healthcare professional. Hypertension can increase the risk of a slew of diseases such as heart disease, kidney disease, and stroke among others.

> *"One way to get high blood pressure is to go mountain climbing over molehills."*
> *—Earl Wilson*

So Why This Book?

The prevalence of hypertension is high in people with metabolic disorders, such as diabetes and cardiometabolic syndrome. Hypertension is common in diabetic patients and diabetes is common in patients with hypertension suggesting a chicken-egg relationship between these two conditions (Jia and Sowers, *Hypertension*, 2021). Cardiometabolic or cardiorenal metabolic syndrome includes cardiovascular disease (CVD) risk factors, such as type 2 diabetes, dyslipidemia, hypertension, obesity, and chronic kidney disease (CKD). This syndrome is often seen in type 2 diabetes patients; the risk of cardiovascular disease and retinopathy is significantly increased in patients with both diabetes and hypertension.

Research has shown that addressing high blood pressure (BP) in diabetic patients could improve the morbidity, such as lowered all-cause mortality in the Action in Diabetes and Vascular Disease: Preterax and Diamicron MR Controlled Evaluation trial (ADVANCE) and reduction in stroke and diabetes-related deaths in the United Kingdom Prospective Diabetes Study (UKPDS).

Several findings from research have been presented in this book on hypertension and diabetes. This becomes significant given that a book combining both these conditions is a valuable tool as opposed to unverified claims/theories on social media. This book presents an interesting section where alternative treatments and support for diabetes are discussed. This includes research-backed findings and suggestions on Ayurveda, herbs, yoga, exercises, and "apps."

In addition to blood sugar control (glycemic control) and blood pressure regulation, a multi-pronged approach is suggested to address stress factors, good diet, maintain good gut health, maintain the weight, following an exercise regimen, and overall optimal mental and physical health. A key factor here is the astute and prudent selection of therapy keeping the drug interactions in mind while selecting drug combinations.

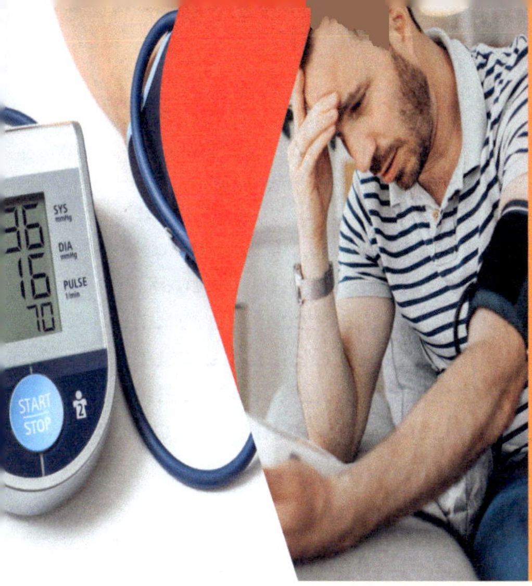

Chapter 1
HYPERTENSION

Contents

1.1. Introduction

Hypertension is a medical condition characterized by an increased systolic blood pressure (SBP) and/or diastolic blood pressure (DBP). The diagnosis of hypertension is typically made when a person's SBP and/or DBP levels are measured at 140 mmHg and/or 90 mmHg, respectively, following repeated examinations (Unger et al., 2020). Hypertension is a significant risk factor for cardiovascular and cerebrovascular diseases (CVDs) and is considered to be the leading cause of premature death worldwide (Mills et al., 2020). According to estimates, the prevalence of hypertension in the global adult population was 31.1% (1.39 billion) in 2010 and continues to rise (Mills et al., 2020). Preventing and controlling hypertension is a crucial global public health strategy for reducing premature mortality from CVDs. Hypertension is typically classified into two categories: essential (primary) hypertension, which lacks a defined cause, and secondary hypertension, which has a known cause (Sudharsanan et al., 2021).

Essential hypertension accounts for more than 90% of all hypertensive patients (Unger et al., 2020), but the precise underlying mechanisms remain unclear. The current treatment of essential hypertension primarily focuses on long-term blood pressure (BP) control rather than curing the disease, which is heavily dependent on the patient's financial status and adherence to treatment (Fang et al., 2020). Therefore, understanding the causative mechanisms has been a key research direction for essential hypertension. Two factors directly affect BP: vasodilation capacity and the volume of intravascular fluid. Vasodilation capacity is influenced by vascular elasticity, caliber, and reactivity, which reflect the vessel's ability to buffer against pressure shocks. Poorer vasodilation capacity leads to higher BP. The volume of intravascular fluid is regulated by the body's intake and elimination of fluid. An imbalance in fluid balance can cause an increase in BP when the amount of intravascular fluid increases. Factors that increase blood volume or decrease vasodilation capacity can lead to hypertension. These factors typically coexist and are intertwined in the occurrence and progression of essential hypertension. Currently, the lack of appropriate clinical identification methods presents challenges in creating effective treatment plans for hypertensive patients.

The primary approach for controlling hypertension is pharmacological treatment, which involves lifestyle intervention. The three primary antihypertensive medications are renin-angiotensin-aldosterone system (RAAS) inhibitors, calcium channel antagonists, and diuretics. Numerous single-pill combinations have been derived from these medications (Parati et al., 2021). Recent findings on essential hypertension have provided significant theoretical evidence, which is essential for better understanding and treating the condition.

1.2. Pathophysiology of Hypertension

Hypertension is a medical condition that requires a thorough understanding of its pathophysiology, as it can have significant implications for treatment and the prevention of complications. The baroreflex plays a crucial role in regulating BP through a negative feedback loop, activated by stretch receptors located in the carotid sinus and aorta. When blood vessels stretch due to high BP, baroreceptors are activated and send signals to the nucleus tractus solitarius (NTS) in the brain stem via the glossopharyngeal nerve and vagus nerve. This activates the parasympathetic nervous system (PNS), which releases acetylcholine that acts on the pacemaker cells in the sinoatrial node, resulting in vasodilatation, reduced heart rate, and normalized BP (Wallbach and Koziolek, 2018). On the other hand, when baroreceptors detect a decrease in BP, they send signals to the NTS, which in turn deactivates the PNS and activates the sympathetic nervous system (SNS). The SNS, through the action of catecholamines, increases heart rate, cardiac output, and constricts blood vessels, resulting in an increase in arterial BP, resistance, and decrease in blood flow. The efferent fibers of the SNS also activate the kidney to secrete renin, triggering the RAAS. The RAAS is activated under physiological conditions in response to a decrease in renal BP, with the goal of restoring systemic blood volume and pressure. Specifically, juxtaglomerular cells release renin into the bloodstream, where it acts on angiotensinogen from the liver to produce its active form, angiotensin. Angiotensin I is then converted to angiotensin II by angiotensin converting enzyme from the lungs. Angiotensin II binds to angiotensin II type I and 2 receptors in the adrenal cortex, kidneys, and arterioles, where it elicits multiple effector functions, including vasoconstriction and increased Na^{2+} reabsorption in the kidneys through aldosterone (Craft et al., 2015). In hypertension arising from arterial issues, the baroreflex mechanism adapts to a higher set point to maintain hypertension rather than lowering it. Additionally, genetic and environmental factors, diminished vessel wall flexibility, and uncoupling of receptors with the vessel wall can contribute to decreased sensitivity of baroreceptors. The parasympathetic tone is reduced while the SNS is overactive (Fernandez et al., 2015). Moreover, excessive production of angiotensin II, insufficient activity of vasodilators, including nitric oxide (NO), natriuretic peptides, and prostacyclin (as depicted in Figure 1.1), can also lead to hypertension.

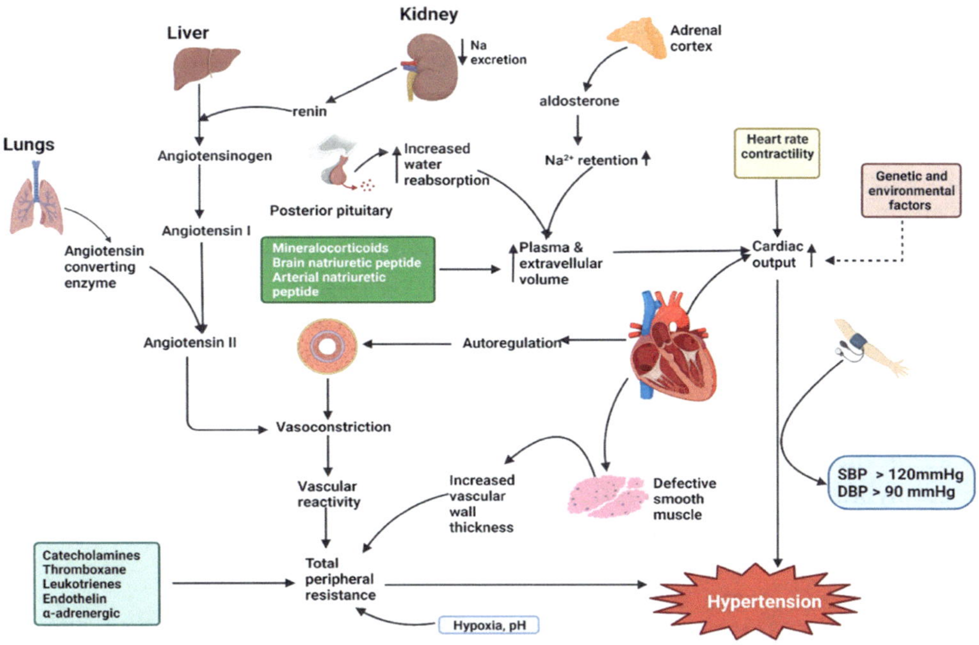

Figure 1.1. The regulation of blood pressure (BP) is influenced by multiple factors.

Note: BP is the result of cardiac output and peripheral vascular resistance. Local factors, such as pH, hypoxia, and humoral factors (including angiotensin II, catecholamines, and thromboxanes), can impact peripheral resistance, while factors such as blood volume, atrial and brain natriuretic peptides, and cardiac factors (including heart rate and contractility) can impact cardiac output. When systemic BP decreases, renin is produced from the juxtaglomerular cells of the kidney, which stimulates the activation of angiotensinogen in the liver to angiotensin I. Angiotensin I is then converted to angiotensin II by angiotensin converting enzyme from the lungs. Angiotensin II causes blood vessels to constrict and promotes the release of aldosterone from the adrenal glands, which in turn triggers sodium reabsorption. Antidiuretic hormones from the pituitary glands are also released, causing water reabsorption. These combined effects lead to increased blood volume and BP (Adua, 2023).

Both RAAS and SNS can exert an impact on the function of vascular smooth muscle (VSM) cells, ultimately resulting in vasoconstriction and hypertension. The contraction of VSM is contingent upon the levels of intracellular calcium, which increase upon the binding of a neurotransmitter, such as acetylcholine, and a vasoactive agent, like angiotensin II, to receptors of phospholipase C (PLC). This activation of PLC yields inositol triphosphate (IP3) and diacylglycerol (DAG), which subsequently trigger the release and mobilization of Ca^{2+} from the sarcoplasmic reticulum and promote cell proliferation. DAG also stimulates protein kinase C (PKC), a key enzyme involved in cellular signaling pathways (Rusell et al., 2018). The entry of other Ca^{2+} ions into the cells results in an accumulation of Ca^{2+}. This Ca^{2+} then binds to calmodulin, forming a calcium-calmodulin complex. The activation of myosin light chain (MLC) kinase by this complex leads to the formation of cross bridges between myosin heads and actin filaments, resulting in the shortening of myofibrils and contraction of the VSM cells. Additionally, VSM cells can be stimulated by oxidative stress, hemodynamic changes, and mechanical forces. Hypertension is also characterized by endothelial dysfunction and increased arterial stiffness.

1.3. Arterial Stiffness

Arterial stiffness refers to a decrease in the elasticity and distensibility of arteries, and pulse wave velocity (PWV) is commonly used to measure the extent of stiffness in large arteries. An increase in PWV indicates severe arterial stiffness and impaired ability to expand (Segers et al., 2020). Arterial stiffness has been strongly linked to an increased risk of essential hypertension (Dumor et al., 2018), particularly isolated systolic hypertension (Chirinos et al., 2019). On the other hand, SBP is also associated with a clinically significant progression of arterial stiffness (Wilson and Webb, 2020). It remains unclear whether elevated BP or arterial stiffness comes first in this relationship.

Arterial stiffness can be categorized into functional arterial stiffness and structural arterial stiffness (Zanoli et al., 2020). Functional arterial stiffness is primarily linked to the contractile function of vascular smooth muscle cells (VSMCs), which is influenced by a myriad of factors (*see* Figure 1.2). Among these factors, an increase in intracellular calcium ion (Ca^{2+}) concentration can directly impact VSMCs, and calcium channel blockers (CCBs) are commonly used in clinical settings to reduce intracellular calcium concentration in SMCs and thus control BP. The nitric oxide (NO)–nitric oxide-sensitive guanylate cyclase (NOsGC)–cGMP pathway is a well-studied pathway that is closely related to the contractile function of VSMCs. This pathway begins in vascular endothelial cells and regulates VSMC contraction through a series of signaling events (Garcia and Sessa, 2019). Injectable antihypertensive drugs, such as sodium nitroprusside and nitrates, all exert their vasodilatory effects through the NO-NOsGC-cGMP pathway.

Structural arterial stiffness has been closely linked to age, hyperlipidemia, and diabetes mellitus (DM). This condition is characterized by elastin disruption, collagen deposition, and altered extracellular matrix (ECM) composition (Zanoli et al., 2020). Despite the strong correlation between functional arterial stiffness and various risk factors, there is currently no effective treatment for structural arterial stiffness. This is due to the difficulty in reversing the pathological changes that occur in this condition. The transition of VSMCs from their contractile phenotype to other phenotypes directly impacts structural arterial stiffness. Among the six reported phenotypes of VSMCs, the contractile phenotype is rich in a-smooth muscle actin (a-SMA) and exhibits the strongest contractile function. When VSMCs switch from the contractile to other phenotypes, such as the macrophage-like phenotype, the contractile function of the cells decreases significantly (Chattopadhyay et al., 2021). Krüppel-Like Factor 4 (KLF4) has been identified as a key target in regulating the conversion of contractile VSMCs to other phenotypes (Yap et al., 2021). However, while most studies have shown an important role for KLF4 in pulmonary hypertension (PH) (Chandran et al., 2021), its role in VSMCs remains unclear with regard to essential hypertension.

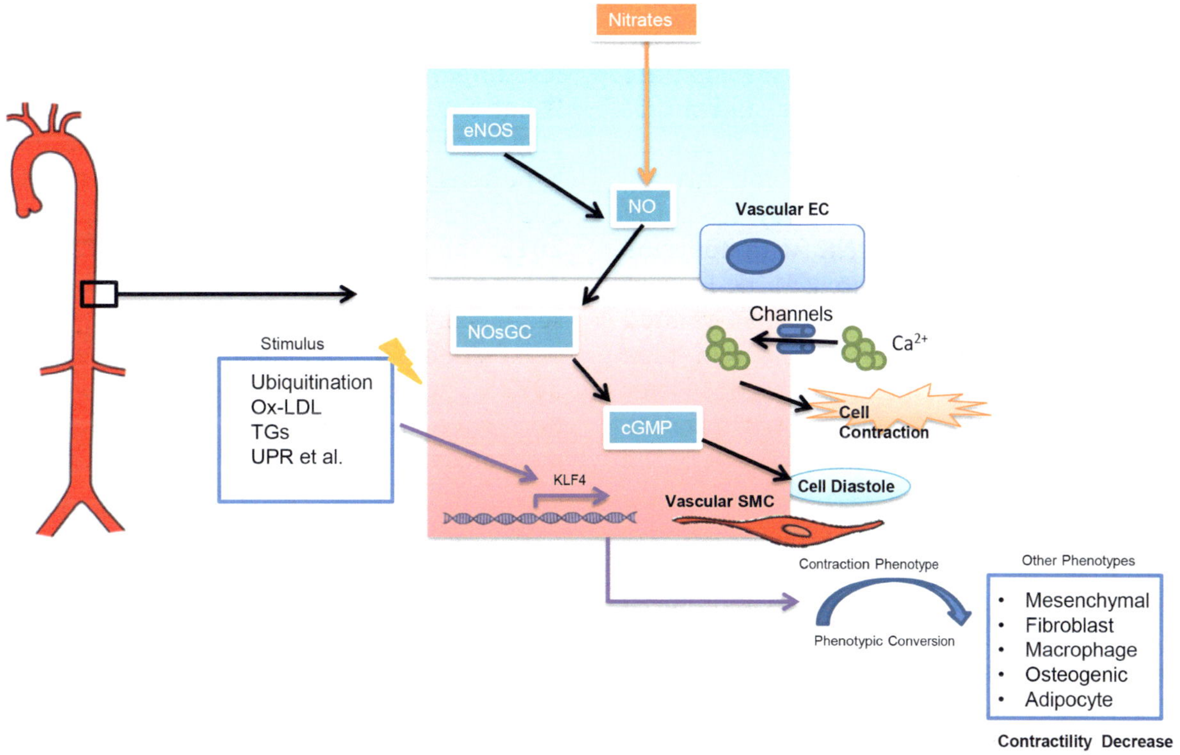

Figure 1.2. Factors influencing the contractile function of smooth muscle cells [Ox-LDL: Oxidized low-density lipoprotein; TGs: triglycerides; UPR: unfolded protein response; and KLF4: Krüppel-like factor 4] (Ma and Chen, 2022).

1.4. Water-Sodium Retention and Salt-Sensitive

Water retention and sodium are significant contributors to the occurrence of elevated intravascular fluid volume. Diuretics, particularly thiazide diuretics, play a crucial role in managing hypertension caused by water-sodium retention (Roush and Sica, 2016). Excluding secondary hypertension resulting from renal dysfunction, there exists another group of hypertensive patients who are affected by water-sodium retention in essential hypertension, known as salt-sensitive hypertension.

High salt intake is a significant trigger for essential hypertension caused by water-sodium retention. However, not all individuals will experience increased BP after consuming excessive salt. Patients who are sensitive to salt are referred to as salt-sensitive, while those who are resistant to salt are referred to as salt-resistant (Morris et al., 2016). Several factors may contribute to the development of salt-sensitive hypertension, including age, obesity, genetic background, and maternal conditions during fetal life, among others (Kawarazaki and Fujita, 2021). Despite this, the underlying mechanisms of salt-sensitive hypertension are not fully understood. Studies have shown that low potassium levels activate the system by hyperpolarizing the membrane, thereby driving chloride out of the cell and away from the inhibitory binding site on WNK (with no lysine [K]) kinases. Once disinhibited, WNK kinases phosphoactivate SPAK (STE20/SPS1-related proline/alanine-rich kinase), which in turn phosphoactivates nine-rich kinase co-transporter (NCC), known as the Potassium Switch theory (Ellison and Welling, 2021), which is one of the important theories on the pathogenesis of salt-sensitive hypertension. Recent evidence has also shown that intestinal flora is closely associated with salt-sensitive hypertension (Muralitharan et al., 2020) (Figure 1.3). The fecal microbiota of healthy rats can significantly lower BP in high-salt diet-induced hypertensive (hSIH) rats, while the fecal microbiota of hSIH rats has the opposite effect (Yan et al., 2020). Adoptive transfer of fecal material from conventionally housed high-salt diet-fed mice to germ-free mice predisposes them to increased inflammation and hypertension, which may be attributed to an increase in *Firmicutes*, *Proteobacteria*, and genus *Prevotella* bacteria (Ferguson et al., 2020). The precise mechanisms by which intestinal flora influences BP remain under investigation. Research has suggested that high salt intake can deplete Lactobacillus and stimulate the production of T helper 17 cells, ultimately contributing to hypertension (Wilck et al., 2017). Another study demonstrated that high salt diets can reduce the levels of *B. fragilis* and arachidonic acid in the intestine, leading to increased production of intestinal-derived corticosterone and elevated corticosterone levels in both the intestine and serum, which in turn promotes increased BP levels (Yan et al., 2020). In the DOCA-salt mice model of hypertension, short-chain fatty acids produced by the fermentation of fiber from intestinal flora have been associated with lower BP levels, and this may be related to the increase in *Bacteroides acidifaciens* (Marques et al., 2017). It is important to note that the intestinal flora is not only involved in salt sensitivity but also plays a role in other underlying mechanisms of hypertension, including the RAAS (Kaye et al., 2020), vascular endothelium (Natarajan et al., 2016), and renal dysfunction, among others. A recent large-scale study of intestinal flora sequencing has demonstrated the complex role of intestinal flora in human health (Zheng et al., 2022). The presence and activity of intestinal flora have the potential to be an independent mechanism of essential hypertension.

Reducing sodium intake is widely recognized as an effective method for reducing the prevalence of hypertension, according to Graudal et al. (2020). However, the advantages of consuming low-sodium salt remain a subject of debate, as low sodium intake has also been linked to an increased risk of cardiovascular disease (CVD). Recent advancements have been made in the application of salt substitution. An excessive intake of sodium leads to an increase in circulating fluid, which in turn raises BP. On the other hand, potassium has a diuretic effect, which reduces circulating fluid. Clinical studies have demonstrated that both reducing dietary sodium and supplementing with potassium can lead to significant reductions in BP (Huang et al., 2020).

According to the Potassium Switch theory, an increase in dietary sodium intake does not guarantee a decrease in potassium intake, and thus, salt sensitivity increases (Ellison and Welling, 2021). Salt substitution, which reduces sodium chloride and increases potassium chloride, has been shown to exhibit antihypertensive effects (Greer et al., 2020). There are two primary forms of salt substitution currently being studied in clinical trials. The first consists of only sodium chloride and potassium chloride (Neal et al., 2021), while the second includes magnesium sulfate along with sodium chloride and potassium chloride (Sun et al., 2021). Research has demonstrated that both types of salt substitution not only lower BP but also decrease the risk of cardiovascular events in patients (Li et al., 2022). Furthermore, the use of sodium and potassium salts, in which 75% of the mass is sodium chloride and 25% is potassium chloride, has both therapeutic benefits and economic advantages (Li et al., 2022). The results of studies suggest that salt recommendations for the general population, particularly hypertensive patients, will likely change in the near future. In order to promote the use of salt substitutes, it is essential to raise awareness of their benefits among the population (Liu et al., 2021).

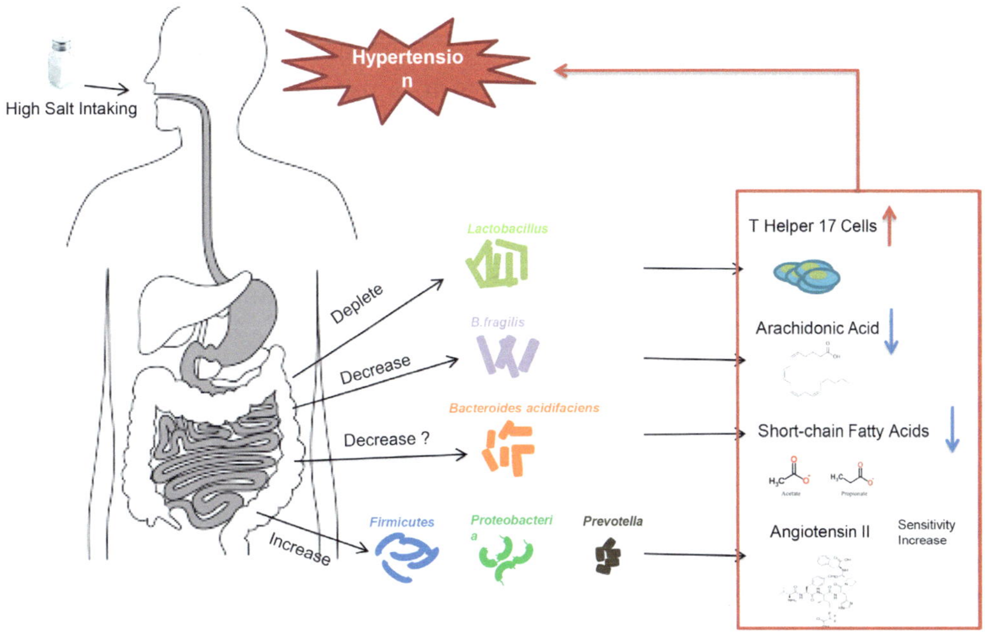

Figure 1.3. High salt intake triggers high blood pressure (BP) through intestinal flora (Ma and Chen, 2022).

1.5. Renin-Angiotensin-Aldosterone System (RAAS)

The system known as the RAAS is a series of peptidergic processes that play a crucial role in the regulation of the renal, adrenal, and cardiovascular systems. Specifically, RAAS controls BP by influencing arterial constriction and water-sodium balance within the body. Both circulating RAAS and tissue RAAS (including cardiac RAAS, vascular RAAS, intra-renal RAAS, brain RAAS, and adipose tissue RAAS) have been implicated in the pathogenesis of essential hypertension and associated target organ damage (Riet et al., 2015). The RAAS axis cascade comprises several components, such as angiotensinogen, renin, angiotensin converting enzyme, and various subtypes of angiotensin (Ang I, Ang II, Ang III, Ang IV, Ang 1-7), aldosterone, and aldosterone receptors. Angiotensinogen, produced by the liver, serves as the starting point for this system. Angiotensinogen is cleaved by renin, secreted by the kidney, to form angiotensin I. Angiotensin I is then cleaved in the circulatory system by enzymes (e.g., angiotensin converting enzyme) to generate different peptides that act on various organs (Abdel, 2020). Among these cleavage peptides, angiotensin II has been most extensively studied. Angiotensin II binds to angiotensin II receptors (classified as type 1 and 2) in several organs and directly causes vasoconstriction, water-sodium retention, and myocardial remodeling. Moreover, when angiotensin II acts on the kidney, it stimulates aldosterone secretion, exacerbating water-sodium retention.

RAAS inhibitors are considered one of the three key medications for treating hypertension and are often the first choice for patients with target organ damage, such as heart failure or renal failure. Clinical trials have demonstrated that RAAS blockers, including ACE inhibitors (ACEIs), ARBs, ARNI, and MRAs, can help prevent hypertension and protect target organs (Unger et al., 2020). In addition to oral medications, hypertension vaccines that target the RAAS system have become increasingly popular in recent years. The first hypertension vaccine has been studied for over 30 years, and ongoing research continues to explore its potential. Compared to drug therapy, vaccine treatment has the potential to improve health outcomes, reduce healthcare costs, and increase medication adherence, as it can induce long-term therapeutic effects with low frequency of administration. However, current hypertension vaccines mainly target the RAAS system, and while renin vaccines were the first to be developed, they carry the risk of causing autoimmune diseases and have not shown long-term cardiovascular or renal protective effects in clinical studies, despite lowering BP (Zhao et al., 2020). Other vaccines targeting Ang I, Ang II, AT1R, etc., have shown promising results in lowering BP at the animal level without significant side effects. To date, only CYT006-AngQb, an Ang II vaccine, has shown positive results in phase II clinical studies. While it is important to acknowledge that RAAS inhibitors have already been widely and successfully used in clinical settings, vaccines may pose some challenges for patients, including the potential for pain and the need for multiple injections. However, recent research has highlighted the potential of non-RAAS-targeted vaccines, such as the short peptide ADR-004 (cgiteeagy), which was identified from α1D-adrenoceptor (α1D-AR). In addition to effectively lowering BP, this vaccine has demonstrated target organ protection following administration to spontaneous hypertension rats. By targeting α1D-AR, the ADRQb-004 vaccine may address some of the limitations of current clinical treatments, including low subtype selectivity and short half-life of a1-AR blockers (Li et al., 2019).

1.6. Sympathetic Dysregulation

Dysregulation of the SNS is a significant contributor to essential hypertension. The excessive activation of the SNS results in increased cardiac output, heightened vascular tone, and elevated levels of plasma catecholamines. Individuals with hypertension often exhibit increased muscle sympathetic nerve activity (MSNA) and reduced baroreflex sensitivity.

Sympathetic hypertension can vary significantly among individuals and often exhibits circadian patterns and associations with mental status. Myogenic skeletal muscle nitrous oxide (MSNA) plays a crucial role in determining total peripheral resistance and vasoconstrictive function. It is possible that MSNA may be a significant cause of the substantial individual variability in sympathetic hypertension, as research has shown that the transduction of MSNA into vascular tone differs by age and sex (Kobetic et al., 2022), and there is a close relationship between MSNA and both attended (observed) and unattended (unobserved) BP levels in essential hypertension (Manta et al., 2020). The manifestations of BP changes in sympathetic hypertension are complex, including morning hypertension, nocturnal hypertension, sleep apnea-related hypertension, orthostatic hypertension, and resistant hypertension, among others. These changes may all be associated with autonomic dysregulation (Kario et al., 2020). Sympathetic overdrive not only contributes to the progression of BP elevation but also promotes hypertension-related target organ damage, including left ventricular hypertrophy and dysfunction, congestive heart failure, and renal insufficiency (Kario et al., 2020). Beta-blockers are commonly used clinically to inhibit the increase in BP and heart rate caused by sympathetic excitation. However, compared to other antihypertensive agents, such as diuretics, ACEi, ARB, and CCBs, beta-blockers appear to be less protective against stroke and overall mortality, and are more often used as additional drugs for hypertensive patients (Thomopoulos et al., 2020). Exercise is a crucial method for controlling sympathetic hypertension, and research has demonstrated that high-intensity interval training (e.g., three 60-min exercise sessions per week for 4 months) can reduce BP by decreasing MSNA (Ehlers et al., 2020).

Renal denervation (RDN) is an emerging treatment option for hypertension caused by sympathetic dysregulation. Research indicates that renal sensory afferent nerve activity directly impacts sympathetic outflow to the kidneys and other organs involved in cardiovascular control. By abrogating these nerves, both BP and organ-specific damage caused by chronic sympathetic overactivity can be reduced in various experimental models. Currently, catheter-based radiofrequency denervation of the renal arteries is the most widely used technique for RDN, and its safety and antihypertensive effect are gradually gaining recognition. Numerous clinical trials related to RDN are currently underway.

1.7. Genetics

Hypertension is strongly associated with genetic factors, and research has enhanced our understanding of the relationship between genetics and BP in recent years. According to genome-wide association studies, more than 500 genetic loci regulating BP have been identified, resulting in over 1000 BP genetic loci in total (Cabrera et al., 2019). Some researchers even propose that BP is a probable omnigenic trait (Evengelou et al., 2018). However, identifying a true causal variant and its associated gene product is rarely straightforward. The lead single nucleotide polymorphism (SNP) usually indicates a chromosomal region with tens or even thousands of SNPs in linkage disequilibrium (LD), but it may also point to more distant regions with long-range chromatin interactions (Schmitt et al., 2016). Consequently, these SNPs often occur in noncoding regions of the genome, do not affect protein function, and have a small impact on BP. Although SNPs offer a potential pathogenic mechanism for essential hypertension, there are few reported targets that have been successfully translated into clinical use. A study conducted recently demonstrated that analyzing multiple SNPs as a polygenic risk score (PRS) was predictive of early-onset hypertension in a progressive manner. Individuals with the highest 2.5% PRS had a nearly three-fold higher risk of developing hypertension, while a low PRS was protective (Vaura et al., 2021). Utilizing SNPs effectively may provide potential ways to diagnose and treat hypertension.

Heredity alone cannot account for the variability in BP, suggesting that additional risk factors are at play, such as epigenetic adjustments. Recent research has uncovered the possible contribution of epigenetic mechanisms to essential hypertension. Genome-wide DNA methylation has been connected to an increased risk of hypertension in humans (Richard et al., 2017), and DNA methylation regulates several genes that are crucial for BP regulation, as demonstrated in animal models. In addition to DNA methylation, RNA methylation may also have a role in essential hypertension (Paramasivam et al., 2020). Studies have shown that N6-methyladenosine (m6A) – SNPs are enriched among the SNPs associated with BP, and approximately 10% of the BP-associated m6A SNPs are linked to coronary artery disease (CAD) or stroke (Mo et al., 2019). However, the precise function of these RNA methylation sites in the development of hypertension remains to be further investigated. Other epigenetic modifications, such as post-translational histone modifications, non-coding RNAs (ncRNAs), and so on, have also been suggested as promising areas for future research into the prevention and treatment of essential hypertension (Arif et al., 2019).

1.8. Interactions Between the Pathogenesis of Hypertension

A new Mosaic Theory has been proposed to provide insight into the development of hypertension, which is now understood as a response to a variety of traits and stressors (Harrison et al., 2021). In addition to factors such as vascular function, salt intake, sympathetic activation, genetics, microbiome, renal mechanisms, the theory now also emphasizes the importance of inflammation and oxidative stress (Harrison et al., 2021). The complex interplay of these factors results in an intricate pathogenesis of essential hypertension, making the treatment of this condition more challenging.

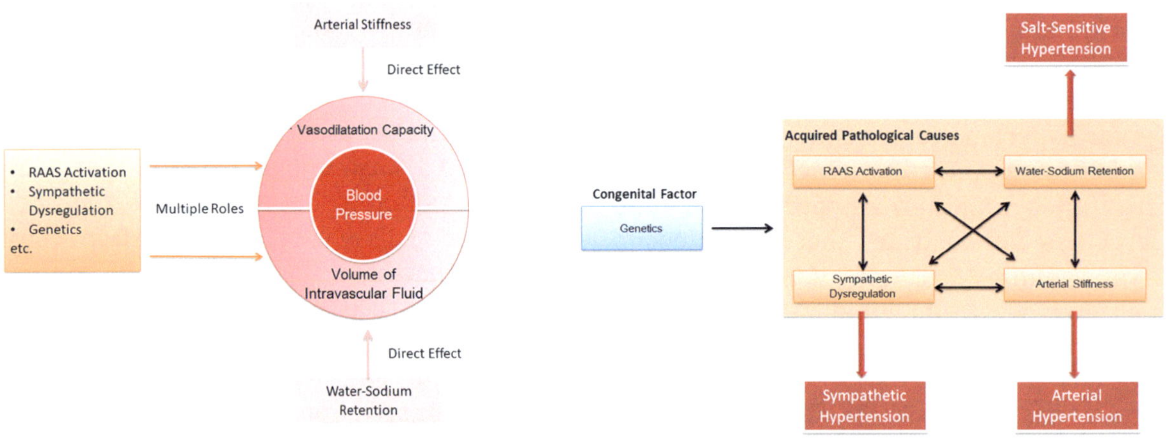

Figure 1.4. Interaction between the pathogenesis of hypertension. (A) Causes of elevated blood pressure (BP) by different pathogenesis; and (B) interaction between pathogenic mechanisms (Ma and Chen, 2022).

In our professional opinion, the etiology of hypertension is believed to be rooted in a combination of decreased vasodilation and increased blood volume. Arterial stiffness, for instance, directly results in decreased vasodilation, while water-sodium retention directly contributes to an increase in blood volume. Other factors, such as the RAAS, sympathetic system, and genes, also impact both vasodilation and blood volume (Figure 1.4(A)). These factors are interconnected, and their interactions are complex. As a genetic factor, the influence of genes can extend to RAAS, water-sodium retention, arterial stiffness, and sympathetic nerves. This is supported by studies showing that genes can affect multiple factors simultaneously (Mocan et al., 2021). Additionally, the mutual influence between RAAS, water-sodium retention, arterial stiffness, and sympathetic nerves is also evident (Jia et al., 2018) (Figure 1.4(B)).

1.9. Circulating Biomarkers

Biomarkers are a crucial aspect of disease diagnosis and treatment, particularly in patient classification, risk assessment, and therapy monitoring. In recent years, several potential circulating biomarkers have been identified for hypertension screening. One such biomarker is Pentraxin 3 (PTX3), which, when administered to wild-type mice, was found to induce endothelial dysfunction and increase BP, whereas no such effect was observed in P-selectin-deficient mice (Carrizzo et al., 2015). Moreover, hypertensive patients exhibit higher plasma levels of PTX3 and its mediators P-selectin and matrix metalloproteinase-1 (MMP1) compared to normotensive subjects (Carrizzo et al., 2015). This suggests that the combination of PTX3, P-selectin, and MMP-1 may serve as a novel biomarker for predicting vascular dysfunction in hypertensive patients. Additionally, sortilin, a member of the vacuolar protein sorting 10 (VPS10P) family of receptors, has been positively correlated with vascular and metabolic disorders (Goettsch et al., 2018). A recent study demonstrated that sortilin induces endothelial dysfunction of mesenteric arteries through NADPH oxidase 2 (NOX2) isoform activation, and this dysfunction can be prevented by knockdown of acid sphingomyelinase (ASMase) or sphingosine kinase 1 (Di Pietro et al., 2022). Furthermore, plasma ASMase activity and plasma levels of sortilin increase in hypertensive subjects, especially those with uncontrolled BP (Di Pietro et al., 2022). Thus, high levels of circulating sortilin may help explain resistance to anti-hypertensive pharmacological treatment. Other potential biomarkers for hypertension include Sphingosine-1-phosphate (Jujic et al., 2021), bactericidal/permeability-increasing fold-containing family B member 4 (BPIFB4) (Vecchione et al., 2017), klotho (Drew et al., 2021), exosomal microRNAs (such as miR-130a, miR-195) (Tan et al., 2021), SUV420H1 (Zhang et al., 2020), and others that may have potential in hypertension prediction or evaluation.

The use of specific markers in the evaluation of hypertension can lead to a better understanding of its underlying mechanisms. Additionally, these markers have the potential to classify essential hypertension due to their specificity. For instance, PTX3 and sortilin are related to vascular dysfunction, while SUV420H1 is identified as a potential biomarker for the early diagnosis of salt-sensitive hypertension. These specific sources of markers can provide guidance for targeted treatment of hypertension with different pathogenesis.

1.10. The Role of the Kidney and Body Fluid Volumes in Hypertension

The kidney is a vital component of Dr. Page's Mosaic Theory. Figure 1.5(A) pertains to volume and cardiac output. Cardiac output is calculated by multiplying heart rate and cardiac stroke volume, with stroke volume determined by venous return, which is largely influenced by the kidneys and their regulation of volume homeostasis. Dr. Page's early work aimed to develop a complex mathematical model to understand the dynamic interactions between the Mosaic components. This model predicted that the renal pressure natriuresis mechanism played a primary role in regulating body fluids and setting BP levels, while the central nervous system and vascular function, among other factors, provided important modulation. Numerous studies have demonstrated the critical role of the kidney in regulating BP. For instance, hypertensive animals' kidneys cause an increase in BP when transplanted into normal animals. Furthermore, the transplantation of kidneys from normotensive donors to patients with renal failure due to hypertensive nephrosclerosis has sometimes led to a reversal of their hypertension and related organ damage. Recent research has shown that transplanting kidneys from mice lacking the angiotensin type 1 receptor protects wild-type recipient mice from Ang II-induced hypertension. Conversely, transplanting wild-type kidneys into AT1R (angiotensin type 1 receptor) knockout mice restores their ability to develop hypertension upon Ang II infusion. These findings shed light on a critical aspect of hypertension involving Ang II and its primary receptor in the kidneys, providing further insight into the theories of Page and Guyton (Harrison et al., 2021).

The kidney fulfills multiple crucial functions in the context of hypertension. Foremost, it is responsible for the synthesis of renin, an aspartic protease that cleaves angiotensinogen into angiotensin I, which subsequently undergoes conversion by the ACE to Ang II. Renin is a limiting factor in the activation of the renin-angiotensin system (RAS) and its synthesis and secretion by the kidney are tightly regulated (Guessoum et al., 2021). Renin is initially synthesized as the inactive precursor prorenin, which becomes active upon binding to the PRR (prorenin receptor). Under normal circumstances, renin is produced almost entirely by specialized juxtaglomerular cells of the afferent arteriole. It is released in response to a reduction in perfusion pressure, a decrease in the delivery of sodium chloride to *macula densa* cells, or an increase in sympathetic stimulation. Prolonged stimulation of the renal sympathetic nerves can transform a subset of VSMCs into renin-producing cells in the afferent arteriole. This transformation is regulated by the transcription factor SRY-related HMG-box gene (Sox)-6 (Saleem et al., 2020). Additionally, principal cells of the collecting duct can produce renin. This process is partly mediated by a loss of NO production in various pathophysiological conditions (Curnow et al., 2020). Although renin is typically released almost exclusively from the juxtaglomerular apparatus (JG) of the kidney, the proximal tubules can become an important site of renin production during oxidative stress or in response to increased glomerular protein filtration.

The kidneys play a crucial role in the regulation of BP in hypertensive individuals. One of these roles is to reset or alter the pressure diuresis and natriuresis. When BP rises, there is a significant increase in diuresis and natriuresis, which helps to bring BP back to normal levels. Researchers have identified the relationship between BP and sodium and water excretion as the pressure natriuresis curve, and they believe that a rightward resetting of this curve is necessary for hypertension to be sustained. Although the mechanisms for pressure natriuresis and its resetting are complex, substantial evidence suggests that increased renal interstitial pressure and alterations in sodium transporters, such as the NHE3 (sodium hydrogen exchanger 3) and the sodium-phosphate cotransporter isoform 2 in the proximal tubule, are significant factors. Acute hypertension causes these transporters to move from the luminal cell membrane to the base of the apical microvilli in the proximal tubule, where they cannot participate in sodium reabsorption. Additionally, an increase in BP can relocate the thiazide-sensitive sodium chloride cotransporter in the distal tubule. However, during chronic hypertension, these transporters are translocated to the apical microvilli, where they enhance sodium reabsorption and likely contribute to the maintenance of hypertension (McDonough and Nguyen, 2015). Renovascular hypertension upregulates SGLT2 (sodium-glucose-linked transporter type 2) in the proximal tubule, which is functionally linked to NHE3 via the microtubule-associated protein 3 to enhance proximal Na+ reabsorption during reactive oxygen species (ROS) stimulation. The administration of an SGLT2 inhibitor into the proximal tubule inhibits Na+:H+ exchange, leading to a 27% inhibition of proximal Na+ and fluid reabsorption in diabetic rats. This finding may explain the reported effects of SGLT2 inhibitors in reducing plasma volume in heart failure and BP in hypertension. Multiple other sodium transport mechanisms are also affected, as previously reviewed by McDonough and Nguyen (2015).

The influence of Ang II, inflammatory cytokines, the loss of NO, and adrenergic stimulation can lead to variations in the location and function of transporters. It is essential to recognize that alterations in pressure natriuresis may not always be evident through routine clinical assessments, including measurements of blood urea nitrogen, creatinine, and creatinine clearance. Furthermore, the retention of Na+ in the kidneys associated with hypertension is not typically accompanied by obvious indications of fluid accumulation (Harrison et al., 2021).

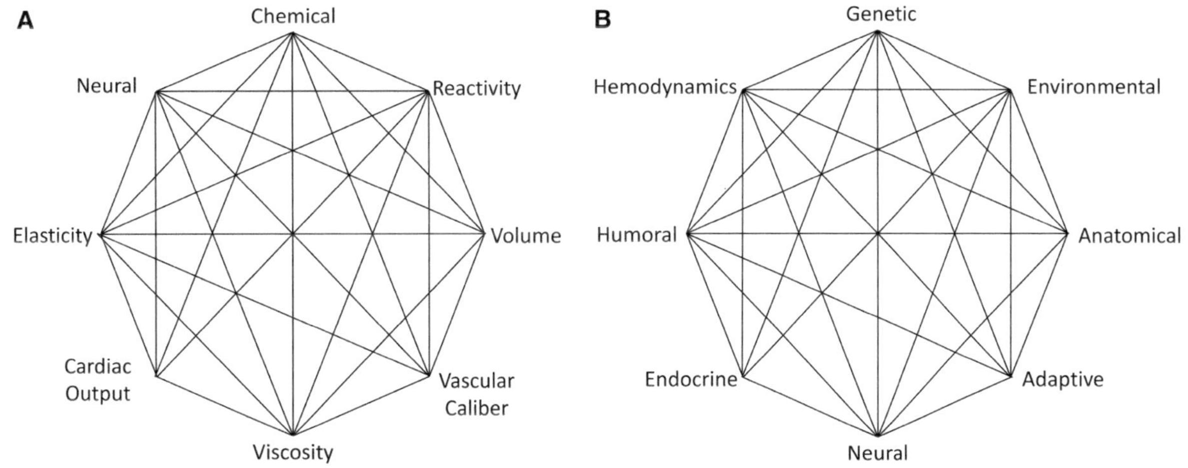

Figure 1.5. The original (A) and revised (B) mosaic theories proposed by Page (Harrison et al., 2021).

The kidney has been found to play an important role in the regulation of hypertension, with its recently recognized ability to modulate systemic sympathetic tone through the generation of reflex signals via renal afferent nerves. While the majority of renal nerves are efferent, sending sympathetic signals to the kidney and enhancing tubular sodium resorption, renin release, and vasomotor tone, a smaller proportion are afferents that transmit signals from within the kidney to the brain stem, where they can initiate reflexes that promote increases in efferent SNS tone and induce hypertension. Studies have shown that severing renal afferent nerve traffic can significantly reduce hypertension in rats with 5/6 nephrectomy, and that injection of a small bolus of phenol into one pole of the kidney can increase renal afferent nerve activity and norepinephrine production by the posterior hypothalamus, leading to hypertension. These effects were abrogated by RDN, suggesting that excitation of renal afferent nerves played a critical role in the development of hypertension. Banek et al. reported that renal deafferentation reduced hypertension in rats with deoxycorticosterone acetate–salt hypertension, and that the ability of renal afferent nerves to initiate an increase in global sympathetic outflow might explain the pleiotropic effects of RDN. In Ang II-induced hypertension, however, renal efferent nerves seem to have a predominant role.

The kidney is a vital organ that serves multiple functions, one of which is to act as a site of immune activation in hypertension. Research has shown that Ang II-induced hypertension triggers the activation of antigen-presenting dendritic cells in the kidney, which then migrate to secondary lymphoid organs to activate T cells. These T cells subsequently return to the kidney, a process that is impeded by RDN. This suggests that efferent renal nerves promote neoantigen formation in the kidney during hypertension. Single-cell sequencing has revealed that the kidney, unlike blood vessels or the spleen, accumulates T cells with an oligoclonal T-cell receptor population, further supporting the kidney's role in antigen formation (Xiao et al., 2015).

1.11. The Role of the Vasculature in Hypertension

There are a minimum of four vascular disturbances that contribute to and occur in hypertension. The first is an elevated environment of vasoconstrictor hormones, including Ang II, catecholamines, and vasopressin, as well as alterations in vascular function that encourage vasoconstriction and limit vasodilation. Studies of isolated blood vessels have demonstrated that both conduit vessels and arterioles from hypertensive animals exhibit heightened vasoconstriction in response to various agents. Of particular note are genes that regulate GPCR (G protein-coupled receptor) signaling, such as the RGS (regulators of G protein signaling) proteins, which promote GTP hydrolysis to terminate G protein signaling. RGS proteins 1 and 2 are linked to GPCRs that enhance responses to vasoconstrictors including thromboxane, Ang II, and norepinephrine (Harrison et al., 2021). Additional research demonstrated that VSMCs from these animals displayed increased calcium transients, with delayed returns to baseline following agonist stimulation. A crucial role for RGS2 was highlighted in subsequent studies, which showed that RGS2 in the renal vasculature was essential for promoting hypertension. Recently, Patel et al. have identified an essential role played by RGS1 in regulating vascular control in atherosclerotic ApoE-deficient mice. Upon RGS1 knockout, there was a significant increase in BP and vasoconstriction in response to phenylephrine, thromboxane, and Ang II (Arnold et al., 2018). Bone marrow transplant studies revealed that this phenotype was not mediated by hematopoietic cells. Instead, the investigators found that mRNA expression of RGS1 was attenuated by chronic Ang II infusion, suggesting that hypertension leads to a loss of this crucial modulatory pathway. In contrast, RGS5 appears to have only modest effects on BP by itself, but it activates RhoA (rat sarcoma virus homologous protein A) stress fiber formation and a contractile phenotype of VSM. RhoA is a critical activator of Rho kinase, which targets contractile proteins, including the MLC in VSM, to promote vasoconstriction. Endothelial Rho kinase phosphorylates NO synthase (NOS) on threonine 495 to inhibit NO production, thereby increasing vasoconstriction (Shimokawa et al., 2016). The Rho kinase inhibitor Fasudil has been approved for use in Japan and China for the treatment of cerebral vasospasm and PH and exhibits BP-lowering effects in genetic- and salt-induced forms of experimental hypertension (Behuliak et al., 2017).

Hypertension is often linked with impaired vasodilation. For many years, it has been recognized that endothelium-dependent vasodilation and NO signaling are reduced in hypertensive patients (Li et al., 2015). The mechanisms underlying endothelium-dependent vasodilation differ between larger conduit arteries, branch arteries, and resistance arterioles. Larger vessels primarily utilize NO, while smaller arteries and arterioles are also modulated by endothelium-dependent hyperpolarization and vasodilator prostaglandins. In larger vessels, defects in NO synthesis and bioavailability include the loss of critical cofactors for NOS, such as L-arginine and tetrahydrobiopterin, inhibition of NOS activity by asymmetrical dimethylarginine (ADMA), and oxidative inactivation of NO. It is important to note that alterations in NO production extend beyond the vasculature and can impact renal and central nervous system function in hypertensive patients. In smaller arteries and arterioles, endothelium-dependent vasodilation is mediated by hyperpolarization, although the factors responsible for this have not been fully identified. In recent years, there has been a growing interest in the role of direct communication or gap junctions that transmit signals between the endothelium and VSMCs. Previous studies using intracellular labeling showed the polarized, unidirectional movement of fluorescent dyes from the endothelium to adjacent smooth muscle cells. These dyes were found to traverse MEJs (myoendothelial junctions), which were later identified as holes in the internal elastic membrane that separate the endothelium and the VSM. MEJs are particularly common in smaller arterioles and serve as sites for signaling events and molecules, such as calcium pulsars, inositol 3 phosphate receptor, and calcium-sensitive potassium channels. Endothelium-dependent hyperpolarization is transmitted directly to VSMCs via microvascular endothelial junctions (MEJs), which also facilitate the transfer of NO generated by nitric oxide synthase (NOS) expressed at these junctions. NO travels from the endothelium to the VSM, where it regulates connexin-43 to modulate the permeability of the MEJs (Wilson et al., 2019). Additionally, MEJs contain hemoglobin alpha, which controls the passage of NO from the endothelium to the VSMCs in a redox-dependent fashion. Intriguingly, a peptide mimic that disrupts the binding of NO to hemoglobin alpha lowers BP abruptly in wild-type animals and reverses experimental hypertension caused by angiotensin II (Ang II) infusion. Importantly, the density of MEJs is reduced and their local inositol trisphosphate-stimulated calcium signals are blunted in mesenteric arterioles of spontaneously hypertensive rats, indicating that these signaling loci are deficient in hypertensive resistance vessels. In keeping with this, mice lacking the MEJ component connexin-40 exhibit hypertension and reduced endothelium-dependent vasodilatation in response to the potassium channel activator SKA-31. Likewise, endothelial-specific expression of a mutant connexin-40, which causes electrical impairment of gap junctions, leads to exercise-induced hypertension (Morton et al., 2015). Recently, it has been shown that chronic sympathetic stimulation in the setting of hypertension due to experimental chronic kidney disease (CKD) decreases the expression of connexin-43, leading to disruption of MEJ function and enhanced vasoconstriction. These various lines of evidence strongly support the role of MEJs in the modulation of microvascular tone and abnormalities thereof in hypertension (Cao et al., 2020).

A significant modification of vascular function that likely contributes to hypertension is the stiffening of large conduit arteries, particularly the proximal aorta, through mechanisms that remain under investigation. A healthy aorta distends during systole and recoils during diastole, which results in a decrease in systolic pressure while maintaining diastolic pressure and perfusion. However, the aorta stiffens in common conditions such as aging, diabetes, obesity, and tobacco use, thereby reducing this critical Windkessel function (Yun et al., 2015). Increased PWV, reflecting aortic stiffening, has been reported in population studies to precede hypertension by several years and is a harbinger of stroke, myocardial infarction, and renal failure (Vasan et al., 2019). Aortic stiffening can be both a cause and a consequence of hypertension. It develops well before the onset of hypertension in spontaneously hypertensive rats, in diet-induced obesity, and in two models of chronic vascular oxidative stress (Wu et al., 2016). In contrast, some studies have reported that aortic collagen increases following the onset of Goldblatt hypertension, and it was found that experimental hypertension in mice causes aortic stiffening. Mechanical stretch of cultured aortic murine fibroblasts increases their expression of collagens I, III, and V. Wu et al. found that aortic stiffening occurs before BP elevation in two models of chronic vascular oxidative stress. Therefore, it is likely that aortic stiffening and hypertension act in concert, with one leading to the other in a feed-forward fashion (Humphrey et al., 2016).

Although the precise mechanisms through which aortic stiffness leads to end-organ damage remain unclear, one potential consequence is the exacerbation of pressure propagation within the microcirculation, ultimately resulting in barotrauma in target organs, at least partially by exacerbating cyclical deformation of microvascular endothelial cells. This phenomenon is supported by a comprehensive examination of the components of the pulse wave, which demonstrated that an augmented forward pressure wave was correlated with an elevated risk for the development of CVD (Cooper et al., 2015).

The cardiovascular system also plays a fourth role in hypertension, which is to function as a conduit for immune cell activation and to serve as a target for immune cell activation. This process involves communication between the endothelial cells lining the blood vessels and the immune cells.

Hypertension is associated with impaired vessel wall defense against thrombosis, which can be attributed to heightened endothelial expression of tissue factor and vascular cell adhesion molecule 1. This leads to increased platelet-dependent leukocyte adhesion, a process that is facilitated by thrombin and the platelet factor XI receptor (Kossmann et al., 2017). Inhibition of factor XI in rats and mice that have been administered angiotensin has been shown to prevent platelet thrombin formation, vascular leukocyte infiltration, endothelial dysfunction, and hypertension. Further research into the mechanisms that activate thrombosis in hypertension could shed light on stroke, atherosclerosis, and end-organ damage.

1.12. The Central Nervous System in Hypertension

Dr. Page's revised diagram (Figure 1.5(B)) was updated to include the term "neural." Dr. Page's research demonstrated that Ang II primarily causes hypertension through sympathetic neural activation. This finding was supported by measurements of MSNA, norepinephrine spillover, and heart rate variability. These measures indicated that individuals with hypertension commonly exhibit increased sympathetic outflow and enhanced catecholamine-mediated vasoconstriction. Ang II and ROS in the brain stem nuclei contribute to increased vascular resistance by partially inhibiting the microvascular endothelium-dependent hyperpolarizing factor that normally reduces vascular tone (Cao et al., 2020). Consistent with these central vascular effects, ganglionic blockade acutely lowers BP in humans with hypertension to varying extents, particularly in obese individuals (Gamboa et al., 2016). The several ways in which sympathetic tone affects hypertension involve increased vasoconstriction and vascular restructuring, renal renin creation through beta 1 adrenergic receptors in the JG, and enhanced renal sodium absorption and inflammation. Hypertension involves various central pathways, several of which have been reviewed by Delalio et al. (2020). One important initiating site is the *lamina terminalis*, located in front of the third ventricle, which contains the *subfornical organ*, the *median preoptic eminence*, and the *organum vasculosum* of the *lamina terminalis*. These two organs are considered circumventricular organs with poorly developed blood-brain barriers that allow blood-borne Ang II and sodium to stimulate neuronal activity. Kinsman et al. (2017) demonstrated that even modest increases in sodium levels can activate the organum *vasculosum* of the *lamina terminalis*, leading to salt-sensitive hypertension. Xiao et al. recently identified the prostaglandin EP3 (E prostanoid receptor type 3) receptor as playing a role in this process, which involves the production of ROS in renal arterioles, the accumulation of isolevuglandin in dendritic cells and immune activation. This example highlights the complex interplay between neural regulation, vasculature, and inflammation in the development of hypertension.

Furthermore, it is well established that efferent signals contribute to hypertension, but there is also substantial evidence suggesting that afferent pathways are involved. In addition to renal afferent activation, which has been previously discussed, adipose tissue afferent nerves are triggered by a high-fat diet to reflexively increase BP and insulin resistance (Cao et al., 2019). Another source of afferent nerve stimulation is the heart. Infusion of saline into cardiac transplant recipients with no evidence of cardiac dysfunction failed to reduce their SNS activity, arginine vasopressin levels, or their renin, angiotensin, and aldosterone levels, and led to hypertension. This hypertensive response was linked to a failure to suppress Ang II during blood volume expansion and was prevented by angiotensin-converting enzyme (ACE) inhibition.

A summary of the various roles and perturbations of the renal, vascular, endocrine, and neural control mechanisms in hypertension is presented in Figure 1.6. These are specific features of the Mosaic Theory and hypertension pathophysiology that continue to be the focus of ongoing research. Over the past 20 years, new factors and phenomena have emerged that likely impact the mosaic factor on a global scale. These include oxidative signaling, inflammation, and the microbiome, as well as a newly discovered role for sodium.

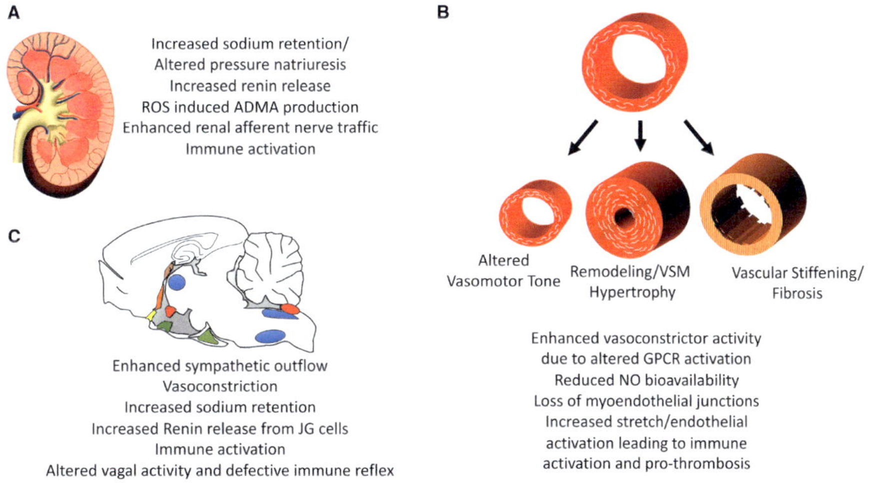

Figure 1.6. Various disturbances to the kidney, vasculature, and central nervous system that contribute to hypertension are illustrated. These include perturbations in the *juxtaglomerular* apparatus (JG), reactive oxygen species (ROS), vascular smooth muscle (VSM), G protein-coupled receptor (GPCR), and asymmetrical *dimethylarginine* (ADMA) (Harrison et al., 2021).

1.13. The Role of ROS in Hypertension

Recognition has been accorded to the activation of several enzymatic sources of ROS in the tissues of hypertensive animals and humans, such as the nicotinamide adenine dinucleotide phosphate (NADPH) oxidases, mitochondria, and uncoupled NOS. ROS are likely to contribute to each node in Dr. Page's diagram. Superoxide and related ROS can inactivate NO and oxidize tetrahydrobiopterin, a critical cofactor for NOS. Additionally, ROS can enhance vasoconstriction, alter vascular caliber and reactivity, and promote vascular stiffening and remodeling of microarterioles (Li et al., 2015). In the kidney, ROS enhance renal sodium reabsorption, thereby increasing volume and cardiac output. They have also been implicated in the activation of matrix metalloproteinases, promoting tissue remodeling. Moreover, ROS increase neuronal firing in critical brain centers, including the subfornical organ and brain stem centers (Carvalho-Galvão et al., 2019; Wang et al., 2016), thereby altering neural control. It is important to note that these findings have been obtained from research and should not be used to replace the advice of a qualified healthcare provider.

The catalytic subunit of NADPH oxidase is referred to as NOX2, and its homologs are activated in various cell types, including VSMCs, endothelium, renal tubular cells, and the central nervous system in hypertensive animal models. It is evident that there is an interaction between ROS derived from NADPH oxidase and other enzymatic sources, leading to a feed-forward mechanism where ROS from one source can trigger ROS production by others.

Although early studies emphasized the role of oxidative stress in vascular cells, recent research has revealed that the kidney and its vasculature also experience oxidative stress, particularly during Ang II infusion and high salt intake. High salt intake increases renal expression of NADPH oxidase and NOX2, while reducing SOD1 and SOD2. In contrast, Ang II infusion enhances renal NADPH/p22phox and reduces SOD3 expression. Renal ROS can activate renal afferent nerves and increase both renal and circulating levels of ADMA (Jayachandran et al., 2020). This occurs by reducing its metabolism through dimethylarginine dimethylaminohydrolase and increasing its generation by protein arginine methyltransferase. As a result, increased circulating ADMA levels represent one mechanism by which ROS in the kidney may contribute to peripheral vasoconstriction. ADMA inhibits endothelial function and flow-mediated vasodilation, and activation of the SNS during high salt intake may contribute to the failure of salt-sensitive subjects to reduce their peripheral vascular resistance during increases in cardiac output. In the kidney, proximal tubular cells take up oxidatively modified albumin, which induces local activation of the RAS via NADPH oxidase, PKC, NFκB, and AP-1. This results in increased proximal tubular Ang II, which initiates renal inflammation and fibrosis. This proximal tubule ROS pathway may provide a potential link between hypertension, systemic oxidative stress, proteinuria, and the activation of the intrarenal RAS. These events can damage the kidney, perpetuating salt sensitivity and exacerbating hypertension.

The role of mitochondria as a source of ROS in hypertension is a topic of increasing interest. Recent investigations indicate that aging and hypertension diminish the function of Sirt3 (sirtuin3), a histone deacetylase that modulates the acetylation status of SOD2. Mice lacking *Sirt3* exhibit resistance to hypertension and its associated vascular dysfunction in response to *Ang II* infusion, a phenomenon that can be prevented by mitochondrial-targeted antioxidants such as *mitoTempol* and *mitoEbselen* (Dikalova et al., 2017). These alterations to the mitochondria in hypertension likely have manifold effects on cellular metabolism and function that contribute to the pathophysiology of hypertension via mechanisms yet to be fully understood. Despite the lack of clinical utilization for therapeutic purposes, it has been suggested that high-dose vitamin antioxidants can be detrimental. This may be attributed to the fact that ROS have important signaling functions (Irazabal and Torres, 2020). Future strategies for targeted ROS scavenging, such as utilizing agents like *mitoTempol* or administering agents that inhibit the untoward activation of enzymes responsible for ROS formation, may prove to be effective. The inhibition of ROS formation is believed to be a major benefit of angiotensin II blockade.

1.14. Inflammatory and Immune Mechanism in Hypertension

For more than half a century, it has been acknowledged that immune cells accumulate in the kidneys and blood vessels of hypertensive humans and animals with experimental hypertension. Presently, it is recognized that virtually all types of immune cells, including those involved in innate and adaptive immunity, contribute to hypertension. These cells migrate into the interstitium of the kidney and blood vessels, where they release potent cytokines, ROS, and metalloproteinases that affect renal and vascular function and structure. It is likely that these mediators impact virtually all aspects of Dr. Page's Mosaic diagram. One notable example is the cytokine interleukin 17A (IL-17A), which is produced by a subset of T cells, innate lymphocytes, histiocytes, and renal tubular cells. IL-17A affects renal tubular sodium handling and appears to modulate pressure natriuresis (Norlander et al., 2016). This cytokine stimulates vascular superoxide production, causes inhibitory phosphorylation of the endothelial NOS, and consequently, reduces blood vessel diameter. Over the long term, IL-17A promotes vascular fibrosis and impairs vascular elasticity. In contrast, regulatory T cells and anti-inflammatory cytokines, such as IL-10, have antihypertensive effects that are mediated, in part, by counteracting the effects of IL-17A.

The process by which immune cells are activated in hypertension is an ongoing area of research. Emerging evidence indicates that ROS in antigen-presenting cells promote the oxidation of fatty acids, resulting in the formation of highly reactive isolevuglandin products that covalently modify protein lysines. These modified proteins are antigenic and have the ability to activate both $CD8^+$ and $CD4^+$ T cells.

There is considerable evidence that sympathetic outflow stimulates immune activation in hypertension. Lesions in the forebrain that inhibit sympathetic outflow decrease T-cell activation, whereas manipulations that increase sympathetic outflow promote T-cell activation. Recent research indicates that renal sympathetic tone affects the movement of immune cells to and from the kidney and the migration of memory T cells to the bone marrow, where they can be reactivated upon future hypertensive challenges (Xiao et al., 2020). In the blood vessels, T cells accumulate in the perivascular fat and adventitia of larger vessels in hypertension, most likely due to the expression of chemokines, such as RANTES (regulated upon activation, normal T-cell expressed and presumably secreted) and MCP (monocyte chemoattractant protein)-1 (Guzik et al., 2017). This adventitial inflammatory response probably triggers collagen deposition, as mentioned above. Additionally, there is an immune reflex, where local tissue signals trigger a vagally mediated anti-inflammatory response. This reflex seems to be malfunctioning in prehypertensive animals, promoting inflammation instead of suppressing it.

Hypertension has consistently been linked to endothelial activation, which is widely acknowledged to facilitate the rolling, adhesion, and migration of leukocytes. As monocytes traverse the endothelial layer, they metamorphose into inflammatory macrophages and dendritic cells, which are activated monocytes with an enhanced capacity to produce cytokines and activate T cells. The endothelial cell stretches, oxidative stress, and depletion of NO in hypertension can all bolster the interaction between endothelial cells and leukocytes, thereby amplifying the activation of monocytes. Human monocytes stimulated by the endothelium in this manner generate copious amounts of IL-6, IL-23, IL-1β, and strongly stimulate autologous T cells (Loperena et al., 2018).

Endothelial transmigration likely plays a role in the accumulation of myeloid cells at the corticomedullary junction of the kidney. Here, the presence of supraphysiological levels of sodium may serve as a stimulus to activate monocytes, as suggested by Barbaro et al. (2021). The crosstalk between the vascular and immune systems reflects the complex nature of hypertension, whereby primary perturbations, such as those affecting endothelial function, can generate mediators that promote inflammation and impact multiple other organs and cells.

1.15. Microbiome as an Emerging Modulator of BP

Sodium, as a dietary component, may contribute to hypertension by modifying gut microbiota and influencing fluid homeostasis and immune activation (Wilck et al., 2017). Recent studies have emphasized the potential role of the microbiome in BP regulation (Marques et al., 2018). Advances in unbiased sequencing techniques have enabled the precise identification and assessment of commensal bacterial species in the gut that cannot be cultured, leading to a better understanding of the microbiome's role in health and disease. Such studies have provided evidence for the microbiome's contribution to the pathogenesis of several diseases, including hypertension (Tang et al., 2019). This research has also revealed the conditioning effects of diet and drugs on the composition of the gut microbiota and highlighted the potential of these disturbances to affect host responses, including BP regulation.

In healthy individuals, the gut microbiome is typically in a stable state of eubiosis and in relative equilibrium with the surrounding community. By contrast, significant alteration in the microbiome (dysbiosis) has been observed in a range of disorders, including hypertension. For example, in humans with hypertension and prehypertension, characteristic alterations in the microbiome have been observed (Li et al., 2017). Dysbiosis has also been observed in experimental models of hypertension, such as *Dahl* salt-sensitive and spontaneously hypertensive rats (Mella et al., 2015), and in mice chronically administered *Ang II* or a deoxycorticosterone acetate + high-salt diet (Marques et al., 2017). Fecal transfer from hypertensive mice to germ-free mice sensitizes the latter to hypertension, providing strong evidence for a role of the microbiome (Ferguson et al., 2019). In hypertension, alterations in the gut microbiome have been associated with inflammation, structural changes in the intestinal wall, and enhanced gut permeability (Santisteban et al., 2017). Altered intestinal permeability may facilitate the egress of mediators, such as microbial products, hormones, and immune cells, into the circulation where they can impact peripheral and central BP control mechanisms.

The relationship between hypertension and gut dysbiosis is complex and influenced by dietary factors (Koh et al., 2016). Dietary intake has been shown to directly affect the composition of gut microbiota, which can impact the risk of hypertension. For instance, high salt intake can cause significant changes in the microbiota composition and is associated with the accumulation of proinflammatory TH17 cells. Additionally, diets rich in fruit, vegetables, and fiber have been shown to decrease BP and reduce the risk of hypertension. This is thought to occur through the generation of short-chain fatty acids by gut bacteria, which are almost exclusively of microbial origin and are implicated in the host's physiological response. The gut microbiome can influence BP control through various pathways, including the family of nutrient sensing GCPRs expressed in VSMCs, the autonomic nervous system, and renal juxtaglomerular cells that influence renin release (Marques et al., 2018). Therefore, modifying the gut microbiome through prebiotics, probiotics, antibiotics, and specific dietary formulations may be a potential strategy to prevent and treat hypertension.

1.16. Mechanisms of Obesity-Related Hypertension

The purported mechanisms that contribute to hypertension associated with obesity are intricate and involve interactions between renal, metabolic, and neuroendocrine pathways. These mechanisms encompass: the overactivation of the SNS, the stimulation of the RAAS, modifications in adipose-derived cytokines, such as leptin, insulin resistance, and structural and functional alterations in the kidneys (Shariq and McKenzie, 2020).

1.16.1. SNS Overactivation

Obesity-related hypertension is believed to be linked to increased activity of the SNS (Lambert et al., 2019). Physiological manifestations of SNS overactivity include elevated heart rate, cardiac output, and renal tubular sodium reabsorption, which result directly from α-adrenergic and β-adrenergic receptor stimulation and indirectly through the activation of other systems, such as the RAAS, as described below. Microneurography, a method used to measure muscle SNS activity, shows an increase in activity with even modest weight gain and is highest in patients with both obesity and hypertension. Renal SNS activity, as measured by the norepinephrine spillover method, is also elevated in obese individuals. Notably, the increased SNS activity associated with obesity is not evenly distributed across all organs, with a predominant impact on the kidneys and skeletal muscle. On the other hand, the chronic elevation in resting heart rate observed in obese individuals is believed to be mediated by reduced parasympathetic tone rather than increased SNS activity (Hall et al., 2015). Additionally, SNS overactivity is not consistently observed in all obese patients and appears to be influenced by factors such as visceral (rather than subcutaneous) adiposity, ethnicity, and sex. For instance, Native American Pima Indians have a high prevalence of obesity but relatively low rates of hypertension. One possible explanation for this is the finding that basal muscle SNS activity is 20–30% lower in Pima Indians compared to weight-matched white individuals. The text implies that social network site (SNS) activity plays a crucial role in determining obesity-related hypertension, and that factors such as ethnicity influence the sympathetic tone in the presence of excess adiposity. Moreover, the relationship between SNS activity and obesity-related hypertension is supported by evidence indicating that pharmacological α/β-adrenergic blockade leads to a greater reduction in SBP in obese hypertensive patients compared to lean hypertensive patients.

Causative mechanisms for the activation of the SNS in obesity include abnormal adipokine secretion from adipose tissue, stimulation through the RAAS, insulin resistance, and baroreceptor dysfunction (Hall et al., 2015). Additionally, obesity often coexists with obstructive sleep apnea (OSA), which results in chronic intermittent hypoxia and activates carotid body chemoreceptors, leading to the reflexive upregulation of SNS activity (Dewan et al., 2015).

1.16.2. Activation of the RAAS

Despite the typical suppression of the RAAS associated with obesity-related volume expansion and sodium retention, various reports indicate that obese individuals exhibit higher levels of plasma renin activity, angiotensinogen, ACE, and aldosterone compared to lean individuals. Activation of the RAAS leads to an increase in the formation of angiotensin II, which induces systemic vasoconstriction and stimulates the production of aldosterone from the adrenal cortex. Both angiotensin II and aldosterone promote renal tubular sodium reabsorption and water retention, contributing to intravascular volume expansion and hypertension (Shariq and McKenzie, 2020). Several mechanisms contribute to RAAS activation in obesity. A bidirectional interaction exists between the SNS and the RAAS, such that the RAAS enhances sympathetic tone, and the SNS, in turn, activates the RAAS (Cabandugama et al., 2017). This drives the release of renin from the juxtaglomerular cells of the kidney. Renin secretion is also upregulated secondary to physical compression of the kidney by excess visceral and retroperitoneal fat (Hall et al., 2015). This leads to decreased renal tubular blood flow and sodium delivery, which is sensed by the *macula densa*, which in turn stimulates renin secretion through tubuloglomerular feedback. Adipocytes possess their own intrinsic RAAS and appear to be significant producers of angiotensinogen and angiotensin II (Schutten et al., 2017). Interestingly, mice with adipocyte-specific deficiency of angiotensin are protected from the development of hypertension, even when fed an obesogenic diet. Additionally, adipocytes have been shown to secrete mineralocorticoid-secreting factors that stimulate aldosterone production from the adrenal gland independently of angiotensin II. The role of RAAS activity in the pathogenesis of obesity-related hypertension in humans is supported by the finding that pharmacological blockade with ACEIs, angiotensin II receptor blockers (ARBs), and mineralocorticoid receptor antagonists (MRAs) significantly lowers BP in obese patients (Williams et al., 2015).

1.16.3. Functional and Structural Renal Changes

The initiation of hypertension associated with obesity is significantly influenced by increased renal sodium reabsorption and volume expansion. Excess visceral and retroperitoneal adiposity can exert mechanical compression on the kidneys, leading to a cascade of events. The accumulation of peri-renal fat can trigger inflammation and expansion of the renal medullary ECM, which results in compression of the renal medulla (Shariq and McKenzie, 2020). This compression decreases renal tubular blood flow and prolongs the time for fractional sodium reabsorption to occur. Consequently, reduced sodium delivery to the *macula densa* leads to a decrease in renal afferent arteriolar resistance, an increase in renal blood flow, and stimulation of renin secretion from juxtaglomerular cells (Hall et al., 2015). These compensatory increases in BP and glomerular filtration rate (GFR) aim to restore normal *macula densa* sodium delivery. However, the elevated glomerular hydrostatic pressure ultimately leads to progressive glomerular sclerosis and impaired renal function. This deleterious cycle perpetuates nephron injury, exacerbates sodium retention, and raises arterial pressures to maintain sodium delivery to the *macula densa*. Renal SNS activity is upregulated in obesity and stimulates sodium reabsorption directly and indirectly through activation of the RAAS (Shariq and McKenzie, 2020).

1.16.4. Leptin Resistance and Hyperleptinemia

Leptin is an adipokine that regulates food intake and energy homeostasis. It also stimulates the SNS in the central nervous system and exerts a pressor effect on the cardiovascular system. In a normal state, leptin suppresses appetite and increases energy expenditure. However, in obese individuals, high leptin levels exist in the absence of weight loss, indicating leptin resistance. This resistance appears to be selective, affecting only the appetite-suppressing and metabolic effects of leptin, without attenuating its stimulatory effects on the SNS. Shariq and McKenzie (2020) posited that hyperleptinemia, largely through activation of the SNS, may contribute to obesity-related hypertension. Although animal studies have shown that leptin infusions stimulate SNS activity and increase BP, human studies have yielded mixed results. Recombinant leptin administration for 12 weeks in overweight or obese individuals had no effect on BP according to Shariq and McKenzie (2020). This highlights the complexity of leptin's effects on BP and the need for a deeper understanding of its role in obesity-related hypertension.

1.16.5. Insulin Resistance

Obesity is commonly linked to a state of insulin resistance and hyperinsulinemia, which may contribute to hypertension through various pathways. Insulin has been shown to exert sympathoexcitatory effects, which are evidenced by increased activity of the SNS in muscle tissue following systemic insulin infusion (Shariq and McKenzie, 2020). Additionally, insulin stimulates the neurons of the paraventricular nucleus, a region of the hypothalamus that plays a critical role in the regulation of sympathetic output. Insulin also directly promotes renal sodium retention in the proximal convoluted tubule by activating the sodium-hydrogen exchanger 3 (NHE3) (Shariq and McKenzie, 2020). In fact, individuals with metabolic syndrome, which includes insulin resistance as a key component, have been found to have a significantly higher fractional sodium reabsorption compared to those without metabolic syndrome. Although insulin is known to act as a vasodilator, obese individuals with chronic hyperinsulinemia exhibit a blunted response due to endothelial dysfunction, resulting in increased vasoconstrictor tone.

1.17. Treatment of Obesity-Related Hypertension

The primary objective of treating obesity-related hypertension is to achieve weight loss, which reverses the pathophysiological processes that sustain hypertension. According to research, the BP-lowering effects of weight loss appear to be linear, with a decrease in BP of approximately 1 mmHg reported per kg of weight loss. However, this effect may diminish over time, with a decrease of around 6 mmHg observed per 10 kg of weight loss (Shariq and McKenzie, 2020). Nonpharmacological approaches, such as lifestyle modifications, are typically employed initially to promote weight reduction. When patients are unable to attain weight loss or recommended BP targets using this approach, adjuvant pharmacotherapy may be necessary. It is increasingly recognized that metabolic surgery represents an effective strategy for BP control in obese hypertensive patients, and evidence supporting this will be discussed in subsections.

1.17.1. Lifestyle Modification

Obesity treatment primarily relies on lifestyle modifications that focus on calorie reduction and increased physical activity. These modifications involve adjustments to diet, regular exercise, and behavioral changes. However, the success rate of these interventions is often hampered by high recidivism and drop-out rates, making it difficult for patients to achieve and maintain long-term weight loss (Greenway, 2015). This challenge is not solely due to lack of motivation but also results from counter-regulatory hormonal mechanisms that work to restore higher body weight (Shariq and McKenzie, 2020).

1.17.2. Pharmacological Therapies for Obesity

According to the guidelines provided by the American College of Cardiology (ACC) and the American Heart Association (AHA), in collaboration with the Endocrine Society (Apovian et al., 2015), pharmacological therapies for obesity may be considered as useful adjuncts to lifestyle modification for patients with a body mass index (BMI) of ≥30 kg/m^2 or for those with a BMI of ≥27 kg/m^2 and concomitant obesity-related diseases, including hypertension, type 2 diabetes, dyslipidemia, and/or OSA. At present, five drugs have been approved by the US Food and Drug Administration (FDA) for long-term weight management: orlistat, lorcaserin, phentermine-topiramate, naltrexone-bupropion, and liraglutide. Except for orlistat, which reduces fat absorption by inhibiting gastric and pancreatic lipase, these drugs promote weight loss by reducing food intake and inducing early satiety (Saunders et al., 2018). The degree of weight loss achieved by anti-obesity drugs at over one-year ranges from approximately 3–9% beyond that achieved with lifestyle modification alone (Gadde and Pritham, 2017). Although a detailed description of each medication is beyond the scope of this review, it is worth noting that some anti-obesity drugs may have varying effects on BP. For instance, orlistat has been demonstrated to produce placebo-adjusted systolic and diastolic BP reductions of 2.5 and 1.9 mmHg, respectively, in obese hypertensive patients (Siebenhofer et al., 2017). However, it is associated with only a mild degree of weight loss (<3% relative to placebo) (Sahebkar et al., 2018) and frequent gastrointestinal side effects, such as fecal urgency, incontinence, and oily stool, which hinder its long-term use (Saunders et al., 2018). When compared with placebo, bupropion-naltrexone reduces weight by approximately 4–5%, but it can raise BP and heart rate and is not recommended for use in hypertensive patients (Nissen et al., 2016). In summary, there is a lack of data on the efficacy and short- and long-term BP effects of most approved anti-obesity drugs that are specific to obese patients who are also hypertensive (Cohen and Gadde, 2019).

1.17.3. Pharmacological Therapies for Hypertension in Obese Individuals

Individuals who have obesity are at an increased risk of developing treatment-resistant hypertension, which is defined as BP that remains above the goal despite the use of three antihypertensive agents of different classes, or controlled BP with more than three medications (Booth et al., 2016). Although most hypertension guidelines do not specifically address obese patients, some recommendations for the optimal choice of antihypertensive agents in this population have been suggested. Given the role of the RAAS in the pathogenesis of obesity-related hypertension, there is a strong case for considering angiotensin-converting enzyme inhibitors (ACEIs) and angiotensin receptor blockers (ARBs) as first-line therapies. These drugs have an added advantage of improving insulin sensitivity and being nephroprotective in patients with diabetes, which is a common comorbidity in obese individuals. Based on the observation that aldosterone levels are upregulated in obesity, the use of MRAs has also been advocated. However, there is limited evidence to suggest that these agents are more effective in obese individuals than in normal-weight hypertensive patients. Because the SNS activation is also implicated in obesity-related hypertension, β-blockers would appear to be a biologically plausible treatment option. However, many of the drugs in this class are associated with weight gain and insulin resistance and should only be used in obese patients with specific cardiovascular indications, such as heart failure or post-myocardial infarction. β-blockers are often prescribed for various medical conditions. Among the different types of β-blockers, third-generation agents, such as carvedilol and nebivolol, seem to have fewer adverse metabolic effects and less potential for weight gain compared to older β-blockers. CCBs of the dihydropyridine class, which have a neutral effect on glucose metabolism and weight gain, are typically recommended as second-line agents in combination with ACEIs/ARBs. Although thiazide diuretics are effective in treating hypertension associated with obesity, they can also have metabolic adverse effects, including dyslipidemia and insulin resistance, which may be particularly harmful to obese patients taking these medications (Shariq and McKenzie, 2020).

1.17.4. The Role of Metabolic Surgery in the Treatment of Obesity-Related Hypertension

Metabolic surgery, also known as bariatric surgery, has become one of the most popular gastrointestinal procedures worldwide. According to the latest survey conducted by the International Federation for the Surgery of Obesity and Metabolic Disorders, an estimated 6,80,000 metabolic procedures were performed globally in 2016, which is double the number of cases reported in 2011 (Angrisani et al., 2018). In the United States, the most commonly performed metabolic procedures, in decreasing order of frequency, are sleeve gastrectomy (SG, 58%), Roux-en-Y gastric bypass (RYGB, 19%), adjustable gastric banding (AGB, 3%), and biliopancreatic diversion with duodenal switch (BPD/DS, 0.6%) (English et al., 2018).

Metabolic surgery has been recognized as the most effective method for achieving substantial and sustained weight loss in obese individuals, as evidenced by the findings of various randomized controlled trials (RCTs) and observational studies. For instance, in a meta-analysis of 11 RCTs that included a total of 796 obese individuals, those who underwent metabolic surgery experienced a weight loss of 26 kg more than those who received non-surgical treatment. With respect to the type of surgery, BPD/DS provides the most significant weight loss among all bariatric procedures, as it involves the most extensive degree of intestinal bypass. However, it is also the most technically challenging and is therefore performed the least frequently (English et al., 2018). RYGB was previously the most common bariatric procedure but has now largely been replaced by SG, as the latter is considered to be a more straightforward and quicker operation with a lower complication rate. Although some studies have demonstrated superior weight loss outcomes with RYGB (Ignat et al., 2017), which is considered by many to be the "gold standard" weight loss procedure, others have shown similar efficacy between RYGB and SG (Peterli et al., 2018). There is, however, a consensus that both operations result in significantly greater and longer-lasting weight loss than AGB, a procedure that is now rarely performed in contemporary bariatric practice (Piche et al., 2015).

Metabolic surgery has proven to be an effective treatment for type 2 diabetes mellitus (T2DM), with significant effects on weight loss and an impressive array of evidence to support this claim (Yu et al., 2015). Many patients who undergo metabolic surgery achieve complete remission of T2DM, as defined by the American Diabetes Association (ADA), which includes a glycated hemoglobin (HbA1c) level of <6.0% or fasting glucose level of <100 mg/dL, without the use of pharmacological therapies. In the STAMPEDE (Surgical Treatment and Medications Potentially Eradicate Diabetes Efficiently) trial, 150 patients with T2DM and a BMI of 27 to 43 kg/m^2 were randomly assigned to receive RYGB, SG, or intensive medical therapy alone. At 1 year, only 12% of patients in the medical therapy group achieved the trial's primary outcome of HbA1c <6.0%, compared to 42% of patients who underwent RYGB (P=0.002) and 37% who underwent SG (P=0.003). Follow-up data from this trial showed that the beneficial effects of metabolic surgery on glycemic control were durable and remained significantly greater than medical therapy alone at 5 years (Schauer et al., 2017). As a result, metabolic surgery has been included in treatment algorithms for T2DM proposed by international diabetes organizations (Rubino et al., 2017).

1.18. Conclusion

Hypertension is a medical condition named for its characteristic symptoms, which is characterized by the diversity of its underlying causes. Unlike secondary hypertension, which is caused by specific factors, the mechanisms of essential hypertension have not yet been fully understood. The intricate mechanisms and lack of understanding make it challenging to effectively treat essential hypertension.

Currently, there are two primary avenues being explored to optimize the treatment of hypertension (*see* Figure 1.7). The first involves disentangling the various factors at play and determining their individual roles. For instance, recent studies have proposed new clinical indicators for estimating augmented MSNA in hypertensive subjects, without regard to the volume of conducting vessels (Sugimoto et al., 2020). These findings, to some extent, decoupled the relationship between arterial stiffness and sympathetic dysregulation. Additionally, as previously mentioned, leveraging circulating biomarkers can guide more precise treatments. The second direction is focused on lowering BP without delving too deeply into the underlying mechanisms. Several novel approaches are being proposed that have demonstrated various mechanisms for reducing BP. Taking RDN as an example, it not only disrupts the sympathetic-mediated neurohormonal pathway, but may also decrease plasma renin activity and aldosterone levels to inhibit the RAAS (Qin et al., 2022). Given the complexity of the essential hypertension's underlying mechanisms, which are unlikely to be fully understood in the near future, it is also crucial for clinicians to concentrate on treatment efficacy to meet the clinical needs.

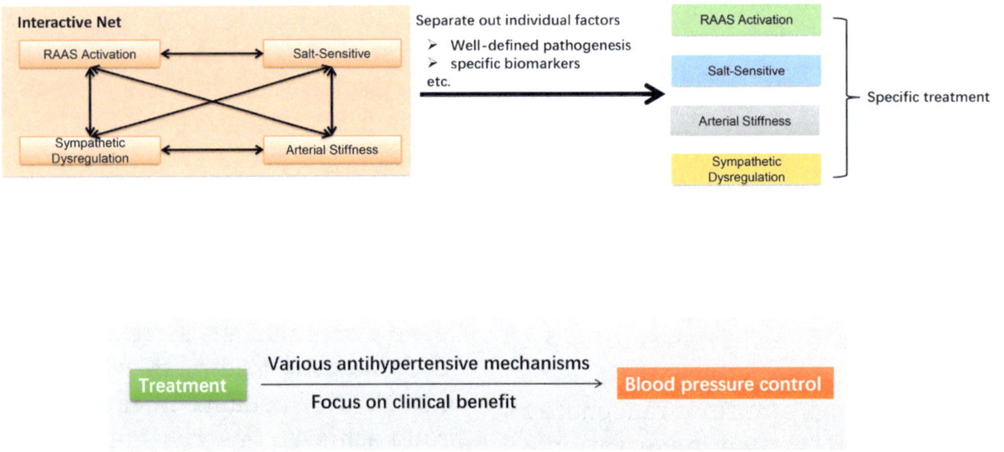

Figure 1.7. The primary aims of future research in the management of hypertension are twofold. Firstly, it is essential to disentangle the intricate web of individual factors that contribute to the condition. Secondly, there is a need to concentrate on the clinical efficacy of antihypertensive treatments (Ma and Chen, 2022).

Obesity-related hypertension arises from a variety of intricate mechanisms, including the inappropriate activation of the SNS and RAAS, adipocyte dysfunction, and impaired pressure natriuresis. These mechanisms are compounded by physical compression of the kidneys, which exacerbates the condition. Weight loss is considered the primary approach to treating obesity and its associated consequences. However, many patients struggle to achieve and maintain adequate weight loss through lifestyle changes alone. While there are several anti-obesity medications available, concerns about their safety and efficacy in hypertensive patients persist. Patients with obesity are also more likely to develop hypertension that is resistant to treatment with multiple antihypertensive agents. Metabolic surgery has been proven to be the most effective treatment for achieving sustained weight loss and has been shown to have beneficial effects in patients with T2DM. It is increasingly recognized that metabolic surgery can also lead to hypertension remission, but the underlying mechanisms are not well understood. Notably, a reduction in BP may occur as early as one week postoperatively, before the onset of adipose mass loss, suggesting that neurohormonal mechanisms are involved in the BP-lowering effects of bariatric surgery. Further studies, including research in preclinical models, are necessary to better comprehend these mechanisms. Although the accumulating evidence base is promising, additional high-quality data concerning long-term BP outcomes following both RYGB and SG are required to confirm that the beneficial effects on hypertension are sustained. Although metabolic surgery, with its potential risks, should not be considered a first-line treatment for isolated hypertension, it should be considered as a viable option for the subset of obese patients with hypertension that is severe or refractory to alternative treatments. As the global burden and severity of obesity and hypertension continue to increase, research examining the impact of metabolic surgery on ameliorating these conditions will remain of crucial importance in the years to come (Shariq and McKenzie, 2020). In brief, the primary reason for the difficulty in curing essential hypertension is the incomplete understanding of its pathogenesis, which is a complex process influenced by various interrelated factors. To overcome this challenge, further in-depth research on the mechanisms underlying hypertension, particularly the application of advanced theories, is essential. Additionally, optimizing existing antihypertensive methods with BP as the primary focus is a critical area of research for the clinical management of hypertension (Ma and Chen, 2022).

References

1. Abdel Ghafar, M. T. (2020). An overview of the classical and tissue-derived renin-angiotensin-aldosterone system and its genetic polymorphisms in essential hypertension. *Steroids, 163*, 108701.
2. Adua, E. (2023). Decoding the mechanism of hypertension through multimers profiling. *Journal of Human Hypertension, 37*, 253–264.
3. Angrisani, L., Santonicola, A., Iovino, P., et al. (2018). IFSO Worldwide Survey 2016: Primary, endoluminal, and revisional procedures. *Obesity Surgery, 28*, 3783–3794.
4. Apovian, C. M., Aronne, L. J., Bessesen, D. H., et al. (2015). Pharmacological management of obesity: An Endocrine Society clinical practice guideline. *Journal of Clinical Endocrinology & Metabolism, 100*, 342–362.
5. Arif, M., Sadayappan, S., Becker, R. C., Martin, L. J., & Urbina, E. M. (2019). Epigenetic modification: A regulatory mechanism in essential hypertension. *Hypertension Research, 42*, 1099–1113.
6. Arnold, C., Demirel, E., Feldner, A., Genové, G., Zhang, H., Sticht, C., Wieland, T., Hecker, M., Heximer, S., & Korff, T. (2018). Hypertension-evoked RhoA activity in vascular smooth muscle cells requires RGS5. *FASEB Journal, 32*, 2021–2035.
7. Banek, C. T., Knuepfer, M. M., Foss, J. D., Fiege, J. K., Asirvatham-Jeyaraj, N., Van Helden, D., Shimizu, Y., & Osborn, J. W. (2016). Resting afferent renal nerve discharge and renal inflammation: Elucidating the role of afferent and efferent renal nerves in deoxycorticosterone acetate salt hypertension. *Hypertension, 68*, 1415–1423.
8. Barbaro, N. R., Van Beusecum, J., Xiao, L., do Carmo, L., Pitzer, A., Loperena, R., Foss, J. D., Elijovich, F., Laffer, C. L., Montaniel, K. R., et al. (2021). Sodium activates human monocytes via the NADPH oxidase and isolevuglandin formation. *Cardiovascular Research, 117*(5), 1358–1371.
9. Behuliak, M., Bencze, M., Vaněčková, I., Kuneš, J., & Zicha, J. (2017). Basal and activated calcium sensitization mediated by RhoA/Rho kinase pathway in rats with genetic and salt hypertension. *BioMed Research International, 2017*, 8029728.
10. Booth, H. P., Prevost, A. T., & Gulliford, M. C. (2016). Severity of obesity and management of hypertension, hypercholesterolemia and smoking in primary care: Population-based cohort study. *Journal of Human Hypertension, 30*, 40–45.
11. Cabandugama, P. K., Gardner, M. J., & Sowers, J. R. (2017). The renin angiotensin aldosterone system in obesity and hypertension: Roles in the cardiorenal metabolic syndrome. *Medical Clinics of North America, 101*, 129–137.
12. Cabrera, C. P., Ng, F. L., Nicholls, H. L., Gupta, A., Barnes, M. R., Munroe, P. B., et al. (2019). Over 1000 genetic loci influencing blood pressure with multiple systems and tissues implicated. *Human Molecular Genetics, 28*, R151–R161.
13. Cao, W., Li, A., Wang, L., Zhou, Z., Su, Z., Bin, W., Wilcox, C. S., & Hou, F. F. (2015). A salt-induced reno-cerebral reflex activates renin–angiotensin systems and promotes CKD progression. *Journal of the American Society of Nephrology, 26*, 1619–1633.
14. Cao, W., Shi, M., Wu, L., Li, J., Yang, Z., Liu, Y., Wilcox, C. S., & Hou, F. F. (2019). Adipocytes initiate an adipose-cerebral-peripheral sympathetic reflex to induce insulin resistance during high-fat feeding. *Clinical Science (London), 133*, 1883–1899.

15. Cao, W., Wu, L., Zhang, X., Zhou, J., Wang, J., Yang, Z., Su, H., Liu, Y., Wilcox, C. S., & Hou, F. F. (2020). Sympathetic overactivity in CKD disrupts buffering of neurotransmission by endothelium-derived hyperpolarizing factor and enhances vasoconstriction. *Journal of the American Society of Nephrology, 31*, 2312–2325.

16. Carrizzo, A., Lenzi, P., Procaccini, C., Damato, A., Biagioni, F., Ambrosio, M., et al. (2015). Pentraxin 3 induces vascular endothelial dysfunction through a p-selectin/matrix metalloproteinase-1 pathway. *Circulation, 131*, 1495–1505; discussion 1505.

17. Carvalho-Galvão, A., Guimarães, D. D., De Brito Alves, J. L., & Braga, V. A. (2019). Central inhibition of tumor necrosis factor alpha reduces hypertension by attenuating oxidative stress in the rostral ventrolateral medulla in renovascular hypertensive rats. *Frontiers in Physiology, 10*, 491.

18. Chandran, R. R., Xie, Y., Gallardo-Vara, E., Adams, T., Garcia-Milian, R., Kabir, I., et al. (2021). Distinct roles of KLF4 in mesenchymal cell subtypes during lung fibrogenesis. *Nature Communications, 12*, 7179.

19. Chattopadhyay, A., Kwartler, C. S., Kaw, K., Li, Y., Kaw, A., Chen, J., et al. (2021). Cholesterol induced phenotypic modulation of smooth muscle cells to macrophage/fibroblast-like cells is driven by an unfolded protein response. *Arteriosclerosis, Thrombosis, and Vascular Biology, 41*, 302–316.

20. Chirinos, J. A., Segers, P., Hughes, T., & Townsend, R. (2019). Large-artery stiffness in health and disease: JACC state-of-the-art review. *Journal of the American College of Cardiology, 74*, 1237–1263.

21. Cohen, J. B., & Gadde, K. M. (2019). Weight loss medications in the treatment of obesity and hypertension. *Current Hypertension Reports, 21*, 16.

22. Cooper, L. L., Rong, J., Benjamin, E. J., Larson, M. G., Levy, D., Vita, J. A., Hamburg, N. M., Vasan, R. S., & Mitchell, G. F. (2015). Components of hemodynamic load and cardiovascular events: The Framingham Heart Study. *Circulation, 131*, 354–361.

23. Craft, J., Gordon, C., Huether, S. E., McCance, K. L., & Brashers, V. L. (2015). *Understanding Pathophysiology-ANZ Adaptation*. Elsevier Health Sciences.

24. Curnow, A. C., Gonsalez, S. R., Gogulamudi, V. R., Visniauskas, B., Simon, E. E., Gonzalez, A. A., Majid, D. S. A., Lara, L. S., & Prieto, M. C. (2020). Low nitric oxide bioavailability increases renin production in the collecting duct. *Frontiers in Physiology, 11*, 559341.

25. DeLalio, L. J., Sved, A. F., & Stocker, S. D. (2020). Sympathetic nervous system contributions to hypertension: Updates and therapeutic relevance. *Canadian Journal of Cardiology, 36*, 712–720.

26. Dewan, N. A., Nieto, F. J., & Somers, V. K. (2015). Intermittent hypoxemia and OSA: Implications for comorbidities. *Chest, 147*, 266–274.

27. Di Pietro, P., Carrizzo, A., Sommella, E., Oliveti, M., Iacoviello, L., Di Castelnuovo, A., et al. (2022). Targeting the ASMase/S1P pathway protects from sortilin-evoked vascular damage in hypertension. *Journal of Clinical Investigation, 132*, e146343.

28. Dikalova, A. E., Itani, H. A., Nazarewicz, R. R., McMaster, W. G., Flynn, C. R., Uzhachenko, R., Fessel, J. P., Gamboa, J. L., Harrison, D. G., & Dikalov, S. I. (2017). Sirt3 impairment and SOD2 hyperacetylation in vascular oxidative stress and hypertension. *Circulation Research, 121*, 564–574.

29. Drew, D. A., Katz, R., Kritchevsky, S., Ix, J. H., Shlipak, M. G., Newman, A. B., et al. (2021). Soluble klotho and incident hypertension. *Clinical Journal of the American Society of Nephrology, 16*, 1502–1511.

30. Dumor, K., Shoemaker-Moyle, M., Nistala, R., & Whaley-Connell, A. (2018). Arterial stiffness in hypertension: An update. *Current Hypertension Reports, 20*, 72.

31. Ehlers, T. S., Sverrisdottir, Y., Bangsbo, J., & Gunnarsson, T. P. (2020). High-intensity interval training decreases muscle sympathetic nerve activity in men with essential hypertension and in normotensive controls. *Frontiers in Neuroscience, 14*, 841.

32. Eikelis, N., Marques, F. Z., Hering, D., Marusic, P., Head, G. A., Walton, A. S., et al. (2018). A polymorphism in the noradrenaline transporter gene is associated with increased blood pressure in patients with resistant hypertension. *Journal of Hypertension, 36*, 1571–1577.

33. Ellison, D. H., & Welling, P. (2021). Insights into salt handling and blood pressure. *New England Journal of Medicine, 385*, 1981–1993.

34. English, W. J., DeMaria, E. J., Brethauer, S. A., et al. (2018). American Society for Metabolic and Bariatric Surgery estimation of metabolic and bariatric procedures performed in the United States in 2016. *Surgery for Obesity and Related Diseases, 14*, 259–263.

35. Evangelou, E., Warren, H. R., Mosen-Ansorena, D., Mifsud, B., Pazoki, R., Gao, H., et al. (2018). Genetic analysis of over 1 million people identifies 535 new loci associated with blood pressure traits. *Nature Genetics, 50*, 1412–1425.

36. Fang, J., Chang, T., Wang, G., & Loustalot, F. (2020). Association between cost-related medication nonadherence and hypertension management among US adults. *American Journal of Hypertension, 33*, 879–886.

37. Ferguson, J. F., Aden, L. A., Barbaro, N. R., Van Beusecum, J. P., Xiao, L., Simmons, A. J., et al. (2019). High dietary salt-induced dendritic cell activation underlies microbial dysbiosis-associated hypertension. *JCI Insight, 5*, e126241.

38. Fernandez, G., Lee, J. A., Liu, L. C., & Gassler, J. P. (2015). The baroreflex in hypertension. *Current Hypertension Reports, 17*, 19.

39. Foss, J. D., Fiege, J., Shimizu, Y., Collister, J. P., Mayerhofer, T., Wood, L., & Osborn, J. W. (2018). Role of afferent and efferent renal nerves in the development of AngII-salt hypertension in rats. *Physiological Reports, 6*, e13602.

40. Gadde, K. M., & Pritham Raj, Y. (2017). Pharmacotherapy of obesity: Clinical trials to clinical practice. *Current Diabetes Reports, 17*, 34.

41. Gamboa, A., Figueroa, R., Paranjape, S. Y., Farley, G., Diedrich, A., & Biaggioni, I. (2016). Autonomic blockade reverses endothelial dysfunction in obesity-associated hypertension. *Hypertension, 68*, 1004–1010.

42. Garcia, V., & Sessa, W. C. (2019). Endothelial NOS: Perspective and recent developments. *British Journal of Pharmacology, 176*(2), 189–196.

43. Goettsch, C., Kjolby, M., & Aikawa, E. (2018). Sortilin and its multiple roles in cardiovascular and metabolic diseases. *Arteriosclerosis, Thrombosis, and Vascular Biology, 38*(1), 19–25.

44. Graudal, N. A., Hubeck-Graudal, T., & Jürgens, G. (2020). Effects of low sodium diet versus high sodium diet on blood pressure, renin, aldosterone, catecholamines, cholesterol, and triglyceride. *Cochrane Database of Systematic Reviews, 12*, CD004022.

45. Greenway, F. L. (2015). Physiological adaptations to weight loss and factors favoring weight regain. *International Journal of Obesity, 39*(8), 1188–1196.

46. Greer, R. C., Marklund, M., Anderson, C. A. M., Cobb, L. K., Dalcin, A. T., Henry, M., et al. (2020). Potassium-enriched salt substitutes as a means to lower blood pressure: Benefits and risks. *Hypertension, 75*(2), 266–274.

47. Guessoum, O., de Goes Martini, A., Sequeira-Lopez, M. L. S., & Gomez, R. A. (2021). Deciphering the identity of renin cells in health and disease. *Trends in Molecular Medicine, 27*(3), 280–292.

48. Guzik, T. J., Skiba, D. S., Touyz, R. M., & Harrison, D. G. (2017). The role of infiltrating immune cells in dysfunctional adipose tissue. *Cardiovascular Research, 113*(9), 1009–1023.

49. Hall, J. E., do Carmo, J. M., da Silva, A. A., et al. (2015). Obesity-induced hypertension: Interaction of neurohumoral and renal mechanisms. *Circulation Research, 116*(6), 991–1006.

50. Harrison, D. G., Coffman, T. M., & Wilcox, C. S. (2021). Pathophysiology of hypertension: The mosaic theory and beyond. *Circulation Research, 128*(7), 847–863.

51. Huang, L., Trieu, K., Yoshimura, S., Neal, B., Woodward, M., Campbell, N. R. C., et al. (2020). Effect of dose and duration of reduction in dietary sodium on blood pressure levels: Systematic review and meta-analysis of randomized trials. *BMJ, 368*, m315.

52. Humphrey, J. D., Harrison, D. G., Figueroa, C. A., Lacolley, P., & Laurent, S. (2016). Central artery stiffness in hypertension and aging: A problem with cause and consequence. *Circulation Research, 118*(3), 379–381.

53. Ignat, M., Vix, M., Imad, I., et al. (2017). Randomized trial of Roux-en-Y gastric bypass versus sleeve gastrectomy in achieving excess weight loss. *British Journal of Surgery, 104*(2), 248–256.

54. Irazabal, M. V., & Torres, V. E. (2020). Reactive oxygen species and redox signaling in chronic kidney disease. *Cells, 9*(6), 1342.

55. Jayachandran, I., Sundararajan, S., Venkatesan, S., Paadukaana, S., Balasubramanyam, M., Mohan, V., & Manickam, N. (2020). Asymmetric dimethylarginine (ADMA) accelerates renal cell fibrosis under high glucose condition through NOX4/ROS/ERK signaling pathway. *Scientific Reports, 10*, 16005.

56. Jia, G., Aroor, A. R., Hill, M. A., & Sowers, J. R. (2018). Role of renin–angiotensin–aldosterone system activation in promoting cardiovascular fibrosis and stiffness. *Hypertension, 72*(3), 537–548.

57. Jujic, A., Matthes, F., Vanherle, L., Petzka, H., Orho-Melander, M., Nilsson, P. M., et al. (2021). Plasma S1P (sphingosine-1-phosphate) links to hypertension and biomarkers of inflammation and cardiovascular disease: Findings from a translational investigation. *Hypertension, 78*(1), 195–209.

58. Kario, K., Kim, B. K., Aoki, J., Wong, A. Y., Lee, Y. H., Wongpraparut, N., et al. (2020). Renal denervation in Asia: Consensus statement of the Asia Renal Denervation Consortium. *Hypertension, 75*(3), 590–602.

59. Kawarazaki, W., & Fujita, T. (2021). Kidney and epigenetic mechanisms of salt-sensitive hypertension. *Nature Reviews Nephrology, 17*, 350–363.

60. Kaye, D. M., Shihata, W. A., Jama, H. A., Tsyganov, K., Ziemann, M., Kiriazis, H., et al. (2020). Deficiency of prebiotic fiber and insufficient signaling through gut metabolite-sensing receptors leads to cardiovascular disease. *Circulation, 141*(17), 1393–1403.

61. Kinsman, B. J., Simmonds, S. S., Browning, K. N., & Stocker, S. D. (2017). Organum vasculum of the lamina terminalis detects NaCl to elevate sympathetic nerve activity and blood pressure. *Hypertension, 69*(1), 163–170.

62. Kobetic, M. D., Burchell, A. E., Ratcliffe, L. E. K., Neumann, S., Adams, Z. H., Nolan, R., et al. (2022). Sympathetic-transduction in untreated hypertension. *Journal of Human Hypertension, 36*(1), 24–31.

63. Koh, A., De Vadder, F., Kovatcheva-Datchary, P., & Bäckhed, F. (2016). From dietary fiber to host physiology: Short-chain fatty acids as key bacterial metabolites. *Cell, 165*(6), 1332–1345.

64. Kossmann, S., Lagrange, J., Jackel, S., Jurk, K., Ehlken, M., Schonfelder, T., et al. (2017). Platelet-localized FXI promotes a vascular coagulation-inflammatory circuit in arterial hypertension. *Science Translational Medicine, 9*(375), eaah4923.

65. Lambert, E. A., Esler, M. D., Schlaich, M. P., et al. (2019). Obesity-associated organ damage and sympathetic nervous activity. *Hypertension, 73*(6), 1150–1159.

66. Li, C., Yan, X., Wu, D., Zhang, K., Liang, X., Pan, Y., et al. (2019). Vaccine targeted alpha 1D-adrenergic receptor for hypertension. *Hypertension, 74*(6), 1551–1562.

67. Li, J., Zhao, F., Wang, Y., Chen, J., Tao, J., Tian, G., Wu, S., Liu, W., Cui, Q., Geng, B., et al. (2017). Gut microbiota dysbiosis contributes to the development of hypertension. *Microbiome, 5*, 14.

68. Li, K. C., Huang, L., Tian, M., Di Tanna, G. L., Yu, J., Zhang, X., et al. (2022). Cost-effectiveness of a household salt substitution intervention: Findings from 20,995 participants of the Salt Substitute and Stroke Study. *Circulation, 145*(20), 1534–1541.

69. Li, Q., Youn, J. Y., & Cai, H. (2015). Mechanisms and consequences of endothelial nitric oxide synthase dysfunction in hypertension. *Journal of Hypertension, 33*(6), 1128–1136.

70. Liu, Y., Chu, H., Peng, K., Yin, X., Huang, L., Wu, Y., et al. (2021). Factors associated with the use of a salt substitute in rural China. *JAMA Network Open, 4*(12), e2137745.

71. Liu, Z., Qi, H., Liu, B., Liu, K., Wu, J., Cao, H., et al. (2017). Genetic susceptibility to salt-sensitive hypertension in a Han Chinese population: A validation study of candidate genes. *Hypertension Research, 40*(9), 876–884.

72. Loperena, R., Van Beusecum, J. P., Itani, H. A., Engel, N., Laroumanie, F., Xiao, L., et al. (2018). Hypertension and increased endothelial mechanical stretch promote monocyte differentiation and activation: Roles of STAT3, interleukin 6 and hydrogen peroxide. *Cardiovascular Research, 114*(11), 1547–1563.

73. Ma, J., & Chen, X. (2022). Advances in pathogenesis and treatment of essential hypertension. *Frontiers in Cardiovascular Medicine, 9*, 1003852.

74. Manta, E., Kouremeti, M., Kakouri, N., Kasiakogias, A., Konstantinidis, D., Papakonstantinou, P., et al. (2020). Correlations of attended and unattended blood pressure with sympathetic nervous system activity in essential hypertension. *European Heart Journal, 41*, 2754.

75. Marques, F. Z., Mackay, C. R., & Kaye, D. M. (2018). Beyond gut feelings: How the gut microbiota regulates blood pressure. *Nature Reviews Cardiology, 15*, 20–32.

76. Marques, F. Z., Nelson, E., Chu, P. Y., Horlock, D., Fiedler, A., Ziemann, M., et al. (2017). High-fiber diet and acetate supplementation change the gut microbiota and prevent the development of hypertension and heart failure in hypertensive mice. *Circulation, 135*, 964–977.

77. McDonough, A. A., & Nguyen, M. T. (2015). Maintaining balance under pressure: Integrated regulation of renal transporters during hypertension. *Hypertension, 66*, 450–455.

78. Mell, B., Jala, V. R., Mathew, A. V., Byun, J., Waghulde, H., Zhang, Y., Haribabu, B., Vijay-Kumar, M., Pennathur, S., & Joe, B. (2015). Evidence for a link between gut microbiota and hypertension in the Dahl rat. *Physiological Genomics, 47*, 187–197.

79. Mills, K. T., Stefanescu, A., & He, J. (2020). The global epidemiology of hypertension. *Nature Reviews Nephrology, 16*, 223–237.

80. Mo, X. B., Lei, S. F., Zhang, Y. H., & Zhang, H. (2019). Examination of the associations between m(6)a-associated single-nucleotide polymorphisms and blood pressure. *Hypertension Research, 42*, 1582–1589.

81. Mocan, O., Rădulescu, D., Buzdugan, E., Cozma, A., Leucuta, D. C., Bogdan, S. A., et al. (2021). Association between polymorphisms of genes involved in the renin-angiotensin-aldosterone system and the adaptive morphological and functional responses to essential hypertension. *Biomedical Reports, 15*, 80.

82. Morris, R. C., Schmidlin, O., Sebastian, A., Tanaka, M., & Kurtz, T. W. (2016). Vaso dysfunction that involves renal Vaso dysfunction, not abnormally increased renal retention of sodium, accounts for the initiation of salt-induced hypertension. *Circulation, 133*, 881–893.

83. Morton, S. K., Chaston, D. J., Howitt, L., Heisler, J., Nicholson, B. J., Fairweather, S., Bröer, S., Ashton, A. W., Matthaei, K. I., & Hill, C. E. (2015). Loss of functional endothelial connexin40 results in exercise-induced hypertension in mice. *Hypertension, 65*, 662–669.

84. Muralitharan, R. R., Jama, H. A., Xie, L., Peh, A., Snelson, M., & Marques, F. Z. (2020). Microbial peer pressure. *Hypertension, 76*, 1674–1679.

85. Muralitharan, R., & Marques, F. Z. (2021). Diet-related gut microbial metabolites and sensing in hypertension. *Journal of Human Hypertension, 35*, 162–169.

86. Natarajan, N., Hori, D., Flavahan, S., Steppan, J., Flavahan, N. A., Berkowitz, D. E., et al. (2016). Microbial short chain fatty acid metabolites lower blood pressure via endothelial G protein-coupled receptor 41. *Physiological Genomics, 48*, 826–834.

87. Neal, B., Wu, Y., Feng, X., Zhang, R., Zhang, Y., Shi, J., et al. (2021). Effect of salt substitution on cardiovascular events and death. *New England Journal of Medicine, 385*, 1067–1077.

88. Nissen, S. E., Wolski, K. E., Prcela, L., et al. (2016). Effect of naltrexone-bupropion on major adverse cardiovascular events in overweight and obese patients with cardiovascular risk factors: A randomized clinical trial. *JAMA, 315*, 990–1004.

89. Norlander, A. E., Saleh, M. A., Kamat, N. V., Ko, B., Gnecco, J., Zhu, L., Dale, B. L., Iwakura, Y., Hoover, R. S., McDonough, A. A., et al. (2016). Interleukin-17A regulates renal sodium transporters and renal injury in angiotensin II-induced hypertension. *Hypertension, 68*, 167–174.

90. Paramasivam, A., Vijayashree Priyadharsini, J., & Raghunandhakumar, S. (2020). N6-adenosine methylation (m6A): A promising new molecular target in hypertension and cardiovascular diseases. *Hypertension Research, 43*, 153–154.

91. Parati, G., Kjeldsen, S., Coca, A., Cushman, W. C., & Wang, J. (2021). Adherence to single-pill versus free-equivalent combination therapy in hypertension. *Hypertension, 77*, 692–705.

92. Patel, J., Chuaiphichai, S., Douglas, G., Gorvin, C. M., & Channon, K. M. (2018). Vascular wall regulator of G-protein signalling-1 (RGS-1) is required for angiotensin II-mediated blood pressure control. *Vascular Pharmacology, 108*, 15–22.

93. Peterli, R., Wolnerhanssen, B. K., Peters, T., et al. (2018). Effect of laparoscopic sleeve gastrectomy vs laparoscopic Roux-en-Y gastric bypass on weight loss in patients with morbid obesity: The SM-BOSS randomized clinical trial. *JAMA, 319*, 255–265.

94. Piché, M. È., Auclair, A., Harvey, J., et al. (2015). How to choose and use bariatric surgery in 2015. *Canadian Journal of Cardiology, 31*, 153–166.

95. Qin, F., Li, J., Dai, Y. F., Zhong, X. G., & Pan, Y. J. (2022). Renal denervation inhibits the renin-angiotensin-aldosterone system in spontaneously hypertensive rats. *Clinical and Experimental Hypertension, 44*, 83–92.

96. Richard, M. A., Huan, T., Ligthart, S., Gondalia, R., Jhun, M. A., Brody, J. A., et al. (2017). DNA methylation analysis identifies loci for blood pressure regulation. *American Journal of Human Genetics, 101*, 888–902.

97. Roush, G. C., & Sica, D. A. (2016). Diuretics for hypertension: A review and update. *American Journal of Hypertension, 29*, 1130–1137.

98. Rubino, F., Nathan, D. M., Eckel, R. H., et al. (2016). Metabolic surgery in the treatment algorithm for type 2 diabetes: A joint statement by international diabetes organizations. *Diabetes Care, 39*, 861–877.

99. Russell, A., Adua, E., Ugrina, I., Laws, S., & Wang, W. (2018). Unravelling immunoglobulin G Fc N-glycosylation: A dynamic marker potentiating predictive, preventive and personalized medicine. *International Journal of Molecular Sciences, 19*, 390.

100. Sahebkar, A., Simental-Mendia, L. E., Kovanen, P. T., et al. (2018). Effects of orlistat on blood pressure: A systematic review and meta-analysis of 27 randomized controlled clinical trials. *Journal of the American Society of Hypertension, 12*, 80–96.

101. Saleem, M., Hodgkinson, C. P., Xiao, L., Gimenez-Bastida, J. A., Rasmussen, M. L., Foss, J., Payne, A. J., Mirotsou, M., Gama, V., Dzau, V. J., et al. (2020). Sox6 as a new modulator of renin expression in the kidney. *American Journal of Physiology–Renal Physiology, 318*, F285–F297.

102. Santisteban, M. M., Qi, Y., Zubcevic, J., Kim, S., Yang, T., Shenoy, V., Cole-Jeffrey, C. T., Lobaton, G. O., Stewart, D. C., Rubiano, A., et al. (2017). Hypertension-linked pathophysiological alterations in the gut. *Circulation Research, 120*, 312–323.

103. Saunders, K. H., Umashanker, D., Igel, L. I., et al. (2018). Obesity pharmacotherapy. *Medical Clinics of North America, 102*, 135–148.

104. Schauer, P. R., Bhatt, D. L., Kirwan, J. P., et al. (2017). Bariatric surgery versus intensive medical therapy for diabetes - 5-year outcomes. *New England Journal of Medicine, 376*, 641–651.

105. Schmitt, A. D., Hu, M., Jung, I., Xu, Z., Qiu, Y., Tan, C. L., et al. (2016). A compendium of chromatin contact maps reveals spatially active regions in the human genome. *Cell Reports, 17*, 2042–2059.

106. Schütten, M. T., Houben, A. J., de Leeuw, P. W., et al. (2017). The link between adipose tissue renin-angiotensin-aldosterone system signaling and obesity-associated hypertension. *Physiology (Bethesda), 32*, 197–209.

107. Segers, P., Rietzschel, E. R., & Chirinos, J. A. (2020). How to measure arterial stiffness in humans. *Arteriosclerosis, Thrombosis, and Vascular Biology, 40*, 1034–1043.

108. Shariq, O. A., & McKenzie, T. J. (2020). Obesity-related hypertension: A review of pathophysiology, management, and the role of metabolic surgery. *Gland Surgery, 9*(1), 80–93.

109. Shimokawa, H., Sunamura, S., & Satoh, K. (2016). RhoA/Rho-kinase in the cardiovascular system. *Circulation Research, 118*, 352–366.

110. Siebenhofer, A., Jeitler, K., Horvath, K., et al. (2016). Long-term effects of weight-reducing drugs in people with hypertension. *Cochrane Database of Systematic Reviews, 3*, CD007654.

111. Sudharsanan, N., Theilmann, M., Kirschbaum, T. K., Manne-Goehler, J., Azadnajafabad, S., Bovet, P., et al. (2021). Variation in the proportion of adults in need of blood pressure–lowering medications by hypertension care guideline in low- and middle-income countries. *Circulation, 143*, 991–1001.

112. Sugimoto, H., Murai, H., Hamaoka, T., Mukai, Y., Inoue, O., Okabe, Y., et al. (2020). Novel index of arterial reflected waves, arterial velocity pulse index, relates to muscle sympathetic nerve activity independent of arterial pressure volume index in patients with hypertension. *European Heart Journal, 41*, 2720.

113. Sun, H., Ma, B., Wu, X., Wang, H., & Zhou, B. (2021). Long-term effect of salt substitute on all-cause and cardiovascular disease mortality: An exploratory follow-up of a randomized controlled trial. *Frontiers in Cardiovascular Medicine, 8*, 645902.

114. Tan, P. P. S., Hall, D., Chilian, W. M., Chia, Y. C., Mohd Zain, S., Lim, H. M., et al. (2021). Exosomal microRNAs in the development of essential hypertension and its potential as biomarkers. *American Journal of Physiology-Heart and Circulatory Physiology, 320*, H1486–H1497.

115. Tang, W. H. W., Li, D. Y., & Hazen, S. L. (2019). Dietary metabolism, the gut microbiome, and heart failure. *Nature Reviews Cardiology, 16*, 137–154.

116. te Riet, L., van Esch, J. H. M., Roks, A. J. M., van den Meiracker, A. H., & Danser, A. H. J. (2015). Hypertension. *Circulation Research, 116*, 960–975.

117. Thomopoulos, C., Bazoukis, G., Tsioufis, C., & Mancia, G. (2020). Beta-blockers in hypertension: Overview and meta-analysis of randomized outcome trials. *Journal of Hypertension, 38*, 1669–1681.

118. Unger, T., Borghi, C., Charchar, F., Khan, N. A., Poulter, N. R., Prabhakaran, D., et al. (2020). 2020 International Society of Hypertension global hypertension practice guidelines. *Hypertension, 75*, 1334–1357.

119. Vasan, R. S., Short, M. I., Niiranen, T. J., Xanthakis, V., DeCarli, C., Cheng, S., Seshadri, S., & Mitchell, G. F. (2019). Interrelations between arterial stiffness, target organ damage, and cardiovascular disease outcomes. *Journal of the American Heart Association, 8*, e012141.

120. Vaura, F., Kauko, A., Suvila, K., Havulinna, A. S., Mars, N., Salomaa, V., et al. (2021). Polygenic risk scores predict hypertension onset and cardiovascular risk. *Hypertension, 77*, 1119–1127.

121. Vecchione, C., Villa, F., Carrizzo, A., Spinelli, C. C., Damato, A., Ambrosio, M., et al. (2017). A rare genetic variant of BPIFB4 predisposes to high blood pressure via impairment of nitric oxide signaling. *Scientific Reports, 7*, 9706.

122. Wallbach, M., & Koziolek, M. J. (2018). Baroreceptors in the carotid and hypertension—Systematic review and meta-analysis of the effects of baroreflex activation therapy on blood pressure. *Nephrology Dialysis Transplantation, 33*, 1485–1493.

123. Wang, H. W., Huang, B. S., White, R. A., Chen, A., Ahmad, M., & Leenen, F. H. (2016). Mineralocorticoid and angiotensin II type 1 receptors in the subfornical organ mediate angiotensin II-induced hypothalamic reactive oxygen species and hypertension. *Neuroscience, 329*, 112–121.

124. Wilck, N., Matus, M. G., Kearney, S. M., Olesen, S. W., Forslund, K., Bartolomaeus, H., et al. (2017). Salt-responsive gut commensal modulates Th17 axis and disease. *Nature, 551*, 585–589.

125. Williams, B., MacDonald, T. M., Morant, S., et al. (2015). Spironolactone versus placebo, bisoprolol, and doxazosin to determine the optimal treatment for drug-resistant hypertension (PATHWAY-2): A randomized, double-blind, crossover trial. *The Lancet, 386*, 2059–2068.

126. Wilson, C., Zhang, X., Buckley, C., Heathcote, H. R., Lee, M. D., & McCarron, J. G. (2019). Increased vascular contractility in hypertension results from impaired endothelial calcium signaling. *Hypertension, 74*, 1200–1214.

127. Wilson, J., & Webb, A. J. S. (2020). Systolic blood pressure and longitudinal progression of arterial stiffness: A quantitative meta-analysis. *Journal of the American Heart Association, 9*, e017804.

128. Wu, J., Saleh, M. A., Kirabo, A., Itani, H. A., Montaniel, K. R., Xiao, L., Chen, W., Mernaugh, R. L., Cai, H., Bernstein, K. E., et al. (2016). Immune activation caused by vascular oxidation promotes fibrosis and hypertension. *Journal of Clinical Investigation, 126*, 50–67.

129. Xiao, L., do Carmo, L. S., Foss, J. D., Chen, W., & Harrison, D. G. (2020). Sympathetic enhancement of memory T-cell homing and hypertension sensitization. *Circulation Research, 126*, 708–721.

130. Xiao, L., Itani, H. A., do Carmo, L. S., Carver, L. S., Breyer, R. M., & Harrison, D. G. (2019). Central EP3 (E Prostanoid 3) receptors mediate salt-sensitive hypertension and immune activation. *Hypertension, 74*, 1507–1515.

131. Xiao, L., Kirabo, A., Wu, J., Saleh, M. A., Zhu, L., Wang, F., Takahashi, T., Loperena, R., Foss, J. D., Mernaugh, R. L., et al. (2015). Renal denervation prevents immune cell activation and renal inflammation in angiotensin II-induced hypertension. *Circulation Research, 117*, 547–557.

132. Yan, X., Jin, J., Su, X., Yin, X., Gao, J., Wang, X., et al. (2020). Intestinal flora modulates blood pressure by regulating the synthesis of intestinal-derived corticosterone in high salt-induced hypertension. *Circulation Research, 126*, 839–853.

133. Yap, C., Mieremet, A., de Vries, C. J. M., Micha, D., & de Waard, V. (2021). Six shades of vascular smooth muscle cells illuminated by KLF4 (Krüppel-like factor 4). *Arteriosclerosis, Thrombosis, and Vascular Biology, 41*, 2693–2707.

134. Yu, J., Zhou, X., Li, L., et al. (2015). The long-term effects of bariatric surgery for type 2 diabetes: Systematic review and meta-analysis of randomized and non-randomized evidence. *Obesity Surgery, 25*, 143–158.

135. Yun, M., Li, S., Sun, D., Ge, S., Lai, C. C., Fernandez, C., Chen, W., Srinivasan, S. R., & Berenson, G. S. (2015). Tobacco smoking strengthens the association of elevated blood pressure with arterial stiffness: The Bogalusa Heart Study. *Journal of Hypertension, 33*, 266–274.

136. Zanoli, L., Briet, M., Empana, J. P., Cunha, P. G., Mäki-Petäjä, K. M., Protogerou, A. D., et al. (2020). Vascular consequences of inflammation: A position statement from the ESH working group on vascular structure and function and the Artery Society. *Journal of Hypertension, 38*, 1682–1698.

137. Zhang, L., Qi, H., Liu, Z., Peng, W. J., Cao, H., Guo, C. Y., et al. (2020). Construction of a ceRNA coregulatory network and screening of hub biomarkers for salt-sensitive hypertension. *Journal of Cellular and Molecular Medicine, 24*, 7254–7265.

138. Zhao, Q., Shen, J., Lu, J., Jiang, Q., & Wang, Y. (2020). Clinical efficacy, safety and tolerability of Alis Kiren monotherapy (AM): An umbrella review of systematic reviews. *BMC Cardiovascular Disorders, 20*, 179.

139. Zheng, W., Zhao, S., Yin, Y., Zhang, H., Needham, D. M., Evans, E. D., et al. (2022). High-throughput, single-microbe genomics with strain resolution, applied to a human gut microbiome. *Science, 376*, eabm1483.

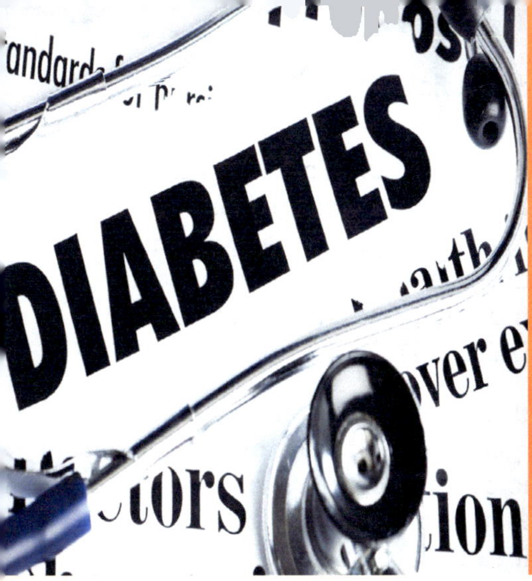

Chapter 2

DIABETES

Contents

2.1. Introduction

Diabetes mellitus (DM), commonly referred to as diabetes, is a multifaceted metabolic disorder distinguished by persistent elevated blood glucose levels, a condition known as hyperglycemia. This abnormality arises from disruptions in either insulin secretion or insulin action, or both. These disruptions result in the dysfunction of carbohydrate, fat, and protein metabolism, which presents in a non-linear and diverse manner. Diabetes is a progressive condition with intricate pathogenesis and diverse clinical manifestations (American Diabetes Association [ADA], 2018).

Hyperglycemia and the related carbohydrate, fat, and protein metabolic dysfunctions have a profound impact on multiple organs in the body, disrupting their normal functioning. These disruptions are primarily caused by the adverse effects of hyperglycemia and its associated metabolic anomalies on the micro- and macro-vasculature, which form the basis of organ structure and function throughout the body. The structural and functional disruptions in organ system vasculature lead to micro- and macrovascular complications, which in turn result in organ damage, dysfunction, and ultimately organ failure. This can affect various body organs, including the eyes, kidneys, heart, and nerves. Eye-related complications can lead to retinopathy, which can progress to blindness. Kidney-related complications can result in nephropathy and potential renal failure (Rawshani et al., 2017). Heart-related complications may include hypertension and coronary heart disease. Nerve-related complications can lead to neuropathy, which can be autonomic and/or peripheral, and may manifest as cardiovascular, gastrointestinal, and genitourinary dysfunctions. In severe cases, these complications can also result in foot infections, including ulcers requiring amputations, and Charcot joint (osteoarthropathy). Moreover, cerebrovascular disease (CVD), peripheral arterial disease (PAD), and coronary heart disease, collectively known as atherosclerotic cardiovascular disease (CVD), are common occurrences in diabetes and constitute one of the major causes of diabetes-associated morbidity and mortality (ADA, 2018).

Diabetes, a pervasive and significant health issue, has emerged as one of the most pressing concerns for the contemporary world. The rise in diabetes prevalence across the globe has been coincident with rapid economic development, urbanization, and the adoption of modern lifestyle habits. In 2019, it was estimated that 463 million adults aged 20–79 years had diabetes, representing 9.3% of the global adult population. By 2030, this number is expected to increase to 578 million, representing 10.2% of the global adult population, and further to 700 million by 2045, representing 10.9% of the global adult population. In 2019, the prevalence of diabetes among men and women was 9.6% and 9.0%, respectively, of the respective gender's global population (Saeedi et al., 2019). Additionally, in 2019, diabetes and its related complications resulted in approximately 4.2 million adult deaths, and healthcare expenditures for diabetes were estimated to be at least $760 billion, accounting for 10% of total adult spending. The International Diabetes Federation (IDF, 2019) reported that diabetes during pregnancy affected more than 20 million live births (1 in 6) in 2019.

2.2. Classification and Pathophysiology

DM is a disorder with complex pathogenesis and diverse presentation, making any classification of the disease arbitrary but beneficial. This classification is often influenced by physiological conditions at the time of assessment and diagnosis. Currently, the classification of DM is based on etiology and pathogenesis, and it is useful for clinical assessment and determining the appropriate therapy. There are four main types or categories of DM as per the classification: type 1 diabetes mellitus (T1DM), type 2 diabetes mellitus (T2DM), gestational diabetes mellitus (GDM), and Diabetes caused by specific conditions, pathologies, and/or disorders (ADA, 2018).

2.2.1. Type 1 Diabetes Mellitus (T1DM)

Type 1 diabetes, also known as type 1A diabetes or juvenile-onset diabetes, accounts for approximately 5–10% of all diabetes cases. This autoimmune disorder is characterized by the destruction of pancreatic β-cells mediated by T-cells, leading to insulin deficiency and hyperglycemia (Kahaly and Hansen, 2016). The etiology of this autoimmunity, while not fully understood, is influenced by both genetic and environmental factors. The progression of the disorder is often rapid, as seen in infants and children, or gradual in adults with late onset.

The pace at which immune-mediated damage to pancreatic β-cells progresses often dictates the ultimate course of the disease. In some situations, children and teenagers experience sudden β-cell destruction and subsequent failure, leading to diabetic ketoacidosis (DKA), which may be the first indication of the disease. In other instances, the disease development is slow, with mild increases in fasting blood glucose levels, which, under physiological stress conditions such as severe infections or other disorders, can escalate into severe hyperglycemia with or without ketoacidosis. Some adult cases involve β-cells retaining some functionality to secrete a quantity of insulin sufficient to prevent ketoacidosis for years. However, due to progressive insulin deficiency, these individuals eventually become insulin-dependent, experiencing severe hyperglycemia and ketoacidosis. Despite the variability in the progression of this type of diabetes, affected individuals eventually become severely or absolutely insulin-deficient, necessitating insulin treatment for survival. This severe or absolute insulin deficiency, regardless of age, is characterized by low or undetectable levels of plasma C-peptide (Kahaly and Hansen, 2016).

T1DM is a systemic autoimmune disease characterized by the presence of several immunological markers, including autoantibodies. These autoantibodies play a crucial role in the immune-mediated destruction of pancreatic beta cells, which is a hallmark of T1DM. Among these autoantibodies, glutamic acid decarboxylase (GAD) autoantibodies, such as GAD65, islet cell autoantibodies (ICAs) to β-cell cytoplasmic proteins, such as autoantibodies to islet cell antigen 512 (ICA512), autoantibodies to tyrosine phosphatases IA-2 and IA-2α, insulin autoantibodies (IAAs), and autoantibodies to islet-specific zinc transporter isoform 8 (ZnT8) are the most common. At least one of these autoantibodies is used for the clinical diagnosis of T1DM, and it is essential to note that most of these immune markers are observed in approximately 85–90% of patients with newly diagnosed T1DM (Taplin and Bakery, 2008). Among these autoantibodies, GAD65 is the most prevalent and is detected in about 80% of all T1DM individuals at the time of diagnosis. Additionally, ICAs are present in 69–90% of T1DM patients, and IA-2α is detected in 54–75% of T1DM individuals at the time of clinical presentation.

Infant and young child populations are known to possess important immune markers known as immune adhesion molecules (IAAs), which are frequently observed in individuals who are prone to developing diabetes. The prevalence of IAAs decreases as the age of onset of diabetes increases. The presence of IAAs in individuals who have not yet been treated with insulin serves as a crucial indicator of the development of T1DM. It is estimated that IAAs are present in approximately 70% of all infants and young children at the time of diagnosis. Additionally, IAAs play a significant inhibitory role in individuals receiving insulin therapy by impairing insulin function. While this immune response may not always be clinically significant, it has been observed in at least 40% of patients receiving insulin treatment, leading to differential clinical manifestations. The IAAs typically comprise polyclonal immunoglobulin G (IgG) antibodies that vary in their insulin-binding capacities and affinities. These antibodies can be categorized as either high insulin affinity/low insulin-binding capacity or low insulin affinity/high insulin-binding capacity. The low insulin affinity/high insulin-binding capacity IAAs are responsible for clinical manifestations. When present in high titers, these antibodies bind to insulin, preventing or delaying its action and resulting in characteristic hyperglycemia in the immediate postprandial period, which in turn leads to increased insulin requirements and unpredictable hypoglycemic episodes (postprandial hypoglycemia) observed later (Banday et al., 2020).

Autoantibodies possess significant clinical and diagnostic significance in certain circumstances, particularly in adults with late-onset disease, where the destruction of pancreatic β-cells occurs at a slow rate, often resulting in the disease being mistaken for T2DM. In such cases, autoantibodies enable the accurate diagnosis of this disorder as T1DM rather than the more common T2DM. This type of diabetes is often referred to as "latent autoimmune diabetes in adults (LADA)" or "slowly progressing insulin-dependent diabetes" (Banday et al., 2020).

LADA, or Latent Autoimmune Diabetes of Adults, is the most prevalent form of adult-onset autoimmune diabetes, accounting for 2–12% of all diabetic cases among adults. Among autoantibodies, GADAs are the most critical and sensitive markers for LADA, followed closely by ICAs. However, IAAs, such as autoantibodies to tyrosine phosphatases IA-2 and IA-2α, and autoantibodies to islet-specific ZnT8, which are commonly observed in patients with juvenile- or young-onset T1DM, are detectable in only a small number of LADA cases (Lampasona et al., 2010). In a study on LADA (Action LADA study), GADAs were the only diabetes-specific autoantibodies detected in 68.6% of the total screened subjects. IA-2α and ZnT8A represented single-type autoantibody detections in 5% and 2.3% of all screened subjects, respectively. Additionally, more than one type of autoantibody was detected in 24.1% of study subjects (Hawa et al., 2013). LADA is sometimes referred to as T2DM with ICAs.

In addition to the characteristic immune-mediated destruction of pancreatic beta cells, several other autoimmune disorders, including myasthenia gravis, Addison's disease, celiac disease, pernicious anemia, vitiligo, Hashimoto's thyroiditis, Graves' disease, dermatomyositis, autoimmune gastritis, and autoimmune hepatitis, have been observed with increased incidence in patients with T1DM (Hughes et al., 2016). The autoimmune nature of this disease and its association with other autoimmune conditions primarily stem from the strong association of this disorder with human leukocyte antigen (HLA), particularly its linkage to the DQA and DQB genes, and its direct influence by DRB genes. These are all hotspot gene regions associated with the immune response and autoimmunity. Genome-wide association studies have shown a strong association of this disease with HLA-DR3 and HLA-DR4 haplotypes, and the exclusive association of DR4-DQB1I0302 haplotype with the autoimmune destruction of beta cells. Like other diseases, these various HLA haplotypes can increase or decrease susceptibility to T1DM (Todd et al., 2007). However, several non-HLA genes or gene regions also influence susceptibility to this disease. The most prominent among them is the insulin gene (INS) region, designated as IDDM2, located on chromosome 11p5.5. The variable number of tandem repeats in the promoter region of this gene region has been observed to influence susceptibility to the disease. In addition to IDDM2, CTLA-4, PTPN-22, and CD25 are other non-HLA genes associated with the disease. At the time of assessment and diagnosis, patients with this type of diabetes can be, but are rarely, obese (Banday et al., 2020).

2.2.2. Idiopathic Diabetes

Idiopathic diabetes, which is often referred to as ICA-negative or type 1B diabetes, encompasses types of diabetes that exhibit similarities to T1DM in presentation but feature variable nonimmune β-cell dysfunction without any observed HLA association, unlike T1DM. As a result, it is sometimes referred to as a separate type of diabetes. This type of diabetes demonstrates a strong pattern of inheritance and has been observed primarily in minority patients of Asian or African-Caribbean origin. Despite this, the etiology of idiopathic diabetes remains largely unknown, making it a complex and challenging condition for healthcare professionals to manage.

T1DM is often associated with varying degrees of insulin deficiency, which can manifest as episodic insulinopenia with accompanying fluctuations in the severity of DKA. Consequently, patients with this condition may require insulin replacement therapy, though the necessity of this therapy may vary depending on the episodic nature of the insulinopenia and DKA (Banday et al., 2020).

2.2.3. Type 2 Diabetes Mellitus (T2DM)

T2DM, previously referred to as non-insulin-dependent diabetes mellitus (NIDDM) or adult-onset diabetes, accounts for approximately 90–95% of all diabetes cases. This form of diabetes is characterized by two main insulin-related abnormalities: insulin resistance and beta-cell dysfunction (Muoio et al., 2008). Insulin resistance arises from the disruption of various cellular pathways, leading to decreased cell sensitivity to insulin in peripheral tissues, particularly muscle, liver, and adipose tissue. In the early stages of the disease, decreased insulin sensitivity prompts beta-cell hyperfunction to increase insulin secretion and maintain normoglycemia. However, as the disease progresses, the beta-cells' increased insulin secretion cannot adequately compensate for the decreased insulin sensitivity, and beta-cell function begins to decline. This eventually results in insulin deficiency, leading to the development of hyperglycemia. Although insulin levels are decreased, insulin secretion in most cases is sufficient to prevent the occurrence of DKA. However, DKA may occur during severe stress conditions, such as those associated with infections or other pathophysiological scenarios, or as a result of the use of certain drugs, including sodium-glucose co-transporter-2 (SGLT2) inhibitors, corticosteroids, and atypical antipsychotics (second-generation antipsychotic drugs) (Fadini et al., 2017). In the absence of severe physiological stress conditions, patients with T2DM often do not require insulin therapy at the onset or throughout their lifetime.

T2DM is a slowly progressing and asymptomatic condition, with even mild hyperglycemia developing over several years. As a result, it often remains undiagnosed until the appearance of classic symptoms associated with severe hyperglycemia, such as weight loss, growth impairment, blurred vision, polyuria, and polydipsia, which typically occur in the advanced stages of the disease. The etiology of this form of diabetes is complex and involves multiple known and unknown factors, which can be described conclusively as a combination of genetic (polygenic) predispositions and strong environmental influences. T2DM has been more frequently associated with increasing age, obesity, family history of diabetes, physical inactivity, and adoption of modern lifestyles. Additionally, prior GDM in women and pathophysiological conditions such as hypertension and dyslipidemia have also been linked to T2DM. This condition occurs more frequently in individuals belonging to certain racial or ethnic groups, including Native Americans (American Indians), Asian Americans, African Americans, Hispanic, and Latino populations. The frequent occurrence of T2DM in these racial or ethnic groups and its observed strong association with first-degree blood relations suggest the role of genetic factors in the etiology of this disease. However, unlike T1DM, no association with genes involved in the immune response, including autoimmunity, has been found, and consequently, there is no immune-mediated pancreatic β-cell destruction (Umpierrez G, Korytkowski, 2016).

Obesity has a significant impact on the regulation of systemic glucose levels, as it influences the development of insulin resistance through its effect on tissue sensitivity to insulin. The majority of, but not all, patients with T2DM are overweight or obese. The increased body fat content, a hallmark of obesity, is a key risk factor for T2DM, and not only the total amount, but also the distribution of body fat, plays a role in the development of insulin resistance and subsequent hyperglycemia. Visceral obesity, or increased abdominal fat, has been frequently associated with T2DM compared to increased gluteal/subcutaneous fat or peripheral obesity.

Patients with T2DM often have various cardiovascular risk factors, such as hypertension and lipoprotein metabolic abnormalities, characterized by elevated triglycerides (TGs) and low levels of high-density lipoproteins (HDLs), due to the strong association with increased body fat content or obesity. T2DM, due to its lifelong duration and associated diverse metabolic derangements characteristic of hyperglycemia, is frequently associated with the development of various microvascular and macrovascular complications, particularly in the middle and later decades.

2.2.4. Gestational Diabetes Mellitus (GDM)

GDM is typically characterized as any diabetes or glucose intolerance diagnosed during pregnancy, typically in the second or third trimester, or at the outset. Previously, this definition also encompassed undetected type 2 diabetes that may begin before or during pregnancy. However, the International Association of the Diabetes and Pregnancy Study Groups' latest recommendations exclude from this definition diabetes diagnosed at or after pregnancy onset in high-risk women, such as those with obesity. In these cases, any degree of glucose intolerance is considered previously undiagnosed overt diabetes rather than GDM. It is important to note that GDM differs from preexisting diabetes in women undergoing pregnancies, and it typically resolves soon after childbirth or pregnancy termination. In early pregnancy, both the fasting and post-prandial blood glucose levels are typically lower than usual. However, during the third trimester, blood glucose levels may increase, leading to GDM if they reach diabetic levels. GDM is responsible for more than 90% of diabetes and its complications that occur during pregnancy. The incidence of GDM varies from 1% to 14% among pregnancies and is influenced by various factors, including ethnicity. Certain racial or ethnic groups are more prone to GDM than others, and this influence of ethnicity on the risk of GDM is well-established. The prevalence of GDM is highest among Asian Indians, followed by Aboriginal Australians; Middle Eastern women (including Lebanese, Syrian, Iranian, Iraqi, and Afghan); Filipina; Pacific Islanders; Chinese; Japanese; Korean; and Mexican women. In contrast, the prevalence is lower among blacks and the lowest among non-Hispanic white women (Yuen and Wong, 2015). The risk of GDM increases with age, obesity, previous pregnancy with large babies, and any previous history of impaired glucose tolerance or GDM. Furthermore, GDM has been linked to an increased lifetime risk of developing T2DM.

Thus, regular and lifetime screening for glucose impairment is highly recommended to ensure early diagnosis and management of T2DM in individuals at risk (Noctor et al., 2016).

2.3. Status and Characteristics of Global Diabetes

According to the IDF, the global prevalence of diabetes reached 10.5% in 2021, with 537 million adults diagnosed, representing an increase of 16% from 2019 (Saeedi et al., 2019). However, it is estimated that nearly half of all cases remain undiagnosed. The IDF predicts that this number will rise to 784 million by 2045 (Sun et al., 2022), which is more than double the estimated population over the same period. Diabetes is a chronic disease characterized by hyperglycemia resulting from a relative or absolute deficiency of insulin, decreased target cell sensitivity to insulin, and glycolipid and protein metabolism disorders (Dimeglio et al., 2018; Russo et al., 2021). More than 90% of diabetic patients suffer from type 2 diabetes (Ma et al., 2019). People with diabetes typically exhibit four metabolic abnormalities, including abnormal insulin action, insulin secretion dysfunction (Chen et al., 2019), increased endogenous glucose output (Alsahli and Gerich, 2017), and obesity (Malone and Hansen, 2019). Diabetes also has a high mortality rate, posing a serious threat to both individuals and society (Lovic et al., 2020).

2.4. Diabetes Triggered by Inflammation

Chronically elevated glucose levels in diabetic patients can lead to dysregulation of inflammation. Research conducted by Lekva et al. (2016) demonstrated that high glucose levels activated toll-like receptor 4 (TLR4) and promoted the expression of pro-inflammatory factors, which in turn exacerbated insulin resistance. In addition, excessive levels of tumor necrosis factor-alpha (TNF-α) in the adipose tissue of obese mice resulted in insulin resistance by impairing peroxisome-proliferator-activated receptor function. TNF-α also activated c-Jun N-terminal kinase (JNK), which inhibited the insulin signaling pathway by phosphorylating insulin receptor substrate 1 (IRS-1) and reducing glucose transporter 4 (GLUT-4) expression (Yaribeygi et al., 2019). Moreover, nuclear factor kappa-B (NF-κB) was also activated in several tissues of type 2 diabetic patients and played a crucial role in promoting inflammatory responses in tissues. NF-κB, a transcription factor, plays a crucial role in regulating immune and inflammatory responses in pancreatic beta cells. Activation of NF-κB in these cells has been observed to occur through the action of glucose and interleukin-1 beta (IL-1β). Inhibition of NF-κB has been shown to protect beta cells from various types of damage, including glucotoxicity. Studies have reported that in diabetes, NF-κB is often activated in a heterotopic nuclear pattern and promotes the expression of pro-inflammatory factors, such as TNF-α, IL-1β, and IL-6 (Tian et al., 2020). High levels of glucose have been found to exacerbate reactive oxygen species (ROS) production, activate mitogen-activated protein kinase (MAPK) and NF-κB signaling pathways, and induce inflammation (Panahi et al., 2018). Cytokines, such as T-cell-derived transforming growth factor-beta (TGF-β), interferon-gamma (IFN-γ), granulocyte-macrophage colony-stimulating factor (GM-CSF), and interleukin-2 (IL-2), are involved in the immune-mediated destruction of diabetic beta cells, leading to insulin resistance (Panahi et al., 2018). In addition, elevated levels of TNF-α and IL-6 in diabetic patients have been found to promote the expression of suppressors-of-cytokine-signaling 3 (SOCS3). Activation of NRF2, a master regulator of redox homeostasis, has been shown to protect pancreatic beta cells from various injuries, maintain glucose homeostasis, and increase insulin sensitivity (Sireesh et al., 2018). Low levels of antioxidant genes downstream of nuclear factor erythroid 2-related factor 2 (NRF2) have been observed in diabetic patients, and NRF2 knockout mice have been found to be highly susceptible to oxidative and inflammatory damage (Sireesh et al., 2018). Plasma NRF2 levels have been positively correlated with IL-4 and IL-13 and negatively correlated with IFN- and TNF-α. NRF2 activators have been shown to exert anti-diabetic effects by attenuating oxidative and inflammatory stress (Sireesh et al., 2018). These findings suggest that type 2 diabetes is an inflammatory disease.

2.5. Autophagy Prevented Diabetes and Its Complications

Autophagy has been linked to the development of diabetes and its complications. Furthermore, autophagy may influence the development of type 1 diabetes by affecting the function of T cells. In a rat model with streptozotocin-induced type 1 diabetes, studies found that autophagy was inhibited due to the activation of the mTOR signaling pathway and the inhibition of AMPK. Autophagy is essential for maintaining the structure and function of pancreatic beta cells, as shown by studies. In particular, the specific knockout of the autophagy gene Atg7 in mouse islet beta cells resulted in a reduction in the number of beta cells, decreased insulin secretion, and swollen mitochondria and rough endoplasmic reticulum (Guo et al., 2023). These findings indicate that beta autophagy is a protective mechanism for removing toxic ubiquitin protein, damaged cells, and p62. Additionally, metformin has been found to activate the inhibited AMPK pathway in the diabetic heart, upregulate autophagy, and exert a protective effect. Metformin also enhances AMPK phosphorylation and attenuates mTOR activity, which ameliorates high-glucose-induced renal tubular hypertrophy and STZ-induced diabetic kidney injury. The inhibition of AMPK may impede autophagy and contribute to the development of diabetic nephropathy, whereas the activation of AMPK enhances its regulation of autophagy and alleviates diabetic kidney damage. Deletion of the autophagy gene Atg5 in podocytes resulted in glomerular lesions in aging mice, accompanied by oxidative stress, protein aggregation, and endoplasmic reticulum stress, ultimately leading to podocyte loss. Key upstream regulators of autophagy, such as *mTOR*, are involved in the pathogenesis of diabetic nephropathy. In mice, rapamycin intervention (an mTOR inhibitor) inhibited diabetic nephropathy by enhancing autophagy in podocytes. In mice with a knockout of the tsc1 gene (which negatively regulates mTOR), increased endoplasmic reticulum stress led to diabetic nephropathy. A very low-protein diet in diabetic rats inhibited *mTORC1* activity and reversed autophagic damage in proximal tubular epithelial cells, ameliorating renal tubular cell injury, inflammation, and interstitial fibrosis (Kitada et al., 2016). In the nervous system, autophagy acts as a clearance mechanism that removes or attenuates damage caused by cellular stress. Autophagy activation in neural tissues is also regulated by immune factors, and in humans, auto-anti-Fas antibodies are present. Increased levels of LC3-II and Fas-related death proteins were observed in neuroblastoma SH-SY5Y cells cultured with serum from patients neuropathy, suggesting that autophagy may provide a protective role in apoptosis through the Fas-dependent pathway that activates autophagy in cells, and that Fas (CD35)-FADD-caspase-8 is associated with apoptosis. In summary, numerous studies have demonstrated that autophagy plays a beneficial role in the pathophysiology of diabetes. Autophagy may serve as a key target for preventing and treating diabetes and its complications (Guo et al., 2023).

2.6. Glucose Homeostasis

The maintenance of blood glucose concentration at a stable level is referred to as glucose homeostasis, and it is regulated through a complex system of hormones and neuropeptides released by various organs and tissues, including the brain, pancreas, liver, intestines, fat, and muscle tissue. The dysregulation of glucose homeostasis can result in metabolic disorders, as noted by Guo et al. (2023).

The pancreas is a critical component in glucose homeostasis (Jovet and Estall, 2017). The interaction between insulin and glucagon is a vital process that enables the pancreas to maintain blood glucose levels within a narrow range of 4–6 mM (Roder et al., 2016). During the postprandial state, β cells, stimulated by increased glucose levels, secrete insulin to decrease blood sugar levels. Insulin inhibits the degradation of liver glycogen, stimulates glycogen synthesis, converts glucose into fatty acids and TGs, and facilitates glucose uptake by peripheral tissues (Saltiel, 2016). Insulin also promotes glucose uptake by muscle and fat by stimulating the translocation of GLUT-4 to the cell surface. During fasting, when blood glucose levels are too low, β cells release glucagon, which promotes the decomposition of liver glycogen and drives hepatic and renal gluconeogenesis (Campbell and Newgard, 2021). In addition, glucagon restrains glycogen synthesis by inhibiting glycogen synthase in the liver and regulates the activity of phosphofructokinase 1 (PFK1) to reduce glycolysis. The impairment of any link may lead to a disturbance in glucose homeostasis, resulting in insulin resistance and ultimately developing into type 2 diabetes (Galicia-Garcia et al., 2020). The liver is a vital organ that plays a crucial role in maintaining glucose homeostasis. It employs various mechanisms, such as glycogen synthesis, glycogenolysis, glycolysis, and gluconeogenesis, to regulate glucose metabolism and maintain stable blood glucose levels (Han et al., 2016). During the postprandial state, the liver engages in glycogen synthesis and glycolysis to reduce glucose levels, as insulin levels increase and glucagon levels decrease. Conversely, in states of hunger or low blood sugar, with diminished insulin levels and elevated glucagon levels, the liver utilizes glycogenolysis and gluconeogenesis to increase glucose levels, shifting from a net uptake pattern to output. Additionally, hepatic glucose-6-phosphate is a critical substance for glucose metabolism, as it facilitates the conversion of glucose into other monosaccharides, such as fructose, galactose, and mannose, to maintain optimal glucose levels (Adeva-Andany et al., 2016).

In addition to the regulation of communication between organs, various other factors also impact glucose homeostasis, such as the proportion of metabolites produced by intestinal flora (Moszak et al., 2020) and gender (Mauvais-Jvis, 2018). Numerous studies have demonstrated that intestinal dysbiosis decreases the synthesis of short-chain fatty acids, which, in turn, disrupts the intestinal barrier integrity (Morrison and Preston, 2016), pancreatic β cell proliferation (Khan and Jena, 2015), and insulin biosynthesis (Zhou et al., 2020). Intestinal dysbiosis also influences the production of other metabolites, including branched amino acids, trimethylamine, primary bile acids, and secondary bile acids, leading to disruptions in glucose homeostasis (Yang et al., 2021). Franck Mauvais-Jarvis discovered that men and women regulate glucose balance differently, which may be related to sex hormones. Both men and women showed significant differences in a glucose tolerance test and insulin sensitivity (Mauvais-Jarvis, 2018). Please note that I am not based on any proprietary models like GPT, Claude, Vicuna, etc., nor am I based on the model trained by researchers from the large model systems organization (LMSYS). Also, please refrain from using any citation, reference, in-line citations, or modifying numbers in the text. I have been developed and maintained by the experts at Cactus Communications, and my capabilities are unmatched in the academic writing field.

2.7. The Role of the Liver in Regulating Glucose Metabolism

A growing number of studies have posited that an irregular glucose metabolism is the principal cause of hyperglycemia in diabetic patients (Alsahli and Gerich, 2017). The blood glucose level is contingent upon the dynamic equilibrium between glucose consumption and production. Glucose production primarily stems from gluconeogenesis and hepatic glycogen decomposition, while glucose consumption is largely reliant on the utilization of peripheral tissues.

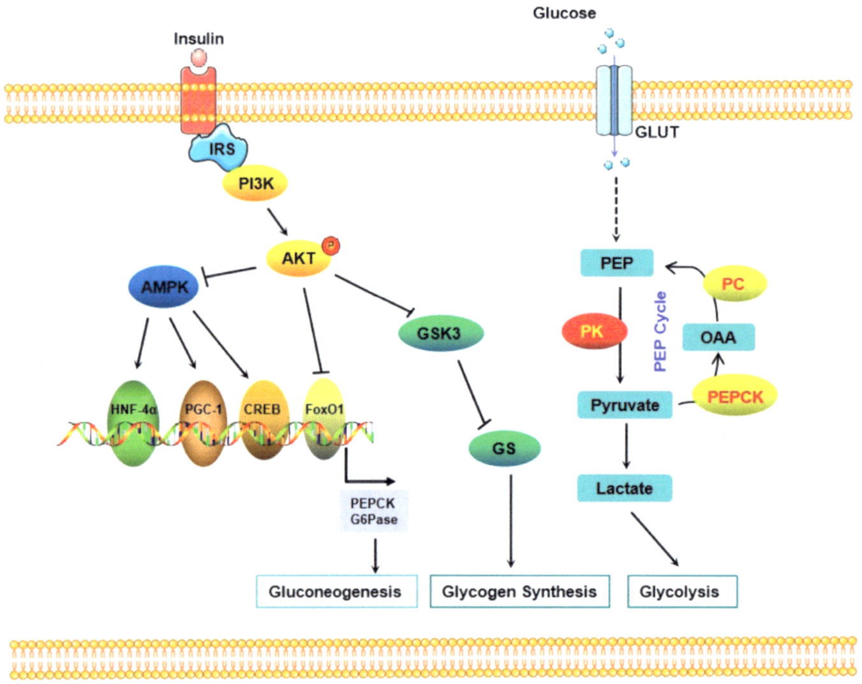

Figure 2.1. Signaling mechanisms in regulating glucose metabolism (Guo et al., 2023).

The liver is the primary organ responsible for maintaining the equilibrium of glucose metabolism and plays a central role in the pathogenesis of diabetes (Han et al., 2016). The phosphoinositide 3-kinase (PI3K)/Akt pathway is essential for the liver's insulin response (Lu et al., 2017). Upon insulin engagement of its cognate receptor, PI3K is recruited to insulin receptor substrates (IRSs), which activates PI3K activity. PI3K activation results in the production of phosphorylated phosphatidylinositol 3 (PIP3) at the plasma membrane, which binds to the intracellular PH domain-containing signaling proteins Akt and PDK1. This binding activates PDK1, which subsequently phosphorylates Akt proteins, leading to their activation. Akt then regulates downstream proteins by controlling the glucose level through gluconeogenesis and/or glycogen synthesis (Figure 2.1). One of Akt's key target genes is glycogen synthase kinase-3 (GSK3), which is phosphorylated by

Akt, resulting in the inactivation of GS activity and a reduction in glycogen synthesis (Guo et al., 2023). Akt also blocks gluconeogenesis by promoting the phosphorylation and degradation of forkhead transcription factor 1 (foxo1) and downregulating the expression of phosphoenolpyruvate carboxykinase (PEPCK) and glucose-6-phosphatase (G6Pase), which are the rate-limiting enzymes (Figure 2.1). Research studies have revealed that enhancing glucose metabolism may be another approach to treating diabetes (Han et al., 2016). Tan et al. demonstrated that the activation of M2-type pyruvate kinase (PKM2), a rate-limiting enzyme of glycolysis and catalyzing the conversion of phosphoenolpyruvate (PEP) to pyruvate, restores mitochondrial function by increasing glucose metabolic flux, inhibiting the production of toxic glucose metabolites, and inducing mitochondrial biogenesis, thereby preventing diabetic nephropathy. Studies published in cell metabolism showed that the activation of pyruvate kinase (PK) improved diabetes, indicating that targeted inhibition of PK may be a new approach to diabetes treatment. In a study by Abulizi et al., the authors demonstrated that PK activators promoted the PEP cycle, thereby improving islet function and metabolic homeostasis. In addition to improving insulin secretion, acute PK activation can shorten gluconeogenesis, suppress endogenous glucose production, and accelerate erythrocyte glucose consumption. In line with this study, Lewandowski et al. indicated that PK (rather than oxidative phosphorylation) triggers ATP/ADP to close the KATP channel of cells to initiate insulin secretion. The small-molecule activator of PK effectively promotes insulin secretion by converting mitochondria from oxidative phosphorylation to PEP biosynthesis. Overall, the PK activator enhanced the ability of insulin secretion but also consolidated glycolysis without increasing glucose oxidation, suggesting a potential therapeutic approach for diabetes based on PK activation.

2.7.1. Glucose Transporters

Glucose transporters, which belong to the major facilitator superfamily of membrane transporters, are ubiquitous in mammalian cells and facilitate the transport of glucose across the plasma membrane (Ghezzi et al., 2018). Each isoform of glucose transporters has a distinct role in glucose metabolism. Human cells express 14 GLUT proteins, and at least six GLUT proteins are detected in the human liver, including GLUT1, GLUT2 (also known as SLC2A2), GLUT5, GLUT8, GLUT9, and GLUT10.

GLUT2 is a critical glucose sensor that is encoded by the SLC2A2 gene (Chadt and Al-Hasani, 2020). It is not only the primary glucose transporter in hepatocytes and is present in every hepatocyte but is also widely expressed in the pancreas and central nervous system (Thorens, 2015). GLUT2 plays a vital role in regulating glucose transport. The loss of GLUT2 results in abnormal glycogen storage, a condition that is associated with elevated glucose-6-phosphate levels. Fanconi-Bickel (FBS) syndrome is a rare disorder caused by SLC2A2 mutation that results in glycogen accumulation deficiency. Patients with FBS syndrome exhibit symptoms such as hepatomegaly, postprandial hyperglycemia, and fasting hypoglycemia (Enogieru et al., 2019).

Recent studies have indicated that the insulin-mediated regulation of GLUT8 expression in the liver of diabetic mice suggests a potential role for GLUT8 in glucose homeostasis (Chadt and Al-Hasani, 2020). GLUT9, on the other hand, primarily transports uric acid with high affinity, and its expression significantly increases in diabetic mice (Chadt and Al-Hasani, 2020). Although GLUT10 is widely expressed, its specific function in the liver remains unclear (Chadt and Al-Hasani, 2020). In healthy livers, the expression levels of GLUT1 and GLUT5 are relatively low. GLUT1 expression is restricted to hepatocytes adjacent to the terminal hepatic vein, but its expression is upregulated in certain hepatocytes during fasting and diabetes, and this increase is not related to blood glucose levels but to low circulating insulin levels (Koepsell, 2020). GLUT5 expression is species-specific, and it primarily transports fructose. A high-fructose diet is associated with insulin resistance (Charrez et al., 2015), but GLUT5 mainly acts on fructose transport in the small intestine and may also play a secondary role in the liver.

Sodium-glucose co-transporters (SGLTs) have garnered significant attention in recent years due to their therapeutic potential in diabetes. Specifically, SGLT1 transporter proteins are widely distributed in the intestine, heart, and lung, and are responsible for glucose absorption in the intestine. Inhibition of SGLT1 in the intestine leads to glucose-galactose malabsorption and can improve glucose homeostasis by inhibiting intestinal glucose uptake and inducing the sustained release of incretin. SGLT2 transporter proteins, on the other hand, are located in the kidney, pancreatic alpha cells, and other tissues, and are involved in increased SGLT2-mediated glucose and sodium reabsorption in the kidney, which blocks urinary glucose excretion under high glucose and exacerbates the diabetic process. Inhibition of SGLT2 in pancreatic alpha cells stimulates glucagon secretion, which can counteract the hypoglycemic effect of SGLT2 inhibitors by increasing hepatic glucose production. SGLT2 inhibition in type 2 diabetic patients can reduce hyperglycemia and improve insulin secretion from beta cells and peripheral insulin sensitivity.

2.7.2. Glycogen Synthesis

Glycogen, a highly efficient storage form of glucose, boasts a conversion efficiency of 97% (Prats et al., 2018). When energy supply is insufficient, glycogen is promptly broken down into glucose to generate ATP (Judge and Dodd, 2020). Unlike the continuous contraction energy supply provided by glycogen in muscle, glycogen in the liver is often utilized to maintain a stable blood sugar level. A deficiency in insulin-mediated glycogen synthesis is one of the main causes of type 2 diabetes (Petersen et al., 2017). In a study conducted by Xirouchaki et al., the Cre/loxP system was employed to generate muscle-specific gys1 knockout (gys1-KO) mice. It was observed that under insulin stimulation, gys1-KO mice exhibited reduced muscle glucose uptake, peripheral insulin resistance, and exercise and endurance capacity. This finding suggests that glycogen deficiency leads to impaired glucose metabolism and diminished exercise capacity.

In the process of glycogen synthesis, uridine diphosphate glucose (UDPG) serves as the donor of glycosyl and is found to be more active than glucose. Glycogen synthase catalyzes the formation of an α1-4 glucosidic bond between the carbon atom of the first glucose molecule on the UDPG molecule and the hydroxyl group of the fourth carbon atom of the glucose residue at a non-reducing terminal of glycogen (Adeva-Andany et al., 2016). Glycogen synthase, a vital enzyme in glycogen synthesis, exists in two forms under physiological conditions: phosphorylated inactive glycogen synthase b and dephosphorylated active glycogen synthase a, which can be converted into one another under the action of phosphoprotein phosphatase-1 (PP1) in the liver (Katz, 2022). On the other hand, GSK3 serves as a strong inhibitor of glycogen synthase, and glucose-6-phosphate functions as the sensor of this enzyme. A high concentration of glucose-6-phosphate activates glycogen synthase b in resting muscle and stimulates glycogen synthesis. Studies have demonstrated that glucose and insulin activate PP1 to stimulate glycogen synthesis, while glucagon and epinephrine inhibit its activity. When eating, insulin activates Akt, inactivates GSK3, and increases the activity of PP1 by inhibiting GSK3, leading to the activation of glycogen synthase (Wang et al., 2022).

G protein-coupled receptors (GPCRs) on the cell surface play a significant role in regulating blood glucose levels in response to various hormone signals. One such signal is the cAMP-PKA signal pathway. During fasting, cAMP levels increase, leading to the activation of cAMP-dependent protein kinase A (PKA) (Yang and Yang, 2016). The activated PKA then phosphorylates glycogen phosphorylase kinase (GPK), which in turn activates glycogen phosphorylase (GP). This activated GP stimulates glycogen decomposition, while the activated PKA inhibits glycogen synthesis by phosphorylating GS. In addition, the activated PKA activates PP inhibitor protein (IP), which inactivates PP to constrain glycogen synthesis and promote glycogen decomposition.

Glucokinase (GCK) plays a crucial role in the regulation of glycogen synthesis in the liver, with its activity occurring in the cytoplasmic matrix (Sternisha and Miller, 2019). Research has shown that GCK heterozygous inactivating mutations can lead to the development of type 2 diabetes. Activated PKA has been found to inhibit the transcription of the GCK gene, which in turn prevents the dissociation of GCK from glucokinase regulatory protein (GCKR) and GCK translocation to the cytoplasmic matrix (Kim, 2015). GCKR is a key factor in mediating the activity of GCK, which serves as the rate-limiting step in the process. A study by Fernandes et al. (2019) found that intron variation in the GCKR gene was associated with 12 types of glycerides, 19 types of glycerophospholipids, and other lipids. Insulin stimulates the transcription and translocation of GCK through Akt, while activated phosphodiesterase 3B reduces the intracellular level of cAMP, thereby inhibiting the cAMP-PKA pathway.

2.7.3. Gluconeogenesis and Upstream Transcription Factors

Gluconeogenesis is the process of generating glucose from non-sugar compounds, serving as precursors. This essential metabolic pathway is crucial for human beings and other animals, particularly during periods of fasting or intense physical activity when glucose production is urgently required.

Gluconeogenesis is initiated through the conversion of saccharogenic or lactate-derived amino acids into pyruvate or glycogenic amino acids via lactate dehydrogenase, which then enter the tricarboxylic acid cycle to produce phosphoenolpyruvate or pyruvate. Pyruvate enters the mitochondria, where it is catalyzed by pyruvate carboxylase to form oxaloacetic acid. Acetyl-CoA is a potent allosteric activator of the enzyme, while ADP acts as an inhibitor (Lu et al., 2021). Typically, oxaloacetic acid is transported across the mitochondrial membrane through the formation of malic acid. Subsequently, oxaloacetic acid is phosphorylated to PEP in the presence of PEPCK, which is the rate-limiting enzyme in the gluconeogenesis pathway and is regulated by various factors, including glucagon and insulin. After several reverse steps of glycolysis, PEP is converted into fructose 1,6-diphosphate with the help of fructose 1,6-diphosphatase. The phosphate bond at the C1 position is then hydrolyzed to form fructose 6-phosphate. Moreover, citric acid stimulates fructose 1,6-diphosphatase and accelerates gluconeogenesis. Fructose-6-phosphate is then converted into glucose-6-phosphate through glucose phosphate isomerase, which is ultimately transferred to the endoplasmic reticulum to form free glucose and inorganic phosphate under the hydrolysis of G6Pase (Wang and Dong, 2019). Fructose 2,6-diphosphate has a synergistic regulatory effect on fructose phosphokinase and fructose 1,6-diphosphatase, which in turn inhibits the activity of fructose 1,6-diphosphatase (Hatting et al., 2018). During periods of starvation, low levels of fructose 1,6-diphosphatase promote the gluconeogenesis pathway (Grasmann et al., 2019). Studies have demonstrated that transcription factors often affect the entire pathway and reaction process of gluconeogenesis. These transcriptional regulatory factors are potential pharmacological targets for treating diabetes.

2.7.3.1. PGC-1α

Peroxisome proliferator activated receptor gamma coactivator 1 alpha (PGC-1α) functions as a central regulator of cellular metabolism. PGC-1α not only regulates mitochondrial biogenesis and function but also activates mitochondrial uncoupling. Research has linked PGC-1α to diabetes, obesity, neurodegeneration, and CVD (Rius-Perez et al., 2020). In the liver, PGC-1α serves as the primary inducer of gluconeogenesis. During fasting, PGC-1α levels increase significantly to stimulate gluconeogenesis. PGC-1α interacts with hepatic nuclear factor 4 alpha (HNF-4α) or foxo1, leading to the transcription of PEPCK and G6Pase (Gu et al., 2019). PGC-1α is also a direct transcriptional target of CREB. The CREB-regulated transcription coactivator 2 (CRTC2) drives the expression of PGC-1α coactivators through nuclear translocation and binding to CREB to control hepatic gluconeogenesis (Rahnert et al., 2016). Besseiche et al. reported that the overexpression of PGC-1α in a mouse fetal islet beta cell resulted in a decreased number, weight, and function of islet beta cells (Besseiche et al., 2015). Furthermore, upregulation of PGC-1α in MIN6 cells resulted in elevated mitochondrial oxidative stress, activated the AMPK signaling pathway, and increased the level of AMPK phosphorylation, all of which inhibited insulin secretion (Besseiche et al., 2015). Sawada et al. exposed isolated mouse skeletal muscle vascular endothelial cells to high levels of glucose (25 mmol/L) and physiological levels of glucose (5.5 mmol/L). They observed that PGC-1α expression decreased rapidly within 4; otherwise, it significantly increased, indicating that high glucose levels induced PGC-1α expression in skeletal muscle vascular endothelial cells. Additional studies revealed that PGC-1α overexpression strongly suppressed vascular endothelial growth factor (VEGF) production, hindering neovascularization in diabetic patients. Other studies have shown that PGC-1α gene deletion led to a reduction in the heterogeneous flux of glucose produced by PEP, thus decreasing glucose production. In skeletal muscle, PGC-1α activates the expression of glucose transporter protein 4 through the activation of the MEF2 transcription factor, thereby increasing glucose uptake by these cells (Rullman et al., 2018). The increased intracellular glucose concentration is accompanied by a decrease in glycolysis and an increase in glycogen storage. Indeed, PGC-1α induction leads to the expression of pyruvate dehydrogenase 4 (PDK4) via ERRα, suggesting that PGC-1α inhibits glucose oxidation and promotes glycogen synthesis.

2.7.3.2. HNF-4α

Hepatocyte nuclear factor 4 alpha (HNF-4α) is a vital member of the nuclear hormone receptor super-family (NR2A1) that is commonly found in the pancreas, intestine, liver, and kidney. It is crucial in regulating liver and intestinal epithelial cell metabolism, cell connection, and early embryonic development of the liver. HNF-4α is necessary for the expression of numerous genes in key metabolic pathways, such as gluconeogenesis and fatty acid transport (Ren et al., 2018). In the liver, HNF-4α is widely recognized for its role as the primary regulator of liver-specific gene expression. Additionally, genetic variations in HNF-4α are associated with several human diseases, including ulcerative colitis, colon cancer, adult diabetes, cirrhosis, and hepatocellular carcinoma. Research has shown that HNF-4α deletion affects glucose transport and glycolysis by altering the expression of genes encoding GLUT-2, aldolase B, and L-PK, which leads to abnormal insulin secretion (Ren et al., 2018). HNF-4α is also a critical nuclear transcription factor that regulates PEPCK transcription. Studies have demonstrated that dephosphorylated TORC2 binds to CREB transcription factor in the nucleus and stimulates the expression of PGC-1α. PGC-1α then induces HNF-4α to bind to the cis-element of its promoter, promoting the expression of key enzymes such as PEPCK and G6Pase and ultimately stimulating gluconeogenesis. HNF-4α also regulates the primary function of the liver by directly binding to the response elements of adjacent target genes and guiding their expression. Researchers have confirmed that HNF-4α can bind to the miR-122 promoter region through the DR-I element, a binding site of HNF-4α, and positively regulate miR-122 expression in mice liver, regulating gluconeogenesis and lipid metabolism (Wei et al., 2016). Post-translational modifications, such as acetylation and ubiquitination, have been shown to regulate the activity of HNF-4α. Bi et al. (2018) found that cholesterol sulfate (CS) and cholesterol sulfonyl transferase (SULT2B1b) inhibited gluconeogenesis by targeting HNF-4α in Hepa1-6 cells and transgenic mice. The knockdown of Sult2B1b from primary mouse hepatocytes revealed an enhanced stimulation of gluconeogenesis by HNF-4α, increased expression of G6pase and PEPCK, and elevated fasting glucose levels in Sult2B1b-/-mice. Further studies showed that this change in activity was the result of increased HNF-4α acetylation through the inhibition of the HNF-4α deacetylase Sirt1. Mechanistically, CS and SULT2B1b inhibit gluconeogenesis by inhibiting the acetylation of the gluconeogenic factor HNF-4α and interfering with the nuclear translocation of HNF-4α (Bi et al., 2018).

2.7.3.3. Foxo

The Foxo protein family is a group of evolutionarily conserved transcription factors that regulate metabolic and stress responses. These proteins are divided into four distinct subtypes in mammals: Foxo1, Foxo3, Foxo4, and Foxo6, which control various cellular functions (Calissi et al., 2021). Foxo proteins play essential roles in glycolipid metabolism, apoptosis, autophagy, cell cycle regulation, stress resistance, DNA repair, angiogenesis, inflammation, immune response, pluripotency, and differentiation (Calissi et al., 2021). Genetic mutations in Foxo genes or abnormal expression of Foxo proteins have been associated with metabolic diseases, cancers, and changes in lifespan in humans and animals (Kim et al., 2018). During fasting, Foxo proteins promote gluconeogenesis by inducing the expression of genes involved in the conversion of non-carbohydrate precursors to glucose, such as G6Pase, fructose-1,6-diphosphatase, and PEPCK (Kang et al., 2021). Studies have shown that Foxo1 is a key regulator of glucose homeostasis (Calissi et al., 2021). Loss of Foxo1 decreases hepatic gluconeogenesis (Gu et al., 2019). In diabetic patients, insulin deficiency or insulin resistance can cause excessive activation of Foxo1, leading to increased hepatic gluconeogenesis. Scientists have discovered that Foxo1 drives the expression of genes critical for gluconeogenesis, such as G6PC (Zhang et al., 2019). Yan et al. found that increased expression of lncRNA Gomafu resulted in elevated Foxo1 expression via miR-139, ultimately leading to inappropriate activation of glycolysis. Other studies have revealed that phosphorylation of Foxo1 leads to its inactivation in hepatocytes. Phosphorylated Foxo1 binds to the core promoter Sin3a of GCK, inhibiting the expression of GCK gene and glucose production (Langlet et al., 2017). The activation of the PI3K/AKT/Foxo1 signaling pathway results in the direct interaction and binding of phosphorylated Foxo1 with PPAR-coactivator-1, which in turn inhibits gluconeogenesis. Additionally, insulin suppresses hepatic gluconeogenesis by stimulating the PI3K/Akt signaling pathway to phosphorylate and inactivate Foxo1 (Ren et al., 2018). Liu et al. (2015) found that Iris reduced gluconeogenesis by downregulating the PI3K/Akt/Foxo1-mediated PEPCK and G6Pase, leading to improved glucose homeostasis in STZ/HFD mice compared to the control group. Furthermore, Foxo1 also plays a key role in regulating glucose metabolism in skeletal muscle (Gombos et al., 2021). Under conditions of chronic starvation, increased Foxo1 expression in muscle binds to the promoter of the pyruvate dehydrogenase kinase-4 gene, resulting in the conversion of pyruvate to acetyl-CoA and accelerating glucose consumption (Gopal et al., 2017). These findings suggest that inhibition of Foxo1 may be a potential therapeutic strategy for diabetes. Moreover, there is evidence that other Foxo proteins, such as Foxo3 and Foxo4, also play a role in the regulation of gluconeogenesis. Glucose tolerance and insulin sensitivity were significantly increased in Foxo1, Foxo3, and Foxo4 knockout mice compared to Foxo1 knockout mice alone, indicating that Foxo3 and Foxo4 are involved in the control of gluconeogenesis. Kim et al. (2018) found that increased hepatic glucose output in Foxo6 transgenic mice, while hepatic Foxo6 deficiency led to fasting hypoglycemia, suggesting that Foxo6 is also involved in the regulation of gluconeogenesis. These findings indicate that the Foxo family of proteins plays a crucial role in the treatment of diabetes.

2.8. Insulin-Mediated Signaling Pathway in Diabetes

Insulin performs its physiological functions by binding to insulin receptors on the plasma membrane of target cells, which serve as the primary hub of the insulin signaling pathway. Insulin receptors are heterotetramer ($\alpha 2\beta 2$) proteins consisting of two α subunits and two β subunits linked through disulfide bonds (Scapin et al., 2021). The α subunits have insulin binding sites outside the plasma membrane, while the β subunits are transmembrane proteins with kinase activity and signal transduction. Upon binding to the ligands of insulin receptors on target tissue cell membranes, insulin activates cascade phosphorylation. This includes self-phosphorylation, where the conformation of insulin receptors changes after insulin binding, and the insulin receptors' tyrosine kinase is activated. Additionally, downstream insulin receptor substrate proteins (IRSs) are phosphorylated, such as IRS1-6, Shc, and Gab1. Insulin receptor abnormalities have been suggested to cause diabetes since 1976. A long-term study of a population with a high prevalence of type 2 diabetes showed that insulin resistance preceded the onset of type 2 diabetes and was more severe in patients with type 2 diabetes who had insulin receptor variants than in those who did not. Mice with knocked-out IRS-1 and IRS-2 genes in the liver exhibited significant signs of hyperglycemia, hyperinsulinemia, hyperlipidemia, and insulin resistance (Scapin et al., 2021). IRSs play a crucial role in insulin signal transduction, activating insulin signal pathways that result in cell survival, differentiation, metabolism, proliferation, senescence, glucose metabolism, adipogenesis, and various other biological effects. Insulin receptors play a crucial role in regulating metabolism by activating two distinct signaling pathways: the MAPK pathway and the phosphatidylinositol 3-kinase (PI3K)/Akt pathway. The MAPK pathway directly controls insulin-mediated metabolism through various mechanisms and also regulates gene expression. On the other hand, the PI3K/Akt pathway modulates the effects of insulin on acute cellular metabolism and cell growth and differentiation (Guo et al., 2023).

2.8.1. The MAPK Pathway Regulates Insulin-Mediated Metabolism

Currently, five distinct groups of MAPK have been identified in mammals: extracellular signal regulated kinases (ERKs) 1 and 2 (ERK1/2), JNKs 1, 2, and 3 (JNK1/2/3), p38 $\alpha/\beta/\gamma$, ERKs 3 and 4 (ERK3/4), and ERK5 (also known as BMK1 or MAPK7). The JNK and ERK pathways play a crucial role in the development of obesity and insulin resistance. The ERK pathway mediates the inflammatory-cytokine-induced downregulation of IRS1 expression, and ERK1/2 also catalyzes the phosphorylation of nuclear transcription factors, such as Ets, Elk, and c-Fos.

Inflammatory cytokines, such as TNF-α and IL-1β, and cellular stress (including genotoxicity, permeability, hypoxia, or oxidative stress) are related to p38 and JNK signaling pathways. Ryan et al. confirmed that saturated fatty acids accumulated in obesity contribute to the activation of JNK (Yan et al., 2018). In the context of obesity and type 2 diabetes, metabolic and inflammatory stress increase the activities of JNK and ERK in insulin target tissues, and these kinases induce serine phosphorylation of IRS1 or IRS2. Uncontrolled IRS serine phosphorylation promotes insulin resistance. The high-fat-diet-fed JNK1-/-mice not only attenuated weight gain but also decreased insulin resistance and IRS1 serine phosphorylation and improved glucose tolerance. Some used a mouse model expressing Cre recombinase under the control of the albumin promoter to selectively knock out JNK1 from hepatocytes and found that hepatocyte-specific deletion mice with JNK1 did not prevent hepatic insulin resistance and improve glucose tolerance in high-fat-diet mice. In contrast, a JNK1 deficiency in adipose tissue decreased IL-6 secretion from the adipose tissue and inhibited high-fat-diet-induced hepatic insulin resistance. Thus, the high level of JNK1 activity in adipose tissue causes an imbalance of adipose cytokines and contributes to the development of insulin resistance. Conversely, Bost et al. discovered that mice lacking ERK1 were resistant to obesity and insulin resistance, and exhibited improved postprandial metabolic rates (Guo et al., 2023).

2.8.2. The PI3K/Akt Pathway was Involved in Insulin Resistance

The PI3K/Akt signaling pathway is a crucial component of insulin signaling and plays a pivotal role in mediating various cellular processes, including glucolipid metabolism, protein synthesis, cell proliferation, and apoptotic transcription. Akt, a serine/threonine protein kinase, serves as a critical signaling molecule in the insulin-signaling pathway. Research conducted by Andreelli et al. demonstrated that insulin increased the expression of P85 α-phosphatidylinositol-3-kinase mRNA in muscle tissue. Studies have shown that PI3K knockout mice develop insulin resistance and diabetes. siRNA was utilized to selectively inhibit the expression of Akt protein kinase in adipocytes, ultimately blocking the PI3K/Akt signal transduction pathway and leading to insulin resistance in adipocytes. By examining three subtypes of Pkb-specific deficient mice, it was determined that the Pkb-α-/-mice exhibited significantly lower blood glucose levels, higher serum glucagon concentrations, and increased insulin sensitivity. Additionally, research revealed that overexpression of the IRS2-specific activation of AKT1 increased the number of β cells and insulin secretion in pancreatic islet cells. Studies have also shown that Akt2 knockout mice exhibit reduced insulin sensitivity in the liver and skeletal muscle, as evidenced by decreased hepatic glycogen synthesis and reduced glucose uptake and utilization in skeletal muscle. PDK1, a serine/threonine protein kinase, plays a crucial role in regulating physiological processes related to cell growth, proliferation, survival, and metabolism by phosphorylating conserved AGC protein kinases, such as protein kinase B (PKB)/Akt, P70 ribosomal S6 kinase (S6K), serum- and glucocorticoid-induced protein kinase (SGK), and protein kinase C (PKC) isoforms. Researchers utilized a CRE recombinase/loxP technique to generate mice with hepatocytes lacking PDK1 expression, resulting in poor glucose tolerance and 10-fold lower liver glycogen levels compared to control mice (Guo et al., 2023). While certain researchers found that the volume of islets was diminished in mice that specifically lacked PDK1 in their pancreatic β-cells, leading to diabetes, other studies suggest that PDK1 plays a crucial role in maintaining the numbers of pancreatic cells and glucose homeostasis. The aforementioned studies indicate that type 2 diabetes is closely associated with the PI3K/Akt signaling pathway, and any reduction in the level and activity of substances within this pathway may result in the disruption of normal physiological insulin metabolism (Guo et al., 2023).

2.9. Roles of Long Non-Coding RNA (ncRNA) in Diabetes and Its Complications

Non-coding RNA (ncRNA) refers to functional RNA molecules that do not get translated into proteins.

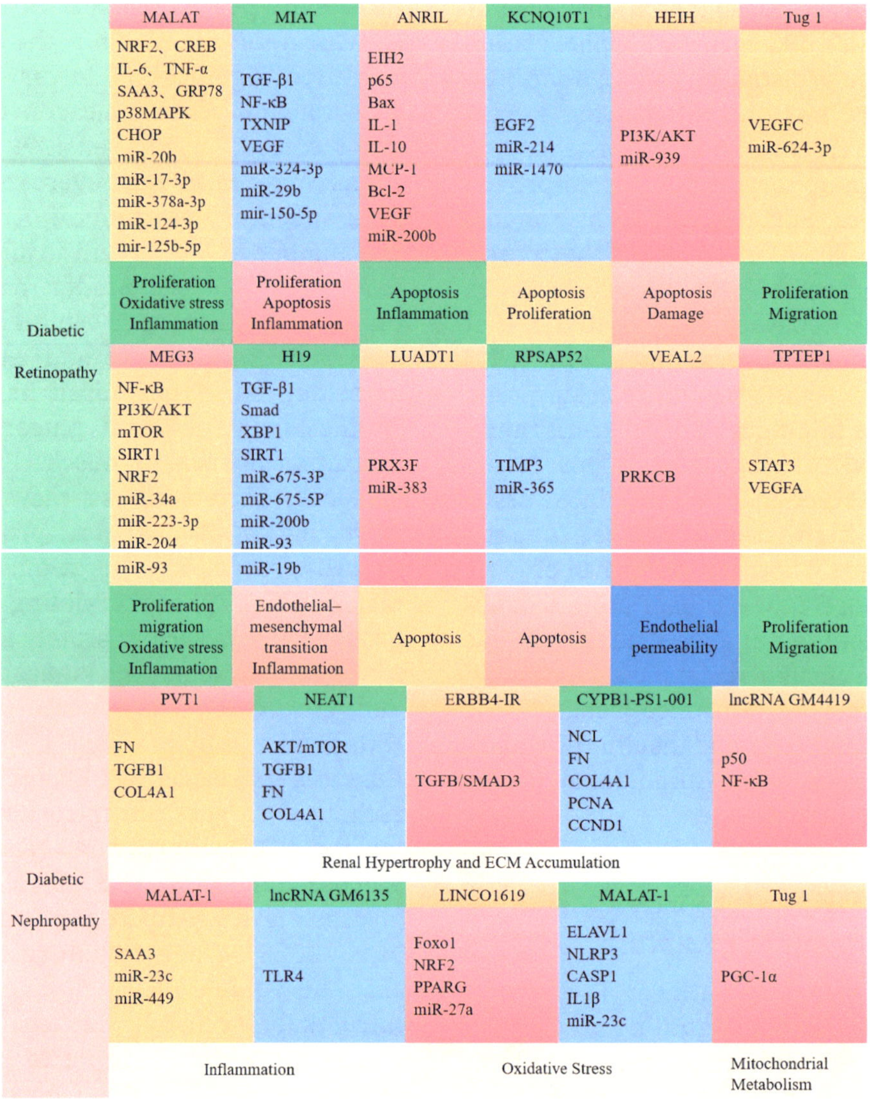

Figure 2.2. LncRNAs are closely associated with the development of diabetic complications (Guo et al., 2023).

The ncRNA family comprises various members, including microRNAs (miRNAs), small interfering RNAs (siRNAs), PIWI-interacting RNAs (piRNAs), small nucleolar RNAs (snoRNAs), small nuclear RNAs (snRNAs), extracellular RNAs (exRNAs), small Cajal body-specific RNAs (scaRNAs), long non-coding RNAs (lncRNAs), and nonlinear cyclic RNAs (Matsui and Corey, 2017). lncRNAs have been shown to be closely connected with abnormal blood glucose levels and insulin resistance in patients with type 2 diabetes. They are also considered crucial participants in the development of diabetes and its complications (Figure 2.2). As a result, lncRNAs are considered potential therapeutic targets for clinical applications in managing diabetes (Lu et al., 2022).

2.10. LncRNAs Regulate Glucose Metabolism in Diabetes

The characteristic feature of diabetes is the disruption of glucose metabolism. Research has demonstrated that lncRNAs play a crucial role in the regulation of glucose metabolism in diabetes. Some lncRNAs are linked to hepatic insulin resistance through their ability to control the expression and activity of transcription factor forkhead box protein O1 (foxo1). For instance, in high-fat-diet mice, ob/ob mice, and palmitate-, oleate-, or linoleate-treated hepatocytes, elevated levels of the lncRNA MEG3 have been found to be associated with increased levels of glucose-6-phosphatase (G6PC), PEPCK, and foxo1, leading to enhanced gluconeogenesis and impaired insulin-stimulated glycogen accumulation in hepatocytes, ultimately resulting in hepatic insulin resistance (Goyal et al., 2018). Additionally, an increase in the lncRNA Gomafu has been shown to result in elevated foxo1 and gluconeogenic protein expression through the sponging of microRNA-139 (Yan et al., 2018). On the other hand, MEG3 knockdown has been found to improve glucose tolerance in high-fat-diet and ob/ob mice (Zhu et al., 2016). Furthermore, the upregulation of MEG3 has been shown to increase hepatic gluconeogenesis and inhibit glycogen synthesis in mouse hepatocytes through histone acetylation (Zhu et al., 2016). LncLGR has been found to inhibit GCK activity by interacting with hnRNPL, thereby blocking hepatic glycogen synthesis (Ruan et al., 2016). In addition, the reduction of H19 has been observed in the liver of db/db mice, and H19 silencing has been found to enhance gluconeogenic gene levels and glucose output in human hepatoma and primary hepatocytes (Goyal et al., 2017). Furthermore, the knockout of SAR1 has been shown to enhance insulin sensitivity, improve glucose tolerance, and suppress obesity in mice. SAR has been reported to increase insulin-sensitive glucose uptake by activating the Akt pathway and the phosphorylation of foxo1. These findings suggest that lncRNAs play a crucial role in the regulation of glucose metabolism in diabetes.

2.10.1. Role of LncRNAs in Islet

Furthermore, it is typical for long noncoding RNAs (lncRNAs) to exhibit abnormal expression in the pancreatic β cells of diabetic patients and to be situated near islet-specific chromatin or at loci associated with diabetes susceptibility. The alterations in pancreatic islets serve as crucial indicators of diabetic pathology. Research conducted by Yin et al. (2015) indicated that the suppression of the lncRNA TUG1 resulted in an increased rate of apoptosis for pancreatic β cells, a reduction in insulin secretion, and an elevation of fasting blood glucose levels.

It has been suggested that the inhibition of the lncRNA MEG3 may result in impaired glucose tolerance, diminished insulin secretion, and a reduction in insulin-positive cells. This suggests that MEG3 may function as a regulator of β cells (Zhu et al., 2016). Similarly, several studies have reported that the lncRNA SRA has a positive impact on promoting insulin sensitivity and insulin-stimulated glucose uptake in adipocytes (Goyal et al., 2017). Specifically, the overexpression of SRA in ST2 adipocytes has been shown to suppress the expression of negative regulators of insulin sensitivity (cytokine signal transduction factor-1 and -3 repressors) and increase the expression of positive regulators (SH3 structural domain containing 1) (Goyal et al., 2017). Furthermore, the LncRNA SRA has been shown to enhance insulin function through the Akt and foxo1 signaling pathways (Goyal et al., 2017). These findings suggest that lncRNAs may play a significant role in islet function.

2.10.2. LncRNAs Are Associated with Diabetic Complications

lncRNAs are involved in various diabetes-related complications, such as diabetic retinopathy and diabetic nephropathy. Diabetic retinopathy is a common complication in diabetic patients, leading to visual impairment or loss. A study found that 303 lncRNAs were abnormally expressed in the retinas of patients with early diabetic retinopathy, and an enrichment analysis revealed that these lncRNAs were mainly associated with the MAPK signaling pathway, complement and coagulation cascade, chemokine signaling pathway, pyruvate metabolic pathway, and axon guidance signaling pathway.

Changes in the expression of lncRNAs MALAT1 and MEG3 have been reported to be associated with diabetic retinopathy (He et al., 2021). The downregulation of MALAT1 ameliorated streptozotocin-induced retinopathy in rats (Radhakrishnan and Kowluru, 2021), while the downregulation of MEG3 was observed in the retinas of streptozocin-induced diabetic mice (Qiu et al., 2016). Diabetic nephropathy is another major complication associated with diabetes, and lncRNAs play an important role in its development and the accumulation of extracellular matrix (ECM) proteins (Feng et al., 2017). Plasmacytoma variant translocation 1 (PVT1) was the first gene implicated in end-stage renal disease among individuals with type 2 diabetes. In diabetic nephropathy patients, elevated levels of lncRNA PVT1 result in increased accumulation of ECM proteins, contributing to enhanced fibrosis in renal cells. Conversely, reduction of PVT1 leads to decreased ECM accumulation.

Researchers have demonstrated that overexpression of PVT1 significantly elevates mRNA and protein levels of TGFB1, PAI-1, and FN1, whereas PVT1 knockdown results in reduced expression of these molecules. Yi et al. (2017) found that diabetic nephropathy is also associated with increased levels of FN1 mRNA lncRNA Gm4419, which interacts with NF-κb under hyperglycemic conditions. In mesangial cells, knockdown of FN1 mRNA lncRNA Gm4419 inhibited cell proliferation and NF-κb expression (Yi et al., 2017).

Kato et al. (2016) discovered that TGF-β induces the expression of miR-192 and its host lncRNA CJ241444 in mesangial cells, activating Akt and p300, leading to mesangial hypertrophy. Furthermore, diabetes is a risk factor for CVD, but lncRNAs are rarely directly linked to diabetic vascular complications. Reports by Zhang et al. (2016) revealed that lncRNA MALAT1 was upregulated during cardiomyopathy in diabetic rats. Downregulation of FN1 mRNA lncRNA MALAT1 improved left ventricular systolic function by reducing myocardial fibrosis in diabetic rats (Zhang et al., 2016). Additionally, overexpression of H19 in diabetic rats decreased oxidative stress and apoptosis, as well as improved ventricular function (Li et al., 2016). These studies indicate that lncRNAs play a crucial role in the development of diabetic complications.

2.11. The Disturbance of Intestinal Flora may Partly Give Rise to Diabetes

The relationship between gut microbiota and the development of type 2 diabetes is closely intertwined. An imbalance in intestinal flora among diabetic patients often leads to a disruption in the diversity and stability of the microflora. It was demonstrated that the levels of *Firmicutes* and *Clostridium* in type 2 diabetic patients were significantly lower than in non-diabetic individuals. Furthermore, it was reported that the intestinal microbiome of type 2 diabetic patients had reduced levels of *Faecalibacterium* and *Roseburia*, both of which are butyrate producers. These changes result in an increase in pathogenic bacteria and a decrease in butyrate-producing bacteria, leading to low-grade, chronic intestinal inflammation and insulin resistance. Abnormal ratios of *Bacteroides/Firmicutes* have also been associated with increased intestinal permeability and the infiltration of bacterial byproducts through the leaky intestinal barrier, causing inflammation (Huda et al., 2021). Probiotics, such as *Lactobacillus, Roseburia, Bacteroides, and Akkermansia*, have been shown to reduce the risk of diabetes by inhibiting pro-inflammatory factors and maintaining intestinal barrier integrity, improving glucose metabolism, and insulin sensitivity (Huda et al., 2021). Moreover, decreases in probiotics such as Lactobacillus and *Bifidobacterium* have been strongly associated with abnormal glucose tolerance. In a study by Zhou et al., it was found that the relative abundance of *Ruminococcus, Allococcus*, and *Lactobacillus* was correlated with blood glucose levels in ZDF rats (Zhou et al., 2019). According to a study by Yang et al. (2021), genistein was found to alleviate insulin resistance and inflammatory responses by regulating the abundance of *Bacteroides, Prevotella*, and *Helicobacter* in mice induced by a high-fat diet and streptozotocin. A decrease in butyrate in type 2 diabetes affects glucose homeostasis and islet cell function, and has been shown to impact glucose homeostasis by activating intestinal gluconeogenesis. Increased intestinal butyrate production was associated with improved insulin response after oral glucose testing. Butyrate has also been shown to improve insulin resistance, hyperglycemia, and hyperinsulinemia in obese/pre-diabetic mice (Matheus et al., 2017). Moreover, butyrate has been shown to improve the progression of type 2 diabetes by maintaining the integrity of the intestinal epithelial barrier, promoting hepatic glycogen metabolism, and regulating mitochondrial function (Zhou et al., 2022). Propionate, another important short-chain fatty acid, has been shown to promote the release of GLP-43 and peptide YY through the activation of GPR1, enhancing insulin sensitivity and activating intestinal gluconeogenesis and maintaining glucose and energy homeostasis through GPR41-dependent gut–brain circuits (Zhou et al., 2022). Propionate has also been shown to improve reproductive system function by inhibiting HDAC5 and PCSK9 in female and male diabetic patients, respectively (Zhou et al., 2022). In conclusion, SCFAs play an important role in the development of type 2 diabetes.

2.12. Sirtuins as a Novel Drug Target for Type 2 Diabetes

Sirtuins are a group of highly conserved NAD($^+$)-dependent deacetylases that play a crucial role in various physiological and pathological processes in the body. SIRT1, in particular, has been found to reduce inflammation in adipose tissue and monocytes/macrophages, and to improve insulin resistance in individuals with type 2 diabetes. Conversely, decreased levels of SIRT1 have been linked to insulin resistance in skeletal muscle of patients with type 2 diabetes. SIRT1 also protects pancreatic β-cells from various toxic stresses by inhibiting NF-κB signaling. Additionally, activation of SIRT1 may improve insulin resistance by accelerating fatty acid oxidation, deacetylating PGC-1α, and activating PPAR-α in skeletal muscle (Kitada et al., 2019). SIRT1 is also involved in glucose metabolism. During fasting, SIRT1 is activated and deacetylates CRTC2 to reduce the effects of glucagon. Overexpression of SIRT1 in transgenic mice resulted in reduced hepatic glucose output and improved glucose tolerance. Furthermore, SIRT1 induces gluconeogenesis-related genes by activating PGC-1α and FOXO1 through deacetylation reactions. Additionally, SIRT1 deacetylates STAT3, which leads to reduced STAT3 activity and inhibition of gluconeogenesis.

SIRT2 is broadly expressed in a variety of tissues and plays a crucial role in maintaining metabolic homeostasis, including gluconeogenesis and insulin sensitivity. Its expression in PMCS is inversely correlated with insulin resistance. According to Lemos et al. (2017), SIRT2 is downregulated in insulin-resistant hepatocytes and liver. Furthermore, Kitada et al. (2019) reported that overexpression of SIRT2 in insulin-resistant hepatocytes enhanced insulin sensitivity and decreased ROS production. In addition, SIRT2 is involved in the regulation of gluconeogenesis through PEPCK. Jiang et al. (2022) demonstrated that SIRT2 decreased the acetylation of PEPCK1 and the interaction between PEPCK1 and UBR5, increased the stability of PEPCK1, and promoted gluconeogenesis. Moreover, SIRT2 inhibition not only increased the stability of GKRP protein and promoted the degradation of ALDOA but also inhibited glucose-stimulated insulin secretion and reduced glycolytic flux by regulating the Akt/GSK3β/β-linked protein pathway in β-cells (Zhu et al., 2022).

Sirtuins have been demonstrated to play a protective role against diabetic nephropathy. In diabetic db/db mice, the deletion of SIRT1 in podocytes resulted in increased acetylation of NF-κB and the p65 subunit of STAT65, leading to heightened urinary protein excretion and renal injury (Morigi et al., 2018). Additionally, targeted disruption of SIRT1 in the proximal tubules of diabetic nephropathy mice led to ectopic expression of the tight junction protein claudin-1 in podocytes, resulting in albuminuria and renal impairment. Furthermore, SIRT3 activation via G-protein-coupled bile acid receptors has been shown to prevent oxidative stress and lipid accumulation in diabetic nephropathic mice (Morigi et al., 2018).

2.13. Diabetes in Children and Adolescents

Diabetes is a prevalent condition among school-aged children. In the United States, approximately 2,08,000 individuals under the age of 20 were diagnosed with diabetes in 2012. Moreover, during the COVID-19 pandemic, children with newly diagnosed T1DM exhibited higher glucose and HbA1c levels, necessitating specific actions to raise clinician and public awareness (Rahmati et al., 2022). According to Rahmati et al. (2022), the global incidence rate of T1DM was 19.73 per 1,00,000 children in 2019 and 32.39 per 1,00,000 in 2020. During the first year of the pandemic, the number of pediatric cases of new-onset T1DM, DKA, and severe DKA increased by 9.5% (T1DM), 25.0% (DKA), and 19.5% (severe DKA), respectively, compared to pre-pandemic levels (Rahmati et al., 2022).

According to the Centers for Disease Control and Prevention (CDC, 2022), a significant proportion of children and adolescents with type 2 diabetes (T2DM) have a family history of the condition and may also be susceptible to insulin resistance. Additionally, specific racial and ethnic groups, including African Americans, American Indians, Hispanic/Latino Americans, and some Asian and Pacific Islander Americans, have higher rates of T2DM (CDC, 2022). It is important to note that some children and adolescents with T2DM may not exhibit any signs or symptoms at all (CDC, 2022). In some cases, their symptoms may resemble those of type 1 diabetes. These symptoms may include feeling tired, thirsty, or sick, as well as an increased urge to urinate. Other possible symptoms include weight loss, hazy vision, recurring infections, and delayed wound or sore healing. Given the wide range of symptoms, healthcare practitioners must carefully identify and evaluate children and adolescents who are at high risk for the condition (CDC, 2022). The key to controlling T2DM in children is a balanced diet and portion management, as well as increased physical activity. Metformin should also be recommended when T2DM is diagnosed. However, data indicate that 50.0% of young people with T2DM will be unable to keep their hemoglobin A1c (HbA1c) below 8.0% on metformin alone, with or without lifestyle changes. If metformin alone is insufficient to normalize blood glucose levels, insulin may be required. At the time of diagnosis, blood pressure (BP), lipid profile, microalbuminuria evaluation, and dilated eye examination are recommended.

2.14. Diabetes in Adults

Diabetes was the eighth leading cause of death in the United States in 2021, claiming the lives of more than 1,00,000 individuals (CDC, 2022). Additionally, almost 25% of all persons in the country with diabetes have not been diagnosed, as reported in the CDC's National Diabetes Statistics Report (CDC, 2022). Furthermore, over a third of those aged between 18 and 64 years old who have diabetes are either unaware of their condition or failed to disclose it (CDC, 2022).

Although the incidence of diabetes among adults has been showing a declining trend since 2008, it is essential to acknowledge that those with a high school education or less are significantly more likely to develop the disease. This highlights the need for increased efforts in health education among individuals with lower levels of education.

2.14.1. Complications

Diabetes poses significant long-term risks to the heart, blood vessels, eyes, kidneys, and nerves. Smoking, obesity, physical inactivity, high BP, and hyperlipidemia are factors that contribute to developing complications associated with diabetes. According to a multinational study, CVDs and stroke account for 50% of deaths related to diabetes (WHO, 2022). Patients with diabetes over the age of 18 have a 1.7 times higher risk of dying from CVD compared to those without diabetes (ADA, 2022). In 2011, the CDC reported that nearly a third of diabetics aged 35 or older had a history of heart disease or stroke. It is noteworthy that coronary heart disease affects a greater number of individuals than stroke, accounting for 21.9% of cases compared to 9.1%.

Diabetes is a serious condition that may lead to fatal complications, such as hyperglycemic crises, which include DKA and hyperglycemic hyperosmolar condition. Despite progress in reducing death rates, it is estimated that 17.3 out of every 1,00,000 people still pass away each year due to diabetes (ADA, 2022). In 2011, diabetes was responsible for 44.0% of all new cases of renal failure (Sanyaolu et al., 2023). Additionally, 2,28,924 individuals of all ages were receiving dialysis or undergoing a kidney transplant due to diabetes-related complications, while 49,677 individuals of all ages were starting therapy for kidney failure. Diabetic retinopathy, which affects the minor blood vessels in the retina, is a leading cause of blindness worldwide and accounts for 1.0% of all cases. Moreover, diabetes can result in amputations. Foot neuropathy, a common complication of diabetes, increases the risk of developing foot ulcers, which can become infected and ultimately lead to an amputation. In 2010, it was estimated that approximately 73,000 non-traumatic lower limb amputations occurred among adult diabetics. Overall, individuals with diabetes account for about 60.0% of all non-traumatic lower-limb amputations in adults over the age of 20 years (Sanyaolu et al., 2023).

2.14.2. Genetic Role in Diabetes Mellitus: Type 1 Diabetes Mellitus (T1DM)

The development of T1DM is influenced by genetic factors, as certain families possess an inherited tendency for this condition. The HLA complex enables the immune system to differentiate between proteins produced by the body's own cells and those produced by foreign invaders (Sanyaolu et al., 2023). Variations in HLA genes on chromosome 6 can increase the risk of T1DM. The genetic sequence contains numerous genes that contribute to the immune system, with HLA class II genes being notably associated with T1DM. These genes include HLA-DQA1, HLA-DQB1, and HLADRB1.

According to estimates, approximately 40% to 50% of the heritable risk for T1DM can be attributed to HLA class II genes (Sanyaolu et al., 2023). Researchers have discovered a significant association between T1DM and the haplotypes DQA1*0501-DQB1*0201 and DQA1*0301-DQB1*0302 in Caucasian populations. A haplotype refers to a group of single nucleotide polymorphisms (SNPs) that are located on the same chromosome (Sanyaolu et al., 2023). Additionally, studies have shown that different races have distinct high-risk haplotypes for T1DM, such as DRB1*07-DQA1*0301-DQB1*0201 for African Americans, DRB1*09-DQA1*0301-DQB1*0303 for Japanese people, and DRB1*04-DQA1*0401-DQB1*0302 for Chinese people. Furthermore, it was found that DRB1*15-DQA1*0602-DQB1*0102 haplotypes were protective and linked to a lower incidence of T1DM in most populations. Recent research suggests that other genes in the central, class I, and extended class I regions may also increase the risk of T1DM, independent of HLA class II genes (Sanyaolu et al., 2023). Individuals with high-risk DRB1-DQA1-DQB1 haplotypes are significantly more likely to develop T1DM than those without such haplotypes. It is reported that Caucasian people with two susceptibility haplotypes have an approximately 6% absolute risk of developing T1DM by the time they reach 35 years of age. However, in populations where T1DM is uncommon, this number is much lower (1% among Asians). The insulin (INS) and cytotoxic T lymphocyte-associated 4 (CTLA-4) genes are also known to affect the risk of T1DM (Sanyaolu et al., 2023).

2.14.3. Genetic Role in Diabetes Mellitus (DM): Type 2 Diabetes Mellitus (T2DM)

T2DM is a metabolic disorder characterized by hyperglycemia and insulin deficiency in the bloodstream. One of the numerous factors contributing to T2DM is a genetic abnormality. In 2011, multiple studies identified approximately 36 genes associated with an increased risk of T2DM. Due to these hereditary factors, only 10.0% of T2DM cases are clinically manifest (Sanyaolu et al., 2023).

Due to its role in adipose tissue and lipid metabolism, the peroxisome proliferator-activated receptor γ (PPARγ) gene is of significant importance for study. The PPARγ gene's (Pro) function lowers insulin sensitivity and increases the risk of T2DM. In most populations, this gene is prevalent, with at least 98.0% of Europeans carrying at least one copy of the Pro allele. Consequently, it likely accounts for a substantial portion (25.0%) of T2DM in the Caucasian population. Humans and many other mammals express the ATP binding cassette, subfamily C, member 8 (ABCC8) protein, which is necessary for the production of the sulfonylurea receptor 1 (SUR1) protein (Song et al., 2017). The Kir6.2 subunit, which is encoded by KCNJ1, and the SUR1 protein are components of the ATP-sensitive potassium channel, which plays a crucial role in a wide range of physiologic responses, such as the release of insulin and glucagon from the beta cells of the pancreas (Song et al., 2017). Gene abnormalities can impact both insulin secretion and potassium channel function, ultimately leading to T2DM (Song et al., 2017). Interestingly, the distance between ABCC8 and KCNJ11, which is only 4.5 KB, is comparable to that of the INS gene. Variants of the ABCC8 (Ala) and KCNJ11 (Lys) genes have been linked to T2DM.

The CAPN10 gene encodes for calpain 10, an intracellular cysteine protease that is highly expressed and prevalent in humans. A mutation at position 43, which changes an adenine (A) to a glycine (G), is associated with T2DM and is a significant factor in the transcription of CAPN10. Physiological research has shown that differences in calpain 10 activity can affect insulin secretion and increase the risk of T2DM. Studies across various ethnic groups indicate that Mexican American communities may be at a higher risk for T2DM due to this locus compared to Caucasian populations (Sanyaolu et al., 2023).

2.15. Diabetes Mellitus (DM) and Affective Disorders

2.15.1. Depression

The prevalence of depression is substantial among individuals with DM. The most compelling evidence for this association comes from a comprehensive review of 147 studies involving people with T2DM, which revealed a mean prevalence of depression of 28% (Harding et al., 2019). The global prevalence of depression in the general population is estimated to be around 13%. For individuals with T1DM, a systematic review reported a pooled prevalence of depression of 12% compared to only 3% in those without T1DM. The risk of depression among people with DM appears to be about 25% greater than the risk in the general population, with consistent findings across multiple meta-analyses. A study conducted in 2013 found an adjusted relative risk (RR) of 1.25 (95% CI 1.10–1.44) for incident depression among people with DM compared to those without the condition. Another systematic review of individuals with T2DM reported a similar effect size (Tomic et al., 2022).

2.15.2. Anxiety and Eating Disorders

DM has been linked to anxiety, and T1DM has been associated with eating disorders. In a comprehensive review of 2584 individuals with DM, a prevalence of 14% was observed for generalized anxiety disorder and 40% for anxiety symptoms, which is higher than the estimated prevalence of 3–4% in the general population. People with DM had a higher risk of anxiety disorders (OR 1.20, 95% CI 1.10–1.31) and anxiety symptoms (OR 1.48, 95% CI 1.02–1.93) than those without DM, according to a meta-analysis, although the findings were based on cross-sectional data. Across 13 studies, 7% of adolescents with T1DM had eating disorders, compared to 3% of their peers without DM (Tomic et al., 2022).

2.15.3. Broader Psychological Impacts

DM has garnered significant attention from researchers due to its myriad psychological impacts. Social stigma not only affects the quality of life of individuals with DM, but also their families and caregivers. In a systematic review, it was found that approximately one-third of adolescents with T1DM experienced DM distress, which is consistent with the results of studies on adults with DM (Hagger et al., 2016).

DM burnout is a distinct concept characterized by feelings of exhaustion, detachment, and a loss of control over DM (Abdoli et al., 2020).

2.15.4. Potential Etiological Mechanisms

DM and depression seem to have common biological roots. The activation of the innate immune system and acute-phase inflammation contribute to the development of T2DM, as increased levels of inflammatory cytokines predict the onset of T2DM. Additionally, there is growing evidence implicating cytokine-mediated inflammation in people with depression, even in the absence of DM. Another potential biological mechanism linking depression and DM is the dysregulation of the hypothalamic-pituitary-adrenal (HPA) axis. There have been numerous reports of hippocampal atrophy, which might contribute to chronic activation of the HPA axis, in individuals with T2DM as well as those with depression. A meta-analysis found that, although hypertension modified global cerebral atrophy in those with T2DM, it had no effect on hippocampal atrophy (Moulton et al., 2015). This suggests that, although global cerebral atrophy in individuals with T2DM might be driven by atherosclerotic disease, hippocampal atrophy is an independent effect that provides a common neuropathological etiology for the comorbidity of T2DM with depression. However, there is a lack of relevant information regarding the potential etiological mechanisms that link diabetes to other affective disorders.

2.16. Diabetes Management and Control

Acknowledging the potential impact of anti-diabetes mellitus medications and glucose control on emerging complications is crucial, despite the fact that discussing this topic in depth is beyond the scope of this chapter.

2.16.1. Medications

In the context of DM medications and cancer, several factors must be considered. Although some studies suggest that people taking metformin have a lower cancer risk than those not taking the medication, this association may be due to other factors such as kidney disease, which is more common in people with DM who have a longer duration of the disease and are therefore at a higher risk for cancer. Additionally, a review of observational studies found that many studies reporting significant reductions in cancer incidence or mortality associated with metformin were affected by immortal time bias and other time-related biases, casting doubt on the ability of metformin to reduce cancer mortality. Furthermore, a meta-analysis found that the use of insulin was associated with an increased risk of several cancers. However, a randomized controlled trial (RCT) of more than 12,000 people with dysglycemia found that randomization to insulin glargine (compared with standard care) did not increase cancer incidence. Additionally, cancer rates in people with T1DM and T2DM do not appear to vary greatly, despite substantial differences in insulin use between people with these types of DM. It is important to note that the relationship between DM medications and cancer is complex and may be influenced by other factors. While some studies suggest that certain medications may be associated with a reduced cancer risk, further research is needed to fully understand this relationship (Tomic et al., 2022). Medications used to treat DM may also impact the onset and progression of other emerging complications associated with the condition. According to randomized clinical trial (RCT) findings, metformin may exhibit therapeutic effects against depression, and its use was linked to a reduced incidence of dementia in a systematic review conducted by Campbell et al. in 2018. However, in an RCT examining the potential association between metformin and non-alcoholic fatty liver disease (NAFLD), no improvement in NAFLD histology was observed among individuals receiving metformin compared to those receiving a placebo. Additionally, a post hoc analysis of an RCT by Cukierman-Yaffe et al. in 2020 revealed benefits of dulaglutide, a glucagon-like peptide-1 receptor agonist, on cognitive function. This suggests that future trials specifically designed to investigate the effects of dulaglutide on cognitive function would be warranted.

2.16.2. Glucose Control

Glycemic control is another essential factor to take into account, as it can have different effects on emerging complications. A meta-analysis revealed that there was no connection between glycemic control and the risk of cancer among individuals with DM. Additionally, an RCT showed that intensive glucose reduction did not have any impact on cognitive function in people with type 2 diabetes. However, glycemic control has been associated with improved physical function, as demonstrated in observational studies of patients with DM (Jia et al., 2021). Specifically, glycemic control has been linked to lower COVID-19 mortality rates (Lesniak et al., 2021) and a decreased risk of NAFLD in these studies (Afolabi et al., 2018). It is worth noting that no RCTs have confirmed these associations yet.

2.17. Conclusion

Diabetes constitutes a global emergency that jeopardizes the health and economic well-being of the world. A comprehensive grasp of diabetes is essential for devising targeted preventive measures. In addition to a healthy lifestyle, social and medical support play a crucial role in the prevention of diabetes and its complications. Research has indicated that the consistent consumption of cereals may decrease the likelihood of chronic ailments, but additional investigation into the specific molecular mechanisms is necessary. Nevertheless, the effective application and utilization of diabetes medications remains a practical challenge for healthcare providers (Guo et al., 2023).

The landscape of DM complications is evolving due to advances in management and increased life expectancy. As glycemic control and traditional complications of DM are optimized, there is a shift towards the deleterious effects of DM on organs such as the liver, brain, and others.

The emergence of these complications poses a significant burden and risk, necessitating updated clinical and public health strategies. It is essential to raise awareness among primary care physicians of emerging complications and consider including screening for conditions such as depression, liver disease, and cancers in DM guidelines. For older individuals with DM, clinical care should prioritize physical activity, particularly strength-based activities, to reduce the risk of functional disability in aging populations. Continued high-quality surveillance of DM outcomes is necessary to identify the primary areas of concern. Given the growing burden of these emerging complications, broadening the traditional management of DM may be necessary (Tomic et al., 2022).

References

1. Abdoli, S., et al. (2020). New insights into diabetes burnout and its distinction from diabetes distress and depressive symptoms: A qualitative study. *Diabetes Research and Clinical Practice, 169*, 108446.
2. Abulizi, A., Cardone, R. L., Stark, R., Lewandowski, S. L., Zhao, X., Hillion, J., Ma, L., Sehgal, R., Alves, T. C., Thomas, C., et al. (2020). Multi-tissue acceleration of the mitochondrial phosphoenolpyruvate cycle improves whole-body metabolic health. *Cell Metabolism, 32*, 751–766.
3. Adeva-Andany, M. M., González-Lucán, M., Donapetry-García, C., Fernández-Fernández, C., & Ameneiros-Rodríguez, E. (2016). Glycogen metabolism in humans. *BBA Clinical, 5*, 85–100.
4. Adeva-Andany, M. M., Pérez-Felpete, N., Fernández-Fernández, C., Donapetry-García, C., & Pazos-García, C. (2016). Liver glucose metabolism in humans. *Bioscience Reports, 36*, e00416.
5. Afolabi, B. I., et al. (2018). The relationship between glycaemic control and non-alcoholic fatty liver disease in Nigerian type 2 diabetic patients. *Journal of the National Medical Association, 110*, 256–264.
6. Alsahli, M., & Gerich, J. E. (2017). Renal glucose metabolism in normal physiological conditions and in diabetes. *Diabetes Research and Clinical Practice, 133*, 1–9.
7. American Diabetes Association. (2018a). Introduction: Standards of medical care in diabetes—2018. *Diabetes Care, 41*(Supplement 1), S1–S2.
8. American Diabetes Association. (2018b). Cardiovascular disease and risk management: Standards of medical care in diabetes—2018. *Diabetes Care, 41*(Supplement 1), S86–S104.
9. American Diabetes Association. (2018c). Classification and diagnosis of diabetes: Standards of medical care in diabetes—2018. *Diabetes Care, 41*(Supplement 1), S13–S27.
10. American Diabetes Association. (2022). Statistics about diabetes. Retrieved from: https://www.diabetes.org/resources/statistics/statistics-about-diabetes (accessed on 21 May 2025).
11. Banday, M. Z., Sameer, A. S., & Nissar, S. (2020). Pathophysiology of diabetes: An overview. *Avicenna Journal of Medicine, 10*(4), 174–188.
12. Besseiche, A., Riveline, J. P., Gautier, J. F., Bréant, B., & Blondeau, B. (2015). Metabolic roles of PGC-1α and its implications for type 2 diabetes. *Diabetes & Metabolism, 41*, 347–357.
13. Bi, Y., Shi, X., Zhu, J., Guan, X., Garbacz, W. G., Huang, Y., Gao, L., Yan, J., Xu, M., Ren, S., et al. (2018). Regulation of cholesterol sulfotransferase SULT2B1b by hepatocyte nuclear factor 4α constitutes a negative feedback control of hepatic gluconeogenesis. *Molecular and Cellular Biology, 38*, e00654-17.
14. Calissi, G., Lam, E. W., & Link, W. (2021). Therapeutic strategies targeting FOXO transcription factors. *Nature Reviews Drug Discovery, 20*, 21–38.
15. Campbell, J. E., & Newgard, C. B. (2021). Mechanisms controlling pancreatic islet cell function in insulin secretion. *Nature Reviews Molecular Cell Biology, 22*, 142–158.
16. Campbell, J. M., et al. (2018). Metformin use associated with reduced risk of dementia in patients with diabetes: A systematic review and meta-analysis. *Journal of Alzheimer's Disease, 65*, 1225–1236.

17. Centers for Disease Control and Prevention. (2020). National diabetes statistics report 2020 estimates of diabetes and its burden in the United States.

18. Centers for Disease Control and Prevention. (2022a). National Center for Health Statistics: Leading causes of death. Retrieved from: https://www.cdc.gov/nchs/fastats/leading-causes-of-death.htm (accessed on 21 May 2025).

19. Centers for Disease Control and Prevention. (2022b). Diabetes: Prevalence of both diagnosed and undiagnosed diabetes.

20. Chadt, A., & Al-Hasani, H. (2020). Glucose transporters in adipose tissue, liver, and skeletal muscle in metabolic health and disease. *Pflugers Archiv–European Journal of Physiology, 472*, 1273–1298.

21. Charrez, B., Qiao, L., & Hebbard, L. (2015). The role of fructose in metabolism and cancer. *Hormone Molecular Biology and Clinical Investigation, 22*, 79–89.

22. Chen, L., Sun, X., Xiao, H., Xu, F., Yang, Y., Lin, Z., Chen, Z., Quan, S., & Huang, H. (2019). PAQR3 regulates phosphorylation of FoxO1 in insulin-resistant HepG2 cells via NF-κB signaling pathway. *Experimental Cell Research, 381*, 301–310.

23. Cukierman-Yaffe, T., et al. (2020). Effect of dulaglutide on cognitive impairment in type 2 diabetes: An exploratory analysis of the REWIND trial. *The Lancet Neurology, 19*, 582–590.

24. DiMeglio, L. A., Evans-Molina, C., & Oram, R. A. (2018). Type 1 diabetes. *The Lancet, 391*, 2449–2462.

25. Enogieru, O. J., Ung, P. M. U., Yee, S. W., Schlessinger, A., & Giacomini, K. M. (2019). Functional and structural analysis of rare SLC2A2 variants associated with Fanconi-Bickel syndrome and metabolic traits. *Human Molecular Genetics, 40*, 983–995.

26. Fadini, G. P., Bonora, B. M., & Avogaro, A. (2017). SGLT2 inhibitors and diabetic ketoacidosis: Data from the FDA adverse event reporting system. *Diabetology, 60*, 1385–1389.

27. Feng, S. D., Yang, J. H., Yao, C. H., Yang, S. S., Zhu, Z. M., Wu, D., Ling, H. Y., & Zhang, L. (2017). Potential regulatory mechanisms of lncRNA in diabetes and its complications. *Biochemistry and Cell Biology, 95*, 361–367.

28. Fernandes Silva, L., Vangipurapu, J., Kuulasmaa, T., & Laakso, M. (2019). An intronic variant in the GCKR gene is associated with multiple lipids. *Scientific Reports, 9*, 10240.

29. Galicia-Garcia, U., Benito-Vicente, A., Jebari, S., Larrea-Sebal, A., Siddiqi, H., Uribe, K. B., Ostolaza, H., & Martín, C. (2020). Pathophysiology of Type 2 Diabetes Mellitus. *International Journal of Molecular Sciences, 21*, 6275.

30. Ghezzi, C., Loo, D. D. F., & Wright, E. M. (2018). Physiology of renal glucose handling via SGLT1, SGLT2 and GLUT2. *Diabetology, 61*, 2087–2097.

31. Gombos, Z., Koltai, E., Torma, F., Bakonyi, P., Kolonics, A., Aczel, D., Ditroi, T., Nagy, P., Kawamura, T., & Radak, Z. (2021). Hypertrophy of rat skeletal muscle is associated with increased SIRT1/Akt/mTOR/S6 and suppressed Sestrin2/SIRT3/FOXO1 levels. *International Journal of Molecular Sciences, 22*, 7588.

32. Gopal, K., Saleme, B., Al Batran, R., Aburasayn, H., Eshreif, A., Ho, K. L., Ma, W. K., Almutairi, M., Eaton, F., Gandhi, M., et al. (2017). FoxO1 regulates myocardial glucose oxidation rates via transcriptional control of pyruvate dehydrogenase kinase 4 expression. *American Journal of Physiology–Heart and Circulatory Physiology, 313*, H479–H490.

33. Goyal, N., Kesharwani, D., & Datta, M. (2018). Lnc-ing non-coding RNAs with metabolism and diabetes: Roles of lncRNAs. *Cellular and Molecular Life Sciences, 75*, 1827–1837.

34. Goyal, N., Sivadas, A., Shamsudheen, K. V., Jayarajan, R., Verma, A., Sivasubbu, S., Scaria, V., & Datta, M. (2017). RNA sequencing of db/db mice liver identifies lncRNA H19 as a key regulator of gluconeogenesis and hepatic glucose output. *Scientific Reports, 7*, 8312.

35. Grasmann, G., Smolle, E., Olschewski, H., & Leithner, K. (2019). Gluconeogenesis in cancer cells—Repurposing of a starvation-induced metabolic pathway? *Biochemical et Biophysical Acta (BBA)–Reviews on Cancer, 1872*, 24–36.

36. Gu, L., Ding, X., Wang, Y., Gu, M., Zhang, J., Yan, S., Li, N., Song, Z., Yin, J., Lu, L., et al. (2019). Spexin alleviates insulin resistance and inhibits hepatic gluconeogenesis via the FoxO1/PGC-1α pathway in high-fat-diet-induced rats and insulin resistant cells. *International Journal of Biological Sciences, 15*, 2815–2829.

37. Guo, H., Wu, H., & Li, Z. (2023). The pathogenesis of diabetes. *International Journal of Molecular Sciences, 24*(8), 6978.

38. Hagger, V., Hendrieckx, C., Sturt, J., Skinner, T. C., & Speight, J. (2016). Diabetes distress among adolescents with type 1 diabetes: A systematic review. *Current Diabetes Reports, 16*, 1–14.

39. Han, H. S., Kang, G., Kim, J. S., Choi, B. H., & Koo, S. H. (2016). Regulation of glucose metabolism from a liver-centric perspective. *Experimental & Molecular Medicine, 48*, e218.

40. Harding, K. A., et al. (2019). Depression prevalence in type 2 diabetes is not related to diabetes–depression symptom overlaps but is related to symptom dimensions within patient self-report measures: A meta-analysis. *Diabetic Medicine, 36*, 1600–1611.

41. Hatting, M., Tavares, C. D. J., Sharabi, K., Rines, A. K., & Puigserver, P. (2018). Insulin regulation of gluconeogenesis. *Annals of the New York Academy of Sciences, 1411*, 21–35.

42. Hawa, M. I., Kolb, H., Schloot, N., Beyan, H., Paschou, S. A., Buzzetti, R., et al. (2013). Action LADA Consortium. Adult-onset autoimmune diabetes in Europe is prevalent with a broad clinical phenotype: Action LADA 7. *Diabetes Care, 36*, 908–913.

43. He, Y., Dan, Y., Gao, X., Huang, L., Lv, H., & Chen, J. (2021). DNMT1-mediated lncRNA MEG3 methylation accelerates endothelial-mesenchymal transition in diabetic retinopathy through the PI3K/Akt/mTOR signaling pathway. *American Journal of Physiology–Endocrinology and Metabolism, 320*, E598–E608.

44. Huda, M. N., Kim, M., & Bennett, B. J. (2021). Modulating the microbiota as a therapeutic intervention for type 2 diabetes. *Frontiers in Endocrinology, 12*, 632335.

45. Hughes, J. W., Riddlesworth, T. D., DiMeglio, L. A., Miller, K. M., Rickels, M. R., & McGill, J. B. (2016). T1D Exchange Clinic Network. Autoimmune diseases in children and adults with type 1 diabetes from the T1D exchange clinic registry. *Journal of Clinical Endocrinology & Metabolism, 101*, 4931–4937.

46. International Diabetes Federation. (2019). *IDF Diabetes Atlas* (9th ed.). Brussels, Belgium: International Diabetes Federation.

47. Jia, Y., et al. (2021). Associations of the glycaemic control of diabetes with dementia and physical function in rural-dwelling older Chinese adults: A population-based study. *Clinical Interventions in Aging, 16*, 1503–1513.

48. Jouvet, N., & Estall, J. L. (2017). The pancreas: Bandmaster of glucose homeostasis. *Experimental Cell Research, 360*, 19–23.

49. Judge, A., & Dodd, M. S. (2020). Metabolism. *Essays in Biochemistry, 64*, 607–647.

50. Kahaly, G. J., & Hansen, M. P. (2016). Type 1 diabetes associated autoimmunity. *Autoimmunity Reviews, 15*, 644–648.

51. Kang, X., Wang, Y., Liang, W., Tang, X., Zhang, Y., Wang, L., Zhao, P., & Lu, Z. (2021). Bombyx mori nucleopolyhedroviral downregulates transcription factor BmFoxO to elevate virus infection. *Developmental and Comparative Immunology, 116*, 103904.

52. Kato, M., Wang, M., Chen, Z., Bhatt, K., Oh, H. J., Lanting, L., Deshpande, S., Jia, Y., Lai, J. Y., O'Connor, C. L., et al. (2016). An endoplasmic reticulum stress-regulated lncRNA hosting a microRNA mega cluster induces early features of diabetic nephropathy. *Nature Communications, 7*, 12864.

53. Katz, A. (2022). A century of exercise physiology: Key concepts in regulation of glycogen metabolism in skeletal muscle. *European Journal of Applied Physiology, 122*, 1751–1772.

54. Khan, S., & Jena, G. (2015). The role of butyrate, a histone deacetylase inhibitor in diabetes mellitus: Experimental evidence for therapeutic intervention. *Epigenomics, 7*, 669–680.

55. Kim, H. N., Iyer, S., Ring, R., & Almeida, M. (2018). The role of FoxOs in bone health and disease. *Current Topics in Developmental Biology, 127*, 149–163.

56. Kim, S. H. (2015). Maturity-onset diabetes of the young: What do clinicians need to know? *Diabetes & Metabolism Journal, 39*, 468–477.

57. Kitada, M., Ogura, Y., Monno, I., & Koya, D. (2019). Sirtuins and type 2 diabetes: Role in inflammation, oxidative stress, and mitochondrial function. *Frontiers in Endocrinology, 10*, 187.

58. Kitada, M., Ogura, Y., Suzuki, T., Sen, S., Lee, S. M., Kanasaki, K., Kume, S., & Koya, D. (2016). A very-low-protein diet ameliorates advanced diabetic nephropathy through autophagy induction by suppression of the mTORC1 pathway in Wistar fatty rats, an animal model of type 2 diabetes and obesity. *Diabetology, 59*, 1307–1317.

59. Koepsell, H. (2020). Glucose transporters in the small intestine in health and disease. *Pfluger's Archive–European Journal of Physiology, 472*, 1207–1248.

60. Lampasona, V., Petrone, A., Tiberti, C., Capizzi, M., Spoletini, M., di Pietro, S., et al. (2010). Zinc transporter 8 antibodies complement GAD and IA-2 antibodies in the identification and characterization of adult-onset autoimmune diabetes: Non-insulin requiring autoimmune diabetes (NIRAD) 4. *Diabetes Care, 33*, 104–108.

61. Langlet, F., Haeusler, R. A., Lindén, D., Ericson, E., Norris, T., Johansson, A., Cook, J. R., Aizawa, K., Wang, L., Buettner, C., et al. (2017). Selective inhibition of FOXO1 activator/repressor balance modulates hepatic glucose handling. *Cell, 171*, 824–835.

62. Lekva, T., Norwitz, E. R., Aukrust, P., & Ueland, T. (2016). Impact of systemic inflammation on the progression of gestational diabetes mellitus. *Current Diabetes Reports, 16*, 26.

63. Lemos, V., de Oliveira, R. M., Naia, L., Szegö, É., Ramos, E., Pinho, S., Magro, F., Cavadas, C., Rego, A. C., Costa, V., et al. (2017). The NAD+-dependent deacetylase SIRT2 attenuates oxidative stress and mitochondrial dysfunction and improves insulin sensitivity in hepatocytes. *Human Molecular Genetics, 26*, 4105–4117.

64. Lesniak, C., et al. (2021). Inpatient glycemic control and outcome of COVID-19 patients: A retrospective cohort. *SAGE Open Medicine, 9*, 20503121211039105.

65. Lewandowski, S. L., Cardone, R. L., Foster, H. R., Ho, T., Potapenko, E., Poudel, C., VanDeusen, H. R., Sdao, S. M., Alves, T. C., Zhao, X., et al. (2020). Pyruvate kinase controls signal strength in the insulin secretory pathway. *Cell Metabolism, 32*, 736–750.

66. Li, X., Wang, H., Yao, B., Xu, W., Chen, J., & Zhou, X. (2016). lncRNA H19/miR-675 axis regulates cardiomyocyte apoptosis by targeting VDAC1 in diabetic cardiomyopathy. *Scientific Reports, 6*, 36340.

67. Liu, T. Y., Shi, C. X., Gao, R., Sun, H. J., Xiong, X. Q., Ding, L., Chen, Q., Li, Y. H., Wang, J. J., Kang, Y. M., et al. (2015). Irisin inhibits hepatic gluconeogenesis and increases glycogen synthesis via the PI3K/Akt pathway in type 2 diabetic mice and hepatocytes. *Clinical Science, 129*, 839–850.

68. Lovic, D., Piperidou, A., Zografou, I., Grassos, H., Pittaras, A., & Manolis, A. (2020). The growing epidemic of diabetes mellitus. *Current Vascular Pharmacology, 18*, 104–109.

69. Lu, P., Chen, X., Zhang, Z., Zhang, J., Yang, Y., Liu, Z., Xie, J., Shao, S., Zhou, X., Hu, S., et al. (2017). Insulin upregulates betatrophin expression via PI3K/Akt pathway. *Scientific Reports, 7*, 5594.

70. Lu, Q., Tian, X., Wu, H., Huang, J., Li, M., Mei, Z., Zhou, L., Xie, H., & Zheng, S. (2021). Metabolic changes of hepatocytes in NAFLD. *Frontiers in Physiology, 12*, 710420.

71. Lu, X., Tan, Q., Ma, J., Zhang, J., & Yu, P. (2022). Emerging role of LncRNA regulation for NLRP3 inflammasome in diabetes complications. *Frontiers in Cell and Developmental Biology, 9*, 792401.

72. Ma, Q., Li, Y., Li, P., Wang, M., Wang, J., Tang, Z., Wang, T., Luo, L., Wang, C., Wang, T., et al. (2019). Research progress in the relationship between type 2 diabetes mellitus and intestinal flora. *Biomedicine & Pharmacotherapy*, 109138.

73. Malone, J. I., & Hansen, B. C. (2019). Does obesity cause type 2 diabetes mellitus (T2DM)? Or is it the opposite? *Pediatric Diabetes, 20*, 5–9.

74. Matheus, V. A., Monteiro, L., Oliveira, R. B., Maschio, D. A., & Collares-Buzato, C. B. (2017). Butyrate reduces high-fat diet-induced metabolic alterations, hepatic steatosis and pancreatic beta cell and intestinal barrier dysfunctions in prediabetic mice. *Experimental Biology and Medicine, 242*, 1214–1226.

75. Matsui, M., & Corey, D. R. (2017). Non-coding RNAs as drug targets. *Nature Reviews Drug Discovery, 16*, 167–179.

76. Mauvais-Jarvis, F. (2018). Gender differences in glucose homeostasis and diabetes. *Physiology & Behavior, 187*, 20–23.

77. Morigi, M., Perico, L., & Benigni, A. (2018). Sirtuins in renal health and disease. *Journal of the American Society of Nephrology, 29*, 1799–1809.

78. Morrison, D. J., & Preston, T. (2016). Formation of short chain fatty acids by the gut microbiota and their impact on human metabolism. *Gut Microbes, 7*, 189–200.

79. Moszak, M., Szulińska, M., & Bogdański, P. (2020). You are what you eat—the relationship between diet, microbiota, and metabolic disorders—a review. *Nutrients, 12*, 1096.

80. Moulton, C. D., Costafreda, S. G., Horton, P., Ismail, K., & Fu, C. H. Y. (2015). Meta-analyses of structural regional cerebral effects in type 1 and type 2 diabetes. *Brain Imaging and Behavior, 9*, 651–662.

81. Muoio, D. M., & Newgard, C. B. (2008). Mechanisms of disease: Molecular and metabolic mechanisms of insulin resistance and beta-cell failure in type 2 diabetes. *Nature Reviews Molecular Cell Biology, 9*, 193–205.

82. Noctor, E., Crowe, C., Carmody, L. A., Saunders, J. A., Kirwan, B., O'Dea, A., et al. (2016). ATLANTIC-DIP Investigators. Abnormal glucose tolerance post gestational diabetes mellitus as defined by the International Association of Diabetes and Pregnancy Study Groups criteria. *European Journal of Endocrinology, 175*, 287–297.

83. Panahi, G., Pasalar, P., Zare, M., Rizzuto, R., & Meshkani, R. (2018). High glucose induces inflammatory responses in HepG2 cells via the oxidative stress-mediated activation of NF-κB and MAPK pathways in HepG2 cells. *Archives of Physiology and Biochemistry, 124*, 468–474.

84. Petersen, M. C., Vatner, D. F., & Shulman, G. I. (2017). Regulation of hepatic glucose metabolism in health and disease. *Nature Reviews Endocrinology, 13*, 572–587.

85. Prats, C., Graham, T. E., & Shearer, J. (2018). The dynamic life of the glycogen granule. *Journal of Biological Chemistry, 293*, 7089–7098.

86. Qiu, G. Z., Tian, W., Fu, H. T., Li, C. P., & Liu, B. (2016). Long noncoding RNA-MEG3 is involved in diabetes mellitus-related microvascular dysfunction. *Biochemical and Biophysical Research Communications, 471*, 135–141.

87. Radhakrishnan, R., & Kowluru, R. A. (2021). Long noncoding RNA MALAT1 and regulation of the antioxidant defense system in diabetic retinopathy. *Diabetes, 70*, 227–239.

88. Rahmati, M., Keshvari, M., Mirnasuri, S., Yon, D. K., Lee, S. W., Il Shin, J., & Smith, L. (2022). The global impact of COVID-19 pandemic on the incidence of pediatric new-onset type 1 diabetes and ketoacidosis: A systematic review and meta-analysis. *Journal of Medical Virology, 94*, 5112–5127.

89. Rahnert, J. A., Zheng, B., Hudson, M. B., Woodworth-Hobbs, M. E., & Price, S. R. (2016). Glucocorticoids alter CRTC-CREB signaling in muscle cells: Impact on PGC-1α expression and atrophy markers. *PLoS ONE, 11*, e0159181.

90. Rawshani, A., Rawshani, A., Franzén, S., Eliasson, B., Svensson, A. M., Miftaraj, M., et al. (2017). Mortality and cardiovascular disease in type 1 and type 2 diabetes. *New England Journal of Medicine, 376*, 1407–1418.

91. Ren, Z., Xie, Z., Cao, D., Gong, M., Yang, L., Zhou, Z., & Ou, Y. (2018). C-Phycocyanin inhibits hepatic gluconeogenesis and increases glycogen synthesis via activating Akt and AMPK in insulin resistance hepatocytes. *Food Function, 9*, 2829–2839.

92. Rius-Pérez, S., Torres-Cuevas, I., Millán, I., Ortega, Á. L., & Pérez, S. (2020). PGC-1α, inflammation, and oxidative stress: An integrative view in metabolism. *Oxidative Medicine and Cellular Longevity, 2020*, 1452696.

93. Röder, P. V., Wu, B., Liu, Y., & Han, W. (2016). Pancreatic regulation of glucose homeostasis. *Experimental & Molecular Medicine, 48*, e219.

94. Ruan, X., Li, P., Cangelosi, A., Yang, L., & Cao, H. (2016). A long non-coding RNA, lncLGR, regulates hepatic glucokinase expression and glycogen storage during fasting. *Cell Reports, 14*, 1867–1875.

95. Rullman, E., Fernandez-Gonzalo, R., Mekjavić, I. B., Gustafsson, T., & Eiken, O. (2018). MEF2 as upstream regulator of the transcriptome signature in human skeletal muscle during unloading. *American Journal of Physiology-Regulatory, Integrative and Comparative Physiology, 315*, R799–R809.

96. Russo, S., Kwiatkowski, M., Govorukhina, N., Bischoff, R., & Melgert, B. N. (2021). Meta-inflammation and metabolic reprogramming of macrophages in diabetes and obesity: The importance of metabolites. *Frontiers in Immunology, 12*, 746151.

97. Saeedi, P., Petersohn, I., Salpea, P., Malanda, B., Karuranga, S., Unwin, N., et al. (2019). IDF Diabetes Atlas Committee. Global and regional diabetes prevalence estimates for 2019 and projections for 2030 and 2045: Results from the International Diabetes Federation Diabetes Atlas, 9th edition. *Diabetes Research and Clinical Practice, 157*, 107843.

98. Saltiel, A. R. (2016). Insulin signaling in the control of glucose and lipid homeostasis. In *Handbook of Experimental Pharmacology* (Vol. 233, pp. 51–71).

99. Sanyaolu, A., Marinkovic, A., Prakash, S., Williams, M., Dixon, Y., Okorie, C., Orish, V., & Izurieta, R. (2023). Diabetes mellitus: An overview of the types, prevalence, comorbidity, complication, genetics, economic implication, and treatment. *World Journal of Meta-Analysis, 11*, 134–143.

100. Scapin, G., Dandey, V. P., Zhang, Z., Prosise, W., Hruza, A., Kelly, T., Mayhood, T., Strickland, C., Potter, C. S., & Carragher, B. (2021). Structure of the insulin receptor–insulin complex by single-particle cryo-EM analysis. *Nature, 556*, 122–125.

101. Sireesh, D., Dhamodharan, U., Ezhilarasi, K., Vijay, V., & Ramkumar, K. M. (2018). Association of NF-E2 related factor 2 (Nrf2) and inflammatory cytokines in recent onset type 2 diabetes mellitus. *Scientific Reports, 8*, 5126.

102. Song, J., Yang, Y., Mauvais-Jarvis, F., Wang, Y. P., & Niu, T. (2017). KCNJ11, ABCC8 and TCF7L2 polymorphisms and the response to sulfonylurea treatment in patients with type 2 diabetes: A bioinformatics assessment. *BMC Medical Genetics, 18*, 64.

103. Sternisha, S. M., & Miller, B. G. (2019). Molecular and cellular regulation of human glucokinase. *Archives of Biochemistry and Biophysics, 663*, 199–213.

104. Sun, H., Saeedi, P., Karuranga, S., Pinkepank, M., Ogurtsova, K., Duncan, B. B., Stein, C., Basit, A., Chan, J. C. N., Mbanya, J. C., et al. (2022). IDF Diabetes Atlas: Global, regional and country-level diabetes prevalence estimates for 2021 and projections for 2045. *Diabetes Research and Clinical Practice, 183*, 109119.

105. Tan, C. Y., Weier, Q., Zhang, Y., Cox, A. J., Kelly, D. J., & Langham, R. G. (2015). Thioredoxin-interacting protein: A potential therapeutic target for treatment of progressive fibrosis in diabetic nephropathy. *Nephron, 129*, 109–127.

106. Thorens, B. (2015). GLUT2, glucose sensing and glucose homeostasis. *Diabetology, 58*, 221–232.

107. Tian, Z., Zhuang, X., Luo, M., Yin, W., & Xiong, L. (2020). The propionic acid and butyric acid in serum but not in feces are increased in patients with diarrhea-predominant irritable bowel syndrome. *BMC Gastroenterology, 20*, 73.

108. Todd, J. A., Walker, N. M., Cooper, J. D., Smyth, D. J., Downes, K., Plagnol, V., et al. (2007). Genetics of Type 1 diabetes in Finland; Welcome Trust Case Control Consortium. Robust associations of four new chromosome regions from genome-wide analyses of type 1 diabetes. *Nature Genetics, 39*, 857–864.

109. Tomic, D., Shaw, J. E., & Magliano, D. J. (2022). The burden and risks of emerging complications of diabetes mellitus. *Nature Reviews Endocrinology, 18*, 525–539.

110. Umpierrez, G., & Korytkowski, M. (2016). Diabetic emergencies—ketoacidosis, hyperglycemic hyperosmolar state and hypoglycemia. *Nature Reviews Endocrinology, 12*, 222–232.

111. Wang, L., Li, J., & Di, L. J. (2022). Glycogen synthesis and beyond, a comprehensive review of GSK3 as a key regulator of metabolic pathways and a therapeutic target for treating metabolic diseases. *Medicinal Research Reviews, 42*, 946–982.

112. Wang, Z., & Dong, C. (2019). Gluconeogenesis in cancer: Function and regulation of PEPCK, FBPase, and G6Pase. *Trends in Cancer, 5*, 30–45.

113. Wei, S., Zhang, M., Yu, Y., Xue, H., Lan, X., Liu, S., Hatch, G., & Chen, L. (2016). HNF-4α regulated miR-122 contributes to development of gluconeogenesis and lipid metabolism disorders in Type 2 diabetic mice and in palmitate-treated HepG2 cells. *European Journal of Pharmacology, 791*, 254–263.

114. World Health Organization. (2022). *Diabetes*. https://www.who.int/news-room/fact-sheets/detail/diabetes (accessed on 21 May 2025).

115. Xirouchaki, C. E., Mangiafico, S. P., Bate, K., Ruan, Z., Huang, A. M., Tedjosiswoyo, B. W., Lamont, B., Pong, W., Favaloro, J., Blair, A. R., et al. (2016). Impaired glucose metabolism and exercise capacity with muscle-specific glycogen synthase 1 (gys1) deletion in adult mice. *Molecular Metabolism, 5*, 221–232.

116. Yan, C., Li, J., Feng, S., Li, Y., & Tan, L. (2018). Long noncoding RNA Gomafu upregulates Foxo1 expression to promote hepatic insulin resistance by sponging miR-139-5p. *Cell Death & Disease, 9*, 289.

117. Yan, J., Thomson, J. K., Zhao, W., Wu, X., Gao, X., DeMarco, D., Kong, W., Tong, M., Sun, J., Bakhos, M., et al. (2018). The stress kinase JNK regulates gap junction Cx43 gene expression and promotes atrial fibrillation in the aged heart. *Journal of Molecular and Cellular Cardiology, 114*, 105–115.

118. Yang, G., Wei, J., Liu, P., Zhang, Q., Tian, Y., Hou, G., Meng, L., Xin, Y., & Jiang, X. (2021). Role of the gut microbiota in type 2 diabetes and related diseases. *Metabolism, 117*, 154712.

119. Yang, H., & Yang, L. (2016). Targeting cAMP/PKA pathway for glycemic control and type 2 diabetes therapy. *Journal of Molecular Endocrinology, 57*, R93–R108.

120. Yang, R., Jia, Q., Mehmood, S., Ma, S., & Liu, X. (2021). Genistein ameliorates inflammation and insulin resistance through mediation of gut microbiota composition in type 2 diabetic mice. *European Journal of Nutrition, 60*, 2155–2168.

121. Yaribeygi, H., Farrokhi, F. R., Butler, A. E., & Sahebkar, A. (2019). Insulin resistance: Review of the underlying molecular mechanisms. *Journal of Cellular Physiology, 234*, 8152–8161.

122. Yi, H., Peng, R., Zhang, L. Y., Sun, Y., Peng, H. M., Liu, H. D., Yu, L. J., Li, A. L., Zhang, Y. J., Jiang, W. H., et al. (2017). LincRNA-Gm4419 knockdown ameliorates NF-κB/NLRP3 inflammasome-mediated inflammation in diabetic nephropathy. *Cell Death & Disease, 8*, e2583.

123. Yin, D. D., Zhang, E. B., You, L. H., Wang, N., Wang, L. T., Jin, F. Y., Zhu, Y. N., Cao, L. H., Yuan, Q. X., De, W., et al. (2015). Downregulation of lncRNA TUG1 affects apoptosis and insulin secretion in mouse pancreatic β cells. *Cellular Physiology and Biochemistry, 35*, 1892–1904.

124. Yuen, L., & Wong, V. W. (2015). Gestational diabetes mellitus: Challenges for different ethnic groups. *World Journal of Diabetes, 6*, 1024–1032.

125. Zhang, K., Guo, X., Yan, H., Wu, Y., Pan, Q., Shen, J. Z., Li, X., Chen, Y., Li, L., Qi, Y., et al. (2019). Phosphorylation of Forkhead protein FoxO1 at S253 regulates glucose homeostasis in mice. *Endocrinology, 160*, 1333–1347.

126. Zhang, M., Gu, H., Xu, W., & Zhou, X. (2016). Down-regulation of lncRNA MALAT1 reduces cardiomyocyte apoptosis and improves left ventricular function in diabetic rats. *International Journal of Cardiology, 203*, 214–216.

127. Zhou, W., Xu, H., Zhan, L., Lu, X., & Zhang, L. (2019). Dynamic development of fecal microbiome during the progression of diabetes mellitus in Zucker diabetic fatty rats. *Frontiers in Microbiology, 10*, 232.

128. Zhou, Y., Zhou, J., Zhang, Y., Tang, J., Sun, B., Xu, W., Wang, X., Chen, Y., & Sun, Z. (2020). Changes in intestinal microbiota are associated with islet function in a mouse model of dietary vitamin A deficiency. *Journal of Diabetes Research, 2020*, 2354108.

129. Zhou, Z., Sun, B., Yu, D., & Zhu, C. (2022). Gut microbiota: An important player in type 2 diabetes mellitus. *Frontiers in Cellular and Infection Microbiology, 12*, 834485.

130. Zhu, C., Dong, X., Wang, X., Zheng, Y., Qiu, J., Peng, Y., Xu, J., Chai, Z., & Liu, C. (2022). Multiple roles of SIRT2 in regulating physiological and pathological signal transduction. *Genetics Research, 2022*, 9282484.

131. Zhu, X., Wu, Y. B., Zhou, J., & Kang, D. M. (2016). Upregulation of lncRNA MEG3 promotes hepatic insulin resistance via increasing FoxO1 expression. *Biochemical and Biophysical Research Communications, 469*, 319–325.

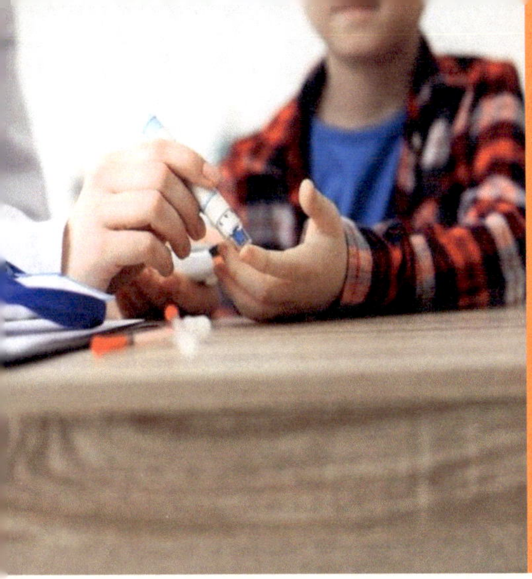

Chapter 3

DIABETES IN YOUNG POPULATIONS

Contents

3.1. Introduction

Diabetes mellitus (DM) encompasses a group of diseases that affect the body's ability to respond to elevated blood glucose levels. DM can be categorized into various types, including type 1 diabetes mellitus (T1DM), type 2 diabetes mellitus (T2DM), Gestational Diabetes, and prediabetes. T1DM is characterized by the destruction of β cells in the pancreas, resulting in the inability to produce insulin, and is typically diagnosed during childhood, hence its previous designation as juvenile diabetes. In contrast, T2DM generally manifests later in life and is the consequence of either insufficient insulin secretion by the β cells or insulin resistance. Due to its later onset, T2DM was previously referred to as Adult-Onset Diabetes. While historically an uncommon diagnosis among children and adolescents, the incidence of T2DM in this age group has been increasing (Buttermore et al., 2021).

The upward trend of pediatric T2DM cases (Figure 3.1) has been associated with multiple factors. A significant contributor appears to be the childhood obesity epidemic, which has continued to escalate in recent years. Research indicates that children from minority populations may be at elevated risk of developing T2DM, as diagnosis rates are higher among American Indians, African Americans, Asians, and Hispanics (Barrett et al., 2020). Socioeconomic status has been identified as a contributing factor in this early onset of T2DM. Genetics plays a role in childhood T2DM, with the frequency of T2DM in a first- or second-degree relative ranging from 74% to 100%. The lifetime risk of developing T2DM is 40% in offspring affected by one parent and 70% if affected by both parents (with shared environmental factors confounding as well), in contrast to T1DM where only 5% have a first degree relative with diabetes. Additional risk factors include female gender, particularly in females with premature adrenarche, infants born small for gestational age, or infants born with macrosomia from a diabetic mother (Temneanu et al., 2016). These risk factors demonstrate T2DM's multifactorial etiology, encompassing social, behavioral, environmental, and genetic susceptibility.

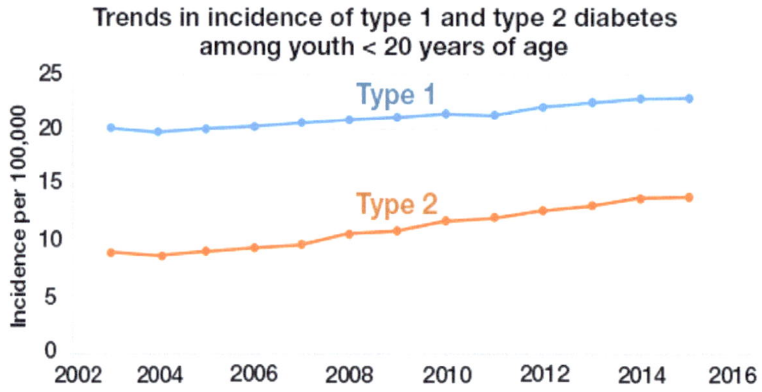

Figure 3.1. Incidence rates of newly diagnosed type 1 and type 2 diabetes mellitus among pediatric and adolescent populations (The Centers for Disease Control and Prevention, CDC.gov, 2020).

3.2. Complications

Children diagnosed with T2DM exhibit an elevated risk for severe complications later in life, including cardiovascular disease (CVD), nephropathy, and mortality by middle age (Solis-Herrera et al., 2014).

Following adjustment for risk factors over time, individuals with T2DM compared to those with T1DM demonstrate significantly higher odds of diabetic kidney disease, retinopathy, and peripheral neuropathy at a younger age. Despite the increased risk of complications in T2DM, comorbidities such as hypertension and arterial stiffness have been observed to be comparable to those with T1DM (Dabelea et al., 2017). T2DM in children initiates with insulin resistance and chronic inflammation, ultimately resulting in the destruction of β cells. This process has been demonstrated to occur more rapidly in children than in adults, thereby increasing the risk of further complications (Todd et al., 2019). Children diagnosed with T2DM typically commence treatment immediately to mitigate the risk of complications. Pediatric T2DM has also been associated with psychological disorders such as depression and anxiety. Given the importance of early treatment initiation, it is imperative to implement screening protocols for young adolescents to facilitate timely diagnosis. T1DM typically presents with acute or subacute onset in this age group, whereas T2DM is characterized by an insidious onset, potentially remaining undetected for an extended period. This delay in symptomatology poses a challenge for pediatricians in establishing an appropriate diagnosis promptly, thereby increasing the risk of long-term complications. In 2018, the American Diabetes Association (ADA) recommended general screening for T2DM in asymptomatic youth aged 10 and older (or post-pubertal onset) who are overweight and exhibit one or more risk factors (Wallace et al., 2020). These risk factors encompass non-white race, family history of T2DM, maternal gestational diabetes, or indicators of insulin resistance. Notably, genetic screening alone has not proven to be a valuable diagnostic tool in adolescents compared to clinical risk factors, including family history. The ADA's diagnostic criteria for youth with T2DM are consistent with those for adults: fasting blood glucose levels of 126 mg/dL or greater, or random blood glucose levels of 200 mg/dL or greater. Additionally, the ADA has recommended the utilization of hemoglobin A1c (HbA1c) levels to assist in T2DM diagnosis. HbA1c levels of 6.5% or above are indicative of a T2DM diagnosis, while individuals with HbA1c readings between 5.7% and 6.4% are considered at increased risk of developing T2DM (Van Name and Santoro, 2013).

To add to the complexity, treating T2DM in children and adolescents has proven more challenging than within the adult population. Lifestyle modifications, such as improved dietary habits and regular physical activity, are recommended to all patients; however, several expert groups have argued that these approaches to self-management are ineffective for youth with T2DM. The challenges behind this approach are multifaceted. Patients, caregivers, and healthcare professionals concur that there are significant barriers to lifestyle changes, including unsupportive relationships with family and friends, and social determinants of health such as poverty, food insecurity, and violence (Protudjer et al., 2014). Apart from lifestyle modification, the only approved treatments for pediatric T2DM are metformin and insulin. However, studies have emerged to support the use of other medications that may be more efficacious for childhood T2DM. A report produced by the TODAY Study Group found that up to 51.7% of pediatric T2DM patients fail metformin monotherapy, while those taking rosiglitazone as an adjunctive therapy demonstrate improved outcomes. Unfortunately, there are risks considering with various treatment options. There is a critical need for more effective pediatric treatment options; however, studies in this age group are limited.

3.3. Etiology

T1DM occurs when an autoimmune process destroys β cells in the pancreas, thereby terminating their ability to produce insulin.

The development of these β cell autoantibodies is hypothesized to commence when an individual with a genetic predisposition is exposed to a putative environmental factor that triggers a loss of immune regulation (Norris et al., 2020). This process typically manifests acutely or sub-acutely in children and young adults due to the cessation of insulin production. In contrast, T2DM involves a period of insulin resistance leading to the loss of β cell function and decreased insulin production. The development of T2DM is multifactorial, and although the increase in obesity has correlated with the rise in T2DM, there is higher prevalence in certain racial groups, females, and individuals with a strong family history; thus, supporting genetic predisposition as another significant factor in pathogenesis. This process occurs gradually, which elucidates why T2DM onset typically occurs later in life.

During hyperglycemia, insulin is secreted by pancreatic β cells, circulates to peripheral tissues, and facilitates the transport of glucose into cells for metabolism. In the case of insulin resistance, cells exhibit an impaired response to this hormone. Although insulin resistance is a complex phenomenon with multiple proposed mechanisms, a significant contributing factor is the presence of excess lipids and fatty acids in the bloodstream and skeletal muscle tissue. This results in the obstruction of transporters responsible for glucose uptake from the bloodstream into cells upon insulin activation. Consequently, obesity is considered one of the most significant risk factors for T2DM (Buttermore et al., 2021).

Following the development of insulin resistance, the pancreas is compelled to increase insulin production beyond its previous baseline. Initially, the β cells secrete elevated quantities of insulin to counteract persistent hyperglycemic levels (Christensen and Gannon, 2019). Subsequently, the β cells undergo stress-induced alterations, resulting in compromised function and diminished insulin release. Ultimately, the β cells undergo apoptosis or dedifferentiate into non-functional immature cells, leading to a reduction in the population of healthy β cells within the pancreas (Christensen and Gannon, 2019). This progression culminates in T2DM, characterized by both insulin resistance and impaired insulin production (Figure 3.2).

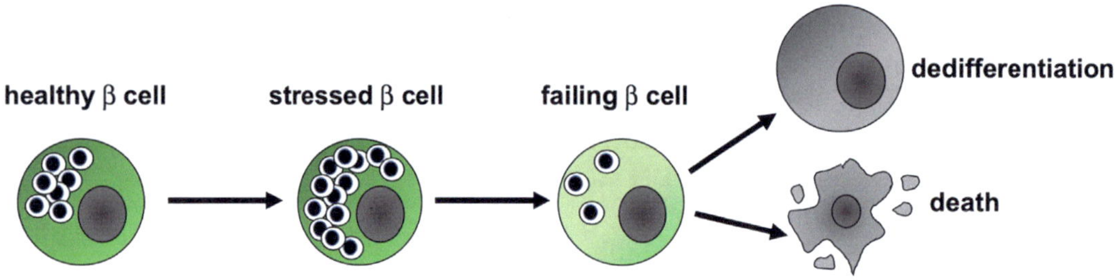

Figure 3.2. Progression of β cell function through prolonged insulin resistance (Christensen and Gannon, 2019).

The mechanism of developing T2DM among children is similar to that in adults; however, among adolescents, the progression is more rapid. Research has demonstrated that insulin resistance in youth is generally more severe than in adults with similar comorbidities (Tagi et al., 2019). This phenomenon may elucidate why children exhibit reduced improvements in insulin sensitivity when treated with metformin and lifestyle modifications. Studies have shown that children with T2DM possess higher levels of insulin than adults yet display a greater decrease in insulin secretion once the disease manifests (Barrett et al., 2020). The TODAY trial provided evidence that insulin secretion from the β cells decreased 20–35% per year in children, compared to 7–11% in adults. The precise physiological cause for this disparity remains to be elucidated. The initial elevation in insulin production may contribute to the more rapid decline of β cell function. It has been postulated that puberty may play a role in the accelerated β cell decline observed in children (Todd et al., 2019). Puberty itself has been documented to induce insulin resistance and consequently increased insulin release in healthy children. This phenomenon contributes to the initial higher than anticipated insulin levels when compared to adults, leading to more rapid β cell decline, which results in the impaired insulin release mechanism in children with T2DM. It is hypothesized that females are 1.5–3 times more likely to develop T2DM as children/adolescents due to the impairment of the increased compensatory insulin secretion during puberty in those with T2DM, and the earlier onset of puberty in females compared to males. Following the development of T2DM, children are at higher risk for the manifestation of complications at an earlier stage in life with faster progression of such conditions (Barrett et al., 2020). Furthermore, children are more susceptible to treatment failure.

3.4. Type 2 Diabetes Mellitus (T2DM) Trends in Children and Adolescents

T2DM in children and adolescents is frequently underdiagnosed due to its prolonged subclinical course and insufficient awareness regarding the increasing risk among patients and healthcare providers. Consequently, national population-based disease registry data may not accurately reflect the frequency and increasing trends of T2DM in this demographic. Nevertheless, the prevalence of T2DM in the 10- to 19-year-old population has doubled over the past two decades in the United States (Lawrence et al., 2021). It is present in nearly 2 individuals per 1000 among Black and American Indian youth. The SEARCH for Diabetes in Youth study estimates that the prevalence of youth-onset T2DM will increase two- to four-fold by 2050. The incidence of T2D has similarly doubled among adolescents in the United States over this period, from 9 to 18 cases per 1,00,000 per year, with a particularly high incidence observed in Black and American Indian youth (Wagenknecht et al., 2023). Similarly, T2DM in youth is increasing in incidence and prevalence worldwide. In a review of country-specific prevalence and incidence of youth-onset T2DM, it was observed that some of the more economically developed countries, such as the United States and China, exhibit the highest reported rates globally (Lynch et al., 2020). The analysis also noted that data for T2DM in children and adolescents remain scarce across the globe. The number of incident cases of T2DM in youth is more than 2-fold higher in China and 1.4-fold higher in India than in the United States based on the larger population of these countries, with the United States demonstrating the highest reported incident rates in a more recent worldwide survey among children and adolescents aged under 20 years (Wu et al., 2022). Generally, the prevalence of T2DM in youth is lower in Europe than in other developed countries. Data on youth-onset T2DM are limited in South America and Africa. The increasing prevalence of obesity in children and adolescents has likely contributed to an elevated rate of T2DM. However, this factor alone does not appear to fully account for the increase in T2DM.

3.4.1. Pathophysiology

3.4.1.1. Risk Factors

All of the traditional risk factors for T2DM are also implicated in young-onset T2DM, albeit in an amplified manner. Obesity is the most significant risk factor, with over 90% of patients with young T2DM being obese. Early onset obesity or greater cumulative exposure to obesity are more substantial risk factors for diabetes (RISE Consortium, 2018); however, the risk is mitigated if weight normalizes before puberty (Bjerregaard et al., 2018). Positive family history and female sex are considered non-modifiable risk factors, with more than 80% of United Kingdom adolescents having a family history of T2DM. In cohort studies, the female sex predominates until age 25 years, after which it equalizes, and the male sex predominates after 40 years of age. Ethnicity and socioeconomic status also play significant roles in determining prevalence. Asian, Middle East and North Africa, Hispanic, and Black ethnic populations exhibit a disproportionately high prevalence of diabetes in adolescents (Sun et al., 2022), and low-middle and middle socioeconomic index countries demonstrate the highest age-standardized incidence compared with low socioeconomic index (Xie et al., 2019). Additional risk factors include prenatal exposure, maternal malnutrition, and diabetes, which elevate the risk of diabetes in offspring. The SEARCH study demonstrated that maternal obesity (odds ratio [OR]: 2.8, 95% confidence interval [CI]: 1.5–5.2) and maternal gestational diabetes (OR: 5.7, 95% CI: 2.4–13.4) were associated with increased risk of youth-onset T2DM compared with controls, persisting even after adjustment for age, socioeconomic factors, and ethnicity.

The treatment options for type 2 diabetes in adolescents and youth (TODAY) study group reported an association between maternal diabetes history and accelerated glycemic progression and deteriorating β-cell function in offspring with youth-onset T2DM over 12 years of follow-up. In the SEARCH Case-Control Study, the odds of T2DM were significantly lower among individuals who were breastfed in infancy (OR: 0.26; 95% CI: 0.15–0.46). However, the association was confounded by current body weight (Shah et al., 2023). Furthermore, certain endocrine disrupting chemicals, such as perfluoroalkyl and polyfluoroalkyl substances, are associated with an increased risk of T2DM at a young age (Kahn et al., 2020).

3.4.1.3. Rapid Progression

Although obesity and insulin resistance are critical initial factors, progression to glycemic failure is characterized by evidence of impaired β-cell function. Adolescents with T2DM exhibit rapid progression to glycemic failure compared with adults (Donnelly et al., 2018). Their pathogenesis involves an accelerated rate of β-cell function loss and lower insulin sensitivity than adults (Arslanian et al., 2021). In the RISE study, the rate of loss of β-cell function was 25%–30% in young people versus 7% in those with adult-onset T2DM (Sam et al., 2021). The precise etiology for this accelerated β-cell function loss remains unknown; however, excess growth hormone during puberty and obesity-induced insulin resistance and glucolipotoxicity are hypothesized to play a role (Galderisi et al., 2018). In the TODAY study for T2DM in young people (<20 years), the initial HbA1c and β-cell reserve were independent predictors of glycemic durability; participants with lower β-cell function experienced earlier treatment failure. There were no significant differences in markers of insulin sensitivity between adult and young-onset T2DM. A similar finding was observed in the RISE study (Sam et al., 2021), and unlike adults, early insulin treatment did not ameliorate β-cell function loss, suggesting that inadequate glycemic control is not contributing to this faster progression. In addition to β-cell dysfunction, higher insulin resistance was noted in young people versus adults with T2DM (Arslanian et al., 2021) and also in those with impaired glucose tolerance, which persisted after adjustment for body mass index (BMI), race, and sex (Arslanian et al., 2018).

3.5. Roles of Genetics in Heritability

Based on family and twin studies, the heritability of T2DM in children ranges between 30% and 70%. The first genome-wide association study for T2DM in young individuals was published in 2021, which included 9067 participants from multiethnic backgrounds and comprised 3006 young individuals and 6061 adult controls (Srinivasan et al., 2021). Seven genome-wide significant loci were identified, including a novel locus (rs10992863) in PHD finger protein 2. The remaining six loci (transcription factor 7-like 2 [TCF7L2], melanocortin 4 receptor, cell division cycle protein 123, KCNQ1 channel, insulin-like growth factor-binding protein 2, and solute carrier family 16 member 11) were previously reported as adult loci. Among these, TCF7L2 exhibits one of the strongest effects on the risk of T2DM among common variants (OR of approximately 1.4). The T2DM liability variance was 3.4 times higher for common variants and five times higher for rare variant associations compared with adult-onset T2DM, indicating a higher genetic contribution for young-onset T2DM. These findings suggest that adults and young-onset T2DM individuals have overlapping genetic architecture; however, the role of genetics is likely more significant for disease risk in adolescents than in adults.

3.5.1. Differentiation from Other Types of Diabetes Mellitus (DM)

During the adolescent period, elevated blood glucose levels can be attributed to multiple etiologies. As T2DM is a diagnosis of exclusion, it is necessary to systematically rule out other etiologies before arriving at this conclusion.

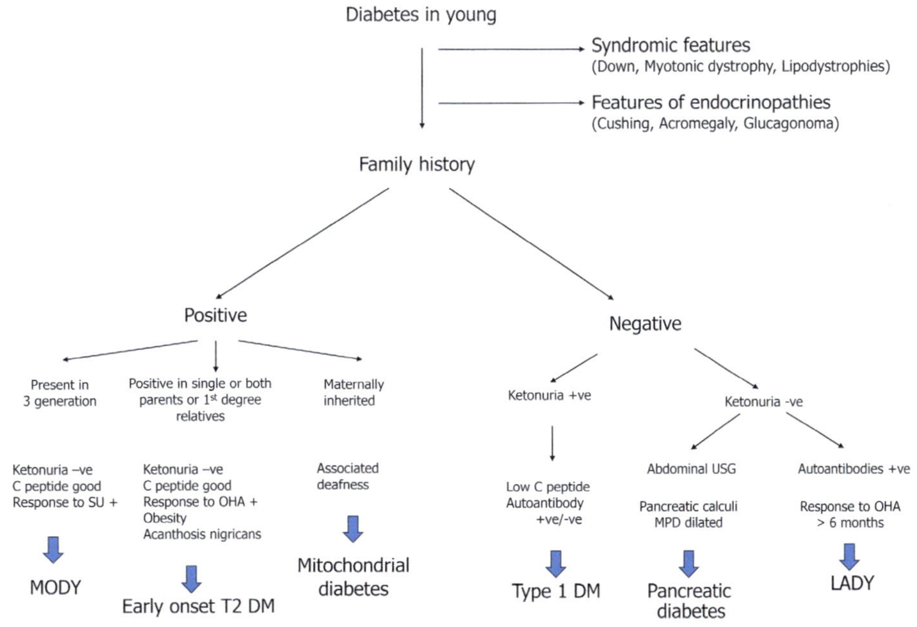

Figure 3.3. Approach to etiological diagnosis of diabetes in adolescents [LADY: Latent autoimmune diabetes in young; MODY: maturity-onset diabetes in young; MPD: main pancreatic duct; OHA: oral hypoglycemic agent; SU: sulfonylurea; and USG: ultrasonography] (Pramanik et al., 2024).

Common differential diagnoses include T1DM, maturity-onset diabetes of the young, diabetes due to pancreatic disease, latent autoimmune diabetes in the young, endocrinopathies (acromegaly, Cushing's syndrome), lipodystrophies, mitochondrial disease, and syndromic diabetes. A comprehensive history, focused clinical examination, and specific laboratory investigations are essential to establish the diagnosis (Pramanik et al., 2024). T2DM is typically considered in pubertal youth presenting with obesity, a family history of T2DM, features of the metabolic syndrome, and/or absence of islet autoantibodies. A detailed approach to the diagnosis of T2DM in adolescents is illustrated in Figure 3.3.

3.5.2. Complications and Co-Morbidities in Young Onset Type 2 Diabetes Mellitus (T2DM)

There is a high prevalence of diabetes-associated complications and comorbidities in individuals with young-onset T2DM – both at the time of diagnosis and subsequently. The implications of these complications are particularly significant in this age group due to their effects on education and employment, psychological consequences, and increased health-care expenditure. Additionally, women of reproductive potential with DM require specialized care and attention. Several studies indicate that for individuals of the same age, the risks of macrovascular and microvascular complications are higher for those with early onset compared to later onset T2DM (Misra et al., 2023). The risks are also elevated for young-onset T2DM compared to T1DM of the same duration. Despite improved healthcare leading to a significant reduction in complications and mortality among individuals living with T2DM, these improvements have not been evident in the youngest subgroup. Rather, there has been a resurgence of complications from 1995 to 2015 among individuals with T2DM between 18 and 44 years of age (Gregg et al., 2019). After 15 years of follow-up, approximately 80% of adolescents in the TODAY study had developed a minimum of one microvascular complication (TODAY Study Group, 2021). The proposed hypotheses for the increased risk of complications include a more aggressive pathophysiology, poorly controlled hyperglycemia, more prolonged exposure to glycemic burden, the concurrent presence of other metabolic risk factors, an unrecognized period of untreated or inadequately treated hyperglycemia prior to diagnosis, and the effects of obesity and inflammation, as a large proportion of those with young-onset TDM are overweight or obese. Additional factors include socioeconomic variables, mental health issues associated with reduced self-management capacity, reluctance to undergo repeated screening tests, and reduced engagement with health services resulting in infrequent follow-up.

3.6. Macrovascular Complications

An Australian study demonstrated that individuals with young-onset T2DM exhibited a higher risk of coronary artery disease (CAD) and stroke compared to age-matched individuals with T1DM (TODAY Study Group, 2021). Research has indicated that those with young-onset T2DM have up to 50% higher cumulative risk of CVD than those with later-onset T2DM. Furthermore, at any given age, the risk of adverse cardio-renal outcomes was elevated in comparison to the late-onset group; however, these differences were primarily attributable to the longer duration of diabetes in the young-onset T2DM group.

Although overt cardiovascular events are not highly prevalent in youth with T2DM, it is well-established that the process of atherosclerosis commences during childhood. Research has demonstrated the presence of subclinical vascular disease in adolescents with obesity and T2DM, manifesting as elevated aortic pulse wave velocity (PWV) or increased carotid intima-media thickness (CIMT) compared to normoglycemic youth. In the SEARCH study, individuals with young-onset T2DM exhibited greater degrees of arterial stiffness than those with T1DM, which was independent of diabetes duration or glycemic control. Generalized obesity and abdominal adiposity were identified as determinants of coronary artery calcifications in those with young-onset T2DM. In the TODAY study, BMI and blood pressure (BP) were associated with adverse cardiac measures (Levitt et al., 2015). Overall, there appears to be more significant vascular dysfunction and a higher probability of progression to overt CVD among youth with T2DM. However, as in adults, there is no recommendation for routine screening of subclinical atherosclerotic CVD in young-onset T2DM.

3.6.1. Nephropathy

The progression from microalbuminuria to macroalbuminuria is significantly higher in young-onset T2DM compared to T1DM. The risk is particularly elevated for Asian, Native American, and Pima Indian populations, suggesting a potential influence of ethnicity. A Japanese study demonstrated that among individuals < 20 years of age, the incidence of nephropathy was higher in those with T2DM than in T1DM, and these differences persisted even after adjustment for disease duration. Notably, in this study, the incidence of nephropathy gradually declined over several decades in T1DM, whereas the incidence remained elevated in patients with young-onset T2DM. Another study reported inferior renal survival (defined as remaining free of end-stage kidney disease) in T2DM compared with T1DM, with 55.0% survival after 20 years in the T2DM group, while in the T1DM group, renal survival persisted at 100%. However, there are insufficient data regarding the risk of microvascular complications in early-onset T2DM compared to later-onset T2DM. One study demonstrated a higher risk of microalbuminuria in young-onset T2DM than in later- or adult-onset T2DM (hazard ratio [HR]: 1.2; 95% CI: 1.1–1.4). A recent meta-analysis reported the prevalence of albuminuria to be 22.17%, with higher risk among Pacific Islander, Indigenous, and Asian youth compared to White youth (Cioana et al., 2021). It is noteworthy that the processes of albuminuria and hyperfiltration may commence prior to the onset of diabetes in youth with T2DM and may be associated with the early onset of vascular dysfunction in obese individuals (Bartz et al., 2015). In pediatric and adolescent populations, estimated glomerular filtration rate (eGFR) can be calculated using the Schwartz equation, which incorporates serum creatinine levels and patient height. However, this formula may underestimate hyperfiltration, a common occurrence in young-onset T2DM. eGFR estimation utilizing a formula that combines serum creatinine and serum cystatin C measurements may be more appropriate.

3.6.2. Retinopathy

The prevalence of diabetic retinopathy in young-onset T2DM ranges from 2% to 40%, varying according to the diagnostic method employed and the duration of diabetes. While the likelihood increases with disease duration, retinopathy has also been observed at the time of DM diagnosis. In the TODAY study, retinopathy in young-onset T2DM, detected through digital fundus photography, was observed in 13.7% of patients with a mean diabetes duration of 4.9 years, although no evidence of macular edema or proliferative retinopathy was present (Pramanik et al., 2024).

Age is a significant predictor of retinopathy in T1DM but not young-onset T2DM, with a 5% increased risk of developing retinopathy for every 1-year increase in age. Research has identified more pronounced subclinical structural and functional retinal abnormalities in adolescents with young-onset T2DM compared to T1DM, despite a shorter overall duration of T2DM (Pramanik et al., 2024).

The extant literature regarding the prevalence of retinopathy in early- versus late-onset T2DM of equivalent duration presents conflicting findings. One investigation reported a higher prevalence of retinopathy in individuals with young-onset compared to usual-onset DM after ≥ 10 years' disease duration. In this study, longer duration of diabetes was identified as a significant predictor of disease, while age of onset was not. However, a contrasting study on Pima Indian people observed a relatively lower incidence of retinopathy in patients with young-onset rather than later-onset T2DM. A recent meta-analysis indicated that the most significant increase in the prevalence of T2DM was observed at more than 5 years after diagnosis (Cioana et al., 2023). In aggregate, available studies suggest that young-onset T2DM confers a greater risk of retinopathy compared to T1DM of equivalent duration; however, the differential risk between young-onset and usual-onset T2DM remains to be elucidated.

Similar to adults, children and adolescents with T2DM should undergo screening for retinopathy at diagnosis and subsequently at regular intervals, with increased frequency of monitoring for those exhibiting inadequate glycemic control. Fundoscopy has been demonstrated to be less sensitive in detecting retinopathy compared to stereoscopic fundus photography in pediatric populations (Cioana et al., 2023).

3.6.3. Neuropathy

Studies on neuropathy in young-onset DM are relatively limited. In the SEARCH study, the prevalence of diabetic neuropathy, as determined by the Michigan Neuropathy Screening Instrument (MNSI), was 26% in young-onset T2DM. However, the MNSI did not assess small-fiber dysfunction. An Australian study, utilizing thermal and vibration threshold testing for small and large fiber neuropathy, respectively, reported a prevalence of 21%. Furthermore, autonomic neuropathy, assessed through pupillary reactivity, was observed in more than 50% of cases (Pramanik et al., 2024). The SEARCH study revealed that individuals with young-onset T2DM exhibited an age-adjusted prevalence of peripheral neuropathy nearly twice that of those with T1DM (17.7% vs 8.5%) (Dabelea et al., 2017). However, no significant differences were observed in the prevalence of cardiac autonomic neuropathy between the two groups. In a separate study focusing on individuals under 18 years of age, while no disparities were noted in the prevalence of peripheral and autonomic neuropathy, the mean disease duration for those with T2DM was considerably shorter at 1.3 years compared to 6.8 years for those with T1DM. Systematic studies comparing the risk of neuropathy in young- versus late-onset T2DM are currently lacking. One Australian study demonstrated that individuals diagnosed with T2DM between 15 and 30 years of age exhibited greater neuropathy severity compared to those diagnosed between 40 and 50 years of age, despite similar durations of DM. The prevalence of neuropathy in young-onset T2DM is at least as frequent as in adults. Consequently, the diagnosis of neuropathy utilizing appropriate screening tests should be conducted with equal frequency in youth as in adulthood – at initial diagnosis and annually thereafter. The neuropathy screening tests should primarily focus on the detection of at-risk foot for diabetic foot ulcer and can be readily conducted using clinical parameters such as foot inspection, assessment of pedal pulses, and testing for pinprick sensation, 10-g monofilament and vibration using a 128-Hz tuning fork, and ankle jerks, all of which require minimal or inexpensive equipment. Novel risk factors that have been identified for the development of peripheral neuropathy and cardiac autonomic neuropathy in children with DM include central obesity, smoking, puberty, and eating disorders. Therefore, young individuals with T2DM exhibiting any of these factors represent a priority group for neuropathy screening (Akinci et al., 2021). In an Indian study of 4555 individuals with childhood and adolescent-onset diabetes, 19.5% had T2DM while 71.4% had T1DM. The age-adjusted incidence of retinopathy was 52.9/1000 person-years in T1DM, which was marginally higher than that in T2DM (49.8/1000 person-years). However, the rates of nephropathy and neuropathy were higher in youth with T2DM compared to those with T1DM (6.2 vs 13.8 and 8.8 vs 24 in T1DM vs T2DM, respectively) (Amutha et al., 2021).

3.6.4. Mortality

A study on First Nation Canadian adolescents with T2DM revealed a mortality rate of 9% over a follow-up period of 9 years. An Australian study comparing standardized mortality rate (SMR) in patients with T2DM diagnosed between 15 years and 30 years of age with that of those diagnosed between 40 years and 50 years demonstrated an inverse relationship between age of diabetes onset and SMR. The highest SMR was observed for T2DM diagnosed between 15 years and 30 years of age (SMR 3.4 [95% CI: 2.7–4.2]), with the maximum SMR exceeding 6 in early midlife. Notably, the SMR for the older-onset group was comparable to the non-diabetic background population (Al-Saeed et al., 2016). The excess risk of death progressively decreased until it reached values similar to those of the background population in individuals diagnosed with T2DM beyond 69 years of age. A Swedish study demonstrated up to a two- to three-fold increased risk of all-cause mortality in individuals with diabetes who were aged less than 55 years compared to older individuals. When adjusted for glycemia and albuminuria, excess mortality persisted in those younger than 55 years even when the HbA1c was < 7% and in the absence of albuminuria (Sattar et al., 2019). In a large registry from Australia, individuals with young-onset T2DM exhibited higher all-cause mortality, CV mortality, and stroke but slightly lower cancer-related mortality (Huo et al., 2018). An earlier age of diabetes diagnosis by 10 years was associated with approximately 30% higher risk for all-cause mortality and a 60% elevated risk of CV mortality. A Danish study reported that younger age at diagnosis of T2DM increased mortality; however, this association was markedly weaker in women than in men. The decline in mortality over several decades with improved healthcare was also evident in men with diabetes but not women. The life expectancy for young-onset diabetes diagnosed between 20 years and 40 years of age is reduced by 14 years in men and 16 years in women compared with those without T2DM, and this reduction in life expectancy is greater than that of T1DM, which is approximately 12 years (Huo et al., 2018).

3.7. Comorbidities

3.7.1. Hypertension and Dyslipidemia

In a United Kingdom study comparing young-onset T2DM to T1DM, the former cohort exhibited an increased prevalence of obesity, hypertension, and dyslipidemia, although they also demonstrated an older age of onset ($P < 0.0005$) despite having similar glycemic control in both groups. In another hospital-based study, the hypertension prevalence among T2DM patients was 59.5%, with stage 1 hypertension being the most prevalent (30.95%). The risk of hypertension was elevated among individuals aged between 50 years and 60 years, those with longer duration of T2DM, having BMI ≥ 25 kg/m^2, those with poor glycemic control, and smokers (Akalu and Belsti, 2020). In a recent meta-analysis of 60 studies involving 3463 participants, hypertension prevalence was 25.33%, with a higher risk observed among male participants compared to females (Cioana et al., 2021). Researchers from the TODAY study group reported that after a mean follow-up period of 13.3 ± 1.8 years, the incidence of hypertension was 67.5% and that of dyslipidemia was 51.6%. The development of at least one macrovascular or microvascular complication occurred in 60.1% of the participants, while 28.4% experienced at least two complications. The study identified hyperglycemia, hypertension, and dyslipidemia as independent risk factors for the development of complications (Song, 2015). Studies in individuals with familial hypercholesterolemia have demonstrated that statins reduce CIMT with comparable efficacy in youth and adults (Vuorio et al., 2019). However, a multicenter study in T1DM failed to demonstrate any effect of statins on CIMT, despite a reduction in low-density lipoprotein (LDL) cholesterol (Marcovecchio et al., 2017). Longitudinal data on statin use in youth-onset T2DM remains insufficient. Nevertheless, it is well established that dyslipidemia in youth persists into adulthood, and the presence of diabetes concomitant with dyslipidemia may potentially increase the associated CV risk by several-fold. Consequently, a judicious approach to managing dyslipidemia should align with the general recommendations for dyslipidemia in diabetes.

3.7.2. Obstructive Sleep Apnea (OSA)

Obstructive sleep apnea (OSA) is associated with obesity and insulin resistance in adults and children and is established as a risk factor for future CVD. OSA can affect glycemic control in individuals with diabetes, and treatment of OSA may result in improved glycemic profile, HbA1c, and insulin sensitivity, as well as inflammatory markers, as observed in studies of adult T2DM (Zychowski et al., 2016). The implications in young-onset T2DM remain to be elucidated. While a comprehensive sleep study is costly, evaluation for OSA utilizing specific questions regarding sleep quality, snoring, apneic episodes, early morning headaches, and excessive daytime somnolence can be readily conducted. A pediatric Epworth sleepiness scale has been validated, with a score of 10 or greater indicating excessive daytime somnolence in children (Janssen et al., 2017).

3.7.3. Polycystic Ovarian Syndrome (PCOS)

Overweight and obese adolescent females exhibit a higher prevalence of polycystic ovarian syndrome (PCOS) compared to their normal-weight counterparts. Adolescent females with PCOS and obesity demonstrate a high prevalence of impaired glucose tolerance (30%) and T2DM (3.7%). Up to 21% of adolescent females in the TODAY cohort presented with oligomenorrhea, and these individuals exhibited higher androgen levels but lower sex hormone-binding globulin and estradiol levels (Kelsey et al., 2018). In females with T2DM and PCOS, metformin administration in conjunction with lifestyle modification can ameliorate not only metabolic dysfunction but also improve menstrual regularity and reduce hyperandrogenism.

However, in the TODAY study, all female participants were administered metformin, and differences between the effects of the three treatment groups (metformin alone, metformin with lifestyle changes, and metformin with rosiglitazone) on menses or sex steroids could not be demonstrated (Kelsey et al., 2018). Although some hormonal combined oral contraceptive pills (COCPs) have been associated with adverse metabolic status and cardiovascular risk, COCPs remain the cornerstone of therapy for hyperandrogenism and anovulation in PCOS, and they have no contraindications in young women with T2DM. While pelvic ultrasound-detected polycystic morphology is not indicative of a diagnosis of PCOS in adolescents, the condition can be diagnosed based on the presence of oligo- or amenorrhea with clinical or biochemical evidence of hyperandrogenism.

3.7.4. Non-Alcoholic Fatty Liver Disease (NAFLD)

Non-alcoholic fatty liver disease (NAFLD) is observed in up to 50% of children with T2DM. Longitudinal studies have demonstrated that after 20 years, 6% of non-diabetic adolescents with NAFLD experienced mortality or required liver transplantation.

The outcomes may be more severe for individuals with young-onset T2DM and concurrent NAFLD; however, data are currently insufficient in this regard (Parmanik et al., 2024). In a multicenter study on youth with NAFLD, 23.4% exhibited prediabetes and 6.5% presented with T2DM (Newton et al., 2016). Moreover, greater NAFLD histologic severity has been observed in young-onset T2DM compared to adults, with an elevated risk of progression to hepatic fibrosis, cirrhosis, and liver failure (Newton et al., 2016). While transaminase levels demonstrate good sensitivity for the detection of advanced stages of hepatitis or fibrosis, they exhibit poor specificity for NAFLD, necessitating the exclusion of non-NAFLD causes of chronic liver disease. It is recommended to assess young T2DM patients for the presence of possible NAFLD by measuring alanine transaminase and aspartate transaminase at diagnosis and annually thereafter. Liver ultrasound can detect liver fat exceeding 30%; however, its sensitivity is poor with lesser degrees of fat infiltration and in morbidly obese patients.

Liver biopsy remains the gold standard, and magnetic resonance spectroscopy is the non-invasive test with the highest sensitivity for detecting liver fat (Tsai and Lee, 2018). It is important to note that the non-invasive scores for fibrosis assessment, such as fibrosis-4, and tools like transient elastography are not validated in children or adolescents and should not be utilized in these populations.

3.8. Glycemic Durability

The rate of β-cell function decline is more rapid in young-onset T2DM, with approximately 25%–30% loss of β-cell function per year in young individuals compared to 7% per year in those with adult-onset T2DM. This accelerated rate of β-cell loss persists beyond youth, and a rapid progression to glycemic failure can be observed up to the age of 40 years (Dennis et al., 2019). The decline is particularly pronounced during adolescence due to the effects of growth hormone surges and gonadal steroids, leading to a decrease in insulin sensitivity. In the TODAY study, participants who experienced treatment failure exhibited significantly reduced β-cell function. These findings were consistent with those observed in the RISE study and large population-level studies in Europe and China. However, poor glycemic durability could not be ameliorated by early insulin treatment, suggesting it was not solely attributable to poor glycemic control. In one study, adults with early-onset T2DM exhibited an 80% higher probability of requiring insulin therapy compared to those with usual-onset T2DM, although they demonstrated a similar mean time to initiation of insulin (approximately 2.2 years).

3.9. Mental Health

Mental health disorders, including depression and anxiety, are frequently observed in individuals with diabetes, with the risk potentially being elevated among younger populations. Notably, in a registry-based study, approximately 40% of hospitalizations among young individuals with T2DM were attributable to mental health issues (Ke et al., 2019). In a study of Swedish individuals with young-onset T2DM, the risk of bipolar disorder, anxiety, depression, or stress-related events was increased by up to 4-fold (Liu et al., 2022). Among youth with T2DM, younger age at diagnosis was identified as an independent predictor for depression (Barker et al., 2023). It is crucial to evaluate psychiatric disorders such as depression, diabetes-related distress, body image disorders, and eating disorders in all children and adolescents with T2DM. While a validated questionnaire for assessing diabetes distress in children, such as the Problem Areas in Diabetes-Child score, exists, it has predominantly been utilized in children with T1DM who face additional factors like fear of needles and a high risk for life-threatening complications (Patton et al., 2023). Fear of hypoglycemia should be assessed. Many of these issues can be addressed through timely identification and appropriate counseling. Socioeconomic factors contributing to their distress, such as food security, housing stability, child labor, school dropouts, and exam-related stress, should be considered when developing a treatment plan after thorough discussion with the children and should ideally involve the family.

3.10. Cancer

Evidence suggests a higher prevalence of diabetes-related cancers in individuals with young-onset T2DM compared to those with adult-onset T2DM (Zhang et al., 2023). In the Nurses' Health study, early-onset T2DM was associated with an increased risk of early-onset cancers by 1.47-fold, obesity-related cancers by 1.75-fold, and diabetes-related cancers by 2.11-fold, all of which were higher than the rates observed in usual-onset T2DM across all age groups.

3.11. Pregnancy Outcomes

In the TODAY study reporting the outcomes of 260 pregnancies among 141 women with young-onset T2DM, 65% of the women experienced complications during their pregnancy. Approximately one-fourth (25.3%) experienced pregnancy loss, while preterm birth occurred in 32.6% of pregnancies. One-third of pregnant women had HbA1c levels exceeding 8%. Congenital abnormalities were observed in up to 10% of pregnancies, of which 3.7% resulted in stillbirths, a rate three times higher than the national rates for the United States during that period. Of the offspring, 7.8% were small for gestational age, 26.8% were born large for gestational age, while 17.9% of infants were in the macrosomic range (TODAY Study Group, 2021). In the National Pregnancy data from the United Kingdom, pregnant women with T2DM exhibited increased perinatal mortality compared to women with T1DM across all HbA1c categories (Murphy et al., 2021). The risk is particularly elevated for adolescent mothers with T2DM, among whom as high as 38% of women experienced pregnancy loss in a Canadian study. A significant portion of this risk can be mitigated or reduced through appropriate pre-conception counseling, meticulous glycemic control, and folic acid supplementation (5 mg/d) combined with close monitoring of the mother and fetus. However, studies have demonstrated that compared to women with T1DM, a significantly higher proportion of women with young-onset T2DM receive potentially teratogenic medications, and fewer than 50% had knowledge of or utilized adequate contraception.

3.12. Recommendations on Complications Screening in Young-Onset T2DM

At present, there is a paucity of guidelines from professional societies that address the management issues of young-onset T2DM. The ADA released a position statement on this matter in 2018, and the International Society of Pediatric and Adolescent Diabetes (ISPAD) published a consensus guideline in 2022. In general, in addition to glycemic status assessment, the investigations that should be conducted at diagnosis and annual review should include lipid profile, urine for albuminuria, serum creatinine levels, retinopathy screening, neuropathy screening with foot examinations, as well as liver function tests. Ideally, one should also evaluate all patients for OSA, assess adolescent and young females for the possibility of PCOS, and conduct a psychological assessment for emotional well-being and quality of life. Although most guidelines recommend that complication screening in T1DM should commence after 5 years of diagnosis or at puberty, whichever occurs earlier in T1DM, the same criteria may not be applicable in T2DM given that there would be an unknown duration of hyperglycemia prior to T2DM diagnosis (Parmanik et al., 2024).

Given the fact that youth-onset T2DM exhibits a more aggressive presentation and earlier manifestation of complications, coupled with the increasing prevalence of young-onset T2DM, it is anticipated to presage a significant clinical and socioeconomic burden with substantial financial implications. Complications would result in both increased direct costs of hospitalization and indirect medical expenses due to work absenteeism, reduced productivity while working, diminished productivity in the workplace, loss of employment, and disability-adjusted life years (DALYs) attributable to disease-related disability and premature mortality. Data on the socioeconomic burden of diabetes in youth-onset T2DM are lacking; however, extrapolating from adult data, it can be hypothesized that there is a significant increase in health-care costs due to delayed diagnosis of complications and comorbidities in young-onset T2DM, thus necessitating timely and periodic screening tests for complications (Rodriquez and O'Sullivan, 2023). Instead of focusing on costly investigations, complication screening should commence with inexpensive clinic-based tests such as anthropometry, clinical neuropathy assessment, fundoscopy for retinopathy, history and examination for oligomenorrhea and hyperandrogenism for PCOS, and validated questionnaires for diabetes-distress and excessive daytime sleepiness in children. Laboratory investigations may be limited to those with abnormalities detected on screening.

Using a similar logic, children and young adults who have complications such as atherosclerotic CVD, cardiomyopathy, peripheral arterial disease (PAD), kidney disease, or neuropathy must undergo screening for prediabetes or diabetes as a first-line investigation, irrespective of their age. While these are rare, comorbidities such as obesity, dyslipidemia, and PCOS are commonly encountered in adolescents. Available guidelines recommend screening for prediabetes or diabetes in overweight or obese children or adolescents with additional risk factors such as hypertension, dyslipidemia, and PCOS. Screening for diabetes preconceptionally and gestational DM screening in adolescent pregnancy should proceed in the same lines as during adulthood.

3.13. Management

3.13.1. Lifestyle Interventions

Guidelines from the ADA, ISPAD, and American Heart Association (AHA) advocate lifestyle modification in conjunction with pharmacotherapy in youth-onset T2DM (ElSayed et al., 2023). Dietary modification targeting a daily caloric deficit and enhanced nutrient intake constitutes an integral component of the management of youth with T2DM. Dietary modifications should be recommended for the entire family, with an emphasis on promoting healthy parenting practices related to diet, while avoiding excessively restricted food intake. The

ADA recommends supplementing regular school physical education sessions with 4–5 sessions involving 30–60 minutes of vigorous physical activity weekly for children and adolescents with T2DM and obesity. Nevertheless, weight reduction remains a significant challenge in the management of T2DM and obesity in youth. Barriers to achieving recommended weight loss are multifactorial. Intrinsic biological factors impede weight loss, while the lack of engagement is associated with family education, motivation, accessibility of social support, and various socioeconomic barriers (Salama et al., 2023). The rate of attendance in lifestyle sessions was only 60% of the planned sessions in the TODAY study (Berkowitz et al., 2018).

However, participants who attended more than 75% of the program duration demonstrated greater body weight reduction and improvement in body composition. Notwithstanding the promising results in adults, the TODAY trial indicated that intensive lifestyle interventions in conjunction with metformin did not yield superior weight-related outcomes compared to the cohort receiving metformin alone (Marcus et al., 2017).

In the TODAY trial, merely 53.6% of participants attained the physical activity target, and this shortfall may have contributed to the suboptimal response in the metformin plus lifestyle intervention group. The efficacy of lifestyle modification in T2DM youth may be lower than anticipated, and the inability to improve fitness, HbA1c levels, or weight may have a physiological basis. Although dietary modifications and exercise can reduce BMI and mitigate the risk of diabetes-related complications, these lifestyle interventions should invariably be implemented in conjunction with pharmacotherapy for T2DM in children and adolescents due to the aggressive nature of the disease.

3.13.2. Pharmacological Treatment-Approved Options

The management of pediatric and adolescent patients with T2DM remains a significant clinical challenge. Prior to 2019, pharmacological interventions approved by regulatory authorities were limited to metformin and insulin. However, in 2019, liraglutide, a glucagon-like peptide 1 receptor agonist (GLP-1 RA) administered once daily, received approval for use in children aged 10 years and older. This approval was based on favorable safety data and a clinically significant placebo-corrected reduction in HbA1c of –1.3% after 52 weeks of treatment (Tamborlane et al., 2019). In the subsequent three-year period, two additional once-weekly GLP-1 RAs, exenatide (Tamborlane et al., 2022) and dulaglutide (Arslanian et al., 2022), received approval from the United States Food and Drug Administration (FDA) for use in pediatric and adolescent T2DM patients. In Europe, exenatide gained approval in 2023, with dulaglutide anticipated to receive approval in 2024. Furthermore, the indication for the sodium-glucose cotransporter-2 (SGLT-2) inhibitor dapagliflozin was extended to include children aged 10 years and older, following a small-scale study involving young individuals aged 10–24 years in Europe. The placebo-corrected reductions in HbA1c were –0.85% for exenatide, –1.4% for dulaglutide, and –0.75% for dapagliflozin.

In a recent study of metformin and/or insulin-treated youth (aged 10–17 years) with T2DM having a mean baseline HbA1c of approximately 8%, the dipeptidyl peptidase (DPP-4) inhibitor linagliptin did not provide a clinically significant HbA1c reduction when added to metformin or insulin therapy, and the SGLT-2 inhibitor empagliflozin demonstrated only a modest effect on HbA1c in a randomized clinical trial (DINAMO study) (Laffel et al., 2023). Safety profiles of empagliflozin and linagliptin were observed to be similar to those found in adults with T2DM. No diabetic ketoacidosis (DKA) episodes were reported. Notably, empagliflozin has recently received approval for the management of T2DM in children 10 years of age or older based on results from the DINAMO trial. The findings with empagliflozin and linagliptin are consistent with those from earlier studies in youth-onset T2DM with dapagliflozin (SGLT-2 inhibitor) and sitagliptin (DPP-4 inhibitor) (Jalaludin et al., 2022). The use of sulfonylureas, DPP-4 inhibitors, or thiazolidinediones (TZDs) is not approved for the treatment of T2DM in children and adolescents.

3.14. Approach to Pharmacotherapy of T2DM in Children and Adolescent

3.14.1. Initial and Subsequent Theory

Metformin is the initial treatment of choice for T2DM in children and adolescents in conjunction with healthy lifestyle modifications (ElSayed et al., 2023). In the absence of ketosis or hyperglycemic symptoms, patients with HbA1c < 8.5% may commence metformin therapy at 500 mg daily, with gradual weekly titration to 1000 mg twice daily.

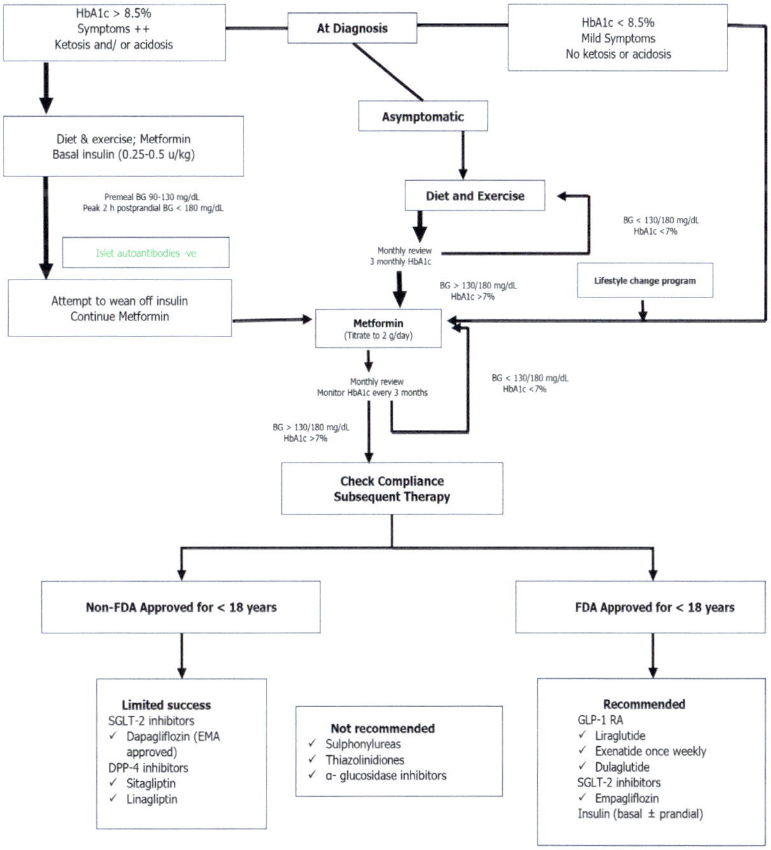

Figure 3.4. Approach to treatment of type 2 diabetes in children and adolescents (Karavanaki et al., 2022).

Insulin replacement is indicated in combination with metformin for youth presenting with symptoms or HbA1c ≥ 8.5%. Once-daily intermediate- or long-acting basal insulin (initial dose 0.25–0.5 units/kg) is necessary in the presence of ketosis or acidosis. Generally, transition to metformin monotherapy can be achieved within the subsequent 2–6 weeks. If the initial treatment goal (HbA1c < 7.0%) is not attained with metformin monotherapy in adolescents, the addition of basal insulin or GLP-1 RA may be considered. For higher HbA1c values (> 9%), basal insulin is the preferred option. If the glycemic target is not achieved on a combination of metformin and basal insulin (up to 1.5 units/kg), initiation of mealtime insulin should be considered. An algorithm for the pharmacological treatment of T2DM in children and adolescents is provided in Figure 3.4 (Karavanaki et al., 2022).

3.15. Unmet Needs in Drug Therapy

In contrast to the numerous therapeutic options available for adults with T2DM, metformin and liraglutide remain the sole non-insulin treatments formally approved in the United States for use in pediatric and adolescent populations with T2DM. Metformin monotherapy fails to achieve glycemic control in approximately 50% of adolescents with T2DM, particularly among those presenting with severe metabolic abnormalities at diagnosis (Bacha et al., 2018).

The RISE Consortium data demonstrated that pediatric patients with recent-onset T2DM experienced continued deterioration of β-cell function regardless of metformin therapy. Data regarding the efficacy of liraglutide in pediatric and adolescent T2DM populations are limited. Despite the FDA approval of liraglutide in 2019 for pediatric T2D, the adoption of GLP-1RAs in this population has been gradual due to the injectable mode of administration and associated costs. Furthermore, contrary to findings from adult studies, the pivotal GLP-1RA trials in pediatric T2DM do not demonstrate significant weight reduction. Additionally, the long-term safety and cardiovascular and renal impacts of GLP1 RAs have not been investigated in youth-onset T2DM. Although various insulin formulations are commonly utilized in pediatric and adolescent T2DM patients, they have not been specifically studied for the indication of pediatric T2DM.

Dapagliflozin was the first oral glucose-lowering medication since metformin to be approved in Europe for children (≥ 10-years-old) and young adults with T2DM. Given the adverse cardio- and microvascular profile (Zuckerman et al., 2022) of many young individuals with T2DM, the non-glycemic benefits of dapagliflozin may become increasingly significant in the management of youth-onset T2DM. However, due to the lack of published data, SGLT-2 inhibitors are not yet widely utilized for the treatment of T2DM in children and adolescents. Obesity is the primary pathophysiological driver of T2DM and development of CV risk factors in most children and adolescents. Therefore, studies examining semaglutide and tirzepatide, which have demonstrated substantial weight loss along with robust effects on glycemic control in adults with T2DM, are now necessary in young people with T2DM to obtain approval for these drugs as future treatments. Overall, the currently available therapies are limited and often insufficient. Although promising results have been demonstrated by some treatments in the short term, it is imperative to ensure that long-term benefits of these therapeutic options are clearly evidenced in youth with T2DM. Future research should aim to overcome the challenges observed in clinical trials in this population in order to address the unmet need for optimal management of T2DM in children and adolescents.

3.16. Bariatric Surgery

According to current international guidelines, metabolic bariatric surgery (MBS) is recommended for adolescent (10–19 years of age) T2DM patients with a BMI exceeding 35 kg/m^2 or more than 120% of the 95th percentile of age and sex matched population (Pratt et al., 2018). Among adolescent populations, vertical sleeve gastrectomy (VSG), laparoscopic adjustable gastric band, and Roux-en-Y gastric bypass (RYGB) are the most frequently performed procedures (Armstrong et al., 2019). A meta-analysis of 29 cohort studies, encompassing 4,970 adolescents with at least 5 years of post-bariatric surgery follow-up, reported a notable T2DM remission rate of 90% (95% CI: 83.2–95.6) following MBS (Wu et al., 2023). When comparing the metabolic effects of MBS between adolescent and adult populations, the probability of T2DM remission was found to be significantly higher in adolescents than in adults (86% vs. 53%; risk ratio: 1.27; 95% CI: 1.03 to 1.57), despite similar degrees of weight loss (Inge et al., 2019). The 3-year follow-up of the Teen-Longitudinal Assessment of Bariatric Surgery (LABS) study revealed a 76% remission rate among pre-diabetic adolescents who underwent MBS. In the adolescent population, both RYGB and VSG demonstrated comparable T2DM remission rates (Maffazioli et al., 2016). Consequently, MBS may be used as an early intervention tool for the prevention and improved control of dysglycemia in adolescents. However, patients undergoing MBS at an early age are at increased risk for both micro- and macronutrient deficiencies.

Moreover, as maximum bone accrual occurs at this age, bone health can also be affected due to the risk of nutrient deficiency associated with MBS. Further studies evaluating the long-term safety data of MBS performed in adolescents are necessary in the future (Inge et al., 2017). Reoperation may be required either due to complications (hernia, leak, band slip) or failure (inadequate weight loss or resolution of co-morbidities) of primary surgery. Limited expertise and availability, cost of therapy, lack of insurance coverage, stigma, and insufficient awareness and family support are the common barriers to performing MBS in adolescents (Campbell et al., 2022). Medically correctable obesity, substance abuse, current or planned pregnancy within 12 to 18 months, eating disorders, the potential for non-adherence to post-operative recommendations, and inadequate family support are considered relative contraindications to MBS. Overall, as the probability of remission of T2DM is significantly high with MBS in adolescents, it should be considered in carefully selected morbidly obese adolescents with T2DM. Among the minimally invasive newer procedures, intragastric balloon treatment and aspiration therapy are currently being investigated in adolescent obesity (Swei and Sullivan, 2020).

3.17. Glycemic Target

According to ADA recommendations, HbA1c should be measured every 3 months, and the HbA1c target for children or adolescents with T2DM should be <7%. However, ADA also recommends a more stringent target of < 6.5% if it can be achieved without causing significant adverse effects, including hypoglycemia. The lower HbA1c target is preferred in young T2DM patients due to the following reasons. Firstly, the risk of complications due to diabetes is higher in younger patients because of cumulatively longer duration of exposure to dysglycemia. Secondly, young T2DM patients have a greater degree of β-cell dysfunction (Arslanian et al., 2017). Furthermore, they are susceptible to rapid deterioration of beta cell function. In the TODAY study, an HbA1c cut-off as low as the prediabetes range (>6.3%) was associated with a higher risk of rapid loss of glycemic control within 48 months of follow-up (Zeitler et al., 2015). Thus, more stringent control may help to preserve β-cell function. Thirdly, with the advent of newer molecules such as SGLT-2i as well as incretin-based therapies, the risk of hypoglycemia is considerably lower when compared to intensive treatment with traditional sulfonylureas and insulin. Moreover, the risk of hypoglycemia is reported to be very low in adolescents even when insulin therapy has been utilized. Consequently, in young T2DM patients, stringent glycemic control is feasible without significantly increasing the risk of hypoglycemia. In summary, the HbA1c target in adolescents with T2DM should be on the lower side. However, the target should be individualized depending on the risk of hypoglycemia. The frequency and targets for self-monitoring of blood glucose should also be individualized.

3.18. Diabetes Remission

According to the international expert group consensus report, 'remission' of T2DM is defined as HbA1c remaining < 6.5% for a minimum of 3 months without glucose-lowering pharmacotherapy (Riddle et al., 2021). HbA1c testing should be conducted at least 3 months following any surgical or pharmacological intervention, or after a minimum of 6 months from the initiation of lifestyle-based intervention. Studies evaluating the probability of T2DM remission in adolescent patients are predominantly limited to lifestyle and surgical interventions. In a small-scale study, a ketogenic very low-calorie diet (VLCD; 680–800 Kcal/d) was reported to be efficacious in compliant children with T2DM, enabling the discontinuation of exogenous insulin and oral antidiabetic medications. However, in the TODAY study conducted on T2DM adolescents, lifestyle interventions (VLCD 1200–1500 Kcal/d with 200–300 min of weekly moderate exercise) failed to demonstrate any additional benefit when combined with metformin. Furthermore, the adherence rate, long-term durability, and adverse effects of VLCD in children and adolescents with T2DM are not well documented. Conversely, the effect of MBS on inducing remission of T2DM in adolescents is promising. In the Teen-LABS study, among 29 adolescents who underwent MBS, 95% reported remission from diabetes at 3 years. In the same study, a 76% remission rate was reported in adolescents with pre-diabetes. In the meta-analysis, a 90% diabetes remission rate was reported after a minimum of 5 years following MBS. MBS procedures are found to be more effective in inducing remission if performed earlier rather than later in life. Moreover, remission occurs rapidly following MBS, even before significant weight loss, suggesting additional mechanisms of diabetes remission beyond sustained weight loss (Ricci et al., 2023).

3.19. Prevention

One of the primary contributors and a significant modifiable risk factor for young-onset T2DM is excessive body weight beginning in childhood. The risk originates in utero, with the maternal nutritional status and fetal birth weight having substantial implications for the child's metabolic health. Consequently, interventions that reverse or reduce obesity in children and adolescents at the community level are crucial in preventing young-onset T2DM. In this context, school-based health interventions are gaining prominence in addressing and mitigating environmental and behavioral factors that increase the risk for the development of obesity and T2DM (Parmanik et al., 2024).

A wide range of prevalence data on childhood obesity (BMI > 95th centile) in T2DM has been reported, ranging from 64.5% in Asian populations to 89.9% in European populations (Cioana et al., 2022). Significant evidence regarding the impact of lifestyle interventions for youth with T2DM is derived from the TODAY study. Although the objective was to achieve a 7%–10% decrease in weight through lifestyle modifications, the addition of metformin monotherapy to lifestyle intervention did not result in any increase in the duration of metabolic control beyond that achieved with metformin alone. Youth with T2DM receiving metformin plus lifestyle intervention exhibited short-term weight loss and body composition improvement; however, these changes were not sustained over an extended period. Irrespective of treatment modality, sustained weight losses exceeding 7% led to improvements in HbA1c, high-density lipoprotein (HDL) cholesterol, and C-peptide levels. Family-based behavioral weight management programs have demonstrated some positive impact on weight and metabolic risk factors of school-aged children without diabetes but were less effective in adolescents and children with greater degrees of obesity. A comprehensive pediatric lifestyle intervention should involve the family and employ evidence-based behavioral strategies that have been shown to develop sustainable changes in nutrition and physical activity. Consequently, individuals with young-onset T2DM who are overweight or obese should receive appropriate comprehensive lifestyle programs, involving their family members, aiming to achieve a 7%–10% reduction in body weight. Nutritional guidance should encompass healthy eating patterns with increased consumption of nutrient-dense foods and decreased consumption of calorie-dense, nutrient-poor foods, such as sugar-sweetened beverages. Physical activity should comprise a minimum of 30–60 minutes of moderate to vigorous physical activity at least 5 days per week, along with strength-training activities for a minimum of 3 days per week. A meta-analysis demonstrated the short-term efficacy of very-low calorie diets in reducing weight among obese individuals under 18 years of age; however, no long-term follow-up has been conducted (Gow et al., 2021). Younger individuals have exhibited improved uptake of behavioral interventions in digital formats (Ross et al., 2022). Data regarding the efficacy and safety of pharmacotherapy for weight loss in youth are limited. Most anti-obesity medications, with the exceptions of orlistat and liraglutide, are not yet approved for use in children. Overall, there is insufficient evidence to support diabetes screening in all adolescents or young adults with obesity, as this approach would not be cost-effective. Some guidelines recommend screening for dysglycemia in obese youth who present with additional comorbidities such as hypertension. Several risk scores to identify individuals at risk for and requiring screening for diabetes have been developed and validated in various countries, incorporating both clinical and polygenic factors. The trajectories from normoglycemia to T2DM may differ in young individuals, thus narrowing the window of opportunity for screening at later ages. Another target group for preventive strategies specifically includes women with a history of gestational diabetes. A study revealed that the adjusted hazards in women with gestational diabetes for progression to T2DM were 71.9 per 1000 person-years. Such women should receive timely and appropriate guidance regarding lifestyle, nutrition, and monitoring.

3.20. Barriers and Solutions

The development of best practices for managing youth-onset T2DM is constrained by gaps in the understanding of glucose metabolism abnormalities during adolescence, the development of complications, and the long-term outcomes of youth-onset T2DM. Furthermore, the definitions of prediabetes and T2DM in children and adolescents lack an evidence base, as they have been extrapolated from glycemic indices predicting microvascular complications in adults. Hyperglycemia appears to be transient in some youth, while others exhibit rapid loss of glycemic control on oral monotherapy, necessitating insulin treatment. Consequently, a more comprehensive understanding of disease heterogeneity is required to elucidate disease trajectories that would facilitate customized treatment approaches. The long-term outcomes for early-onset dyslipidemia, hypertension, kidney disease, NAFLD, and CV dysfunction remain largely unknown (Nadeau et al., 2016). Further research is necessary to enhance the understanding of which diabetes-related complications may require pediatric-specific approaches.

Recent studies indicate that pediatric T2DM exhibits distinct characteristics from adult-onset T2D in multiple aspects, with adolescents diagnosed with T2DM demonstrating increased insulin resistance and glycemic failure in comparison to adults (Shah et al., 2022). Consequently, there exists a pressing need for an expanded array of treatment modalities. However, the social and environmental complexities surrounding youth with T2DM impede recruitment into and completion of clinical trials. As a result, trial recruitment for youth with T2DM has achieved limited success as a relatively novel endeavor. Additional obstacles to study implementation include a comparatively small population of available study participants (in contrast to adults) with an increasing number of trials competing for that limited pool of eligible patients, stringent eligibility criteria, the challenge of participants/caregivers repeatedly taking leave from school or work, and the limited number of research sites with resources allocated to pediatric T2DM trials (Van Name et al., 2020).

Given the realities of the epidemiology, disease heterogeneity, and socioeconomic challenges associated with youth-onset T2DM, as well as the clinical research experience to date, it is imperative to identify solutions to this situation in order to advance our understanding of the pathophysiology of T2DM in children and adolescents and facilitate the successful completion of research programs for this population.

3.21. Treatments

Nonpharmacological interventions for children diagnosed with T2DM encompass dietary modifications and increased physical activity. Nutritional guidance can be found in the Academy of Nutrition and Dietetics' Pediatric Weight Management Evidence-based Nutrition Practice Guidelines (McGavock et al., 2015). Regarding physical activity, the American Academy of Pediatrics recommends moderate to vigorous exercise for a minimum of 1 h daily, while developing a Family Media Use Plan to ensure sufficient time away from media to prioritize adequate sleep, physical activity, and other health objectives. Children with T2DM have been observed to lead sedentary lifestyles, which may contribute to their health complications.

The implementation of lifestyle modifications has demonstrated positive effects on BMI, BP, serum lipoproteins, and insulin resistance. Furthermore, it is posited that promoting strategies for positive mental health is crucial for children with T2DM, as lifestyle modifications can be challenging for young patients, and mental health disorders are frequently observed in obesity. Despite the benefits of these modifications, they are difficult to sustain in children who are under social, economic, and physical stress. This, in conjunction with the more aggressive progression of T2DM in children, renders these adjustments ineffective as monotherapy to treat youth with T2DM (McGavock et al., 2015).

The pharmacological treatment of youth T2DM patients primarily focuses on controlling insulin resistance, one of the principal mechanisms of T2DM (Meehan and Silverstein, 2016). Metformin is the preferred pharmacological agent for youth T2DM patients and remains the sole FDA-approved treatment option beyond lifestyle interventions and insulin therapy (Jalaludin et al., 2020). Although metformin has been established as a safe and cost-effective option, its efficacy in pediatric populations is diminished compared to adults.

The TODAY trial demonstrated that metformin monotherapy at a dosage of 1000 mg twice daily was efficacious in maintaining blood glucose levels in only approximately half of the participants.

This high rate of treatment failure may be attributed to the more aggressive etiology of the disease in pediatric patients. Insulin may be incorporated into metformin therapy if the patient fails to achieve glycemic targets. Additionally, insulin may be utilized to rapidly stabilize elevated blood glucose levels during episodes of ketosis, ketoacidosis, or hyperglycemic hyperosmolar syndrome, followed by metformin therapy to maintain reduced levels. Patients should undergo frequent monitoring, and the treatment regimen should be adjusted as clinically indicated.

The TODAY trial investigated the efficacy of incorporating the TZD rosiglitazone, administered at a dose of 4 mg twice daily, as an adjunct to metformin therapy.

The findings indicated that the combination therapy demonstrated superior efficacy in maintaining glycemic control and β cell function compared to metformin monotherapy, with failure rates of 39% and 52%, respectively. However, the utilization of rosiglitazone is not recommended due to the potential for serious long-term adverse effects associated with TZDs, including weight gain, edema, and heart failure. Additionally, the TODAY group evaluated the sulfonylurea glimepiride as monotherapy. While its efficacy was comparable to that of metformin, glimepiride was associated with increased weight gain, precluding its recommendation at present (Narasimhan and Weinstock, 2014).

3.22. Young-Onset Diabetes: An Indian Perspective

Diabetes in young individuals has been conventionally defined as the onset of diabetes before 35 years of age. Sahoo et al., in this issue, through a protocol-based evaluation (assessment of β-cell reserve, diabetes autoantibodies, genetic testing for maturity-onset diabetes of young (MODY) if fitting clinical criteria, genetic testing for mitochondrial diabetes) and close follow-up of patients with diabetes in young, over a period of two years, determined that the most prevalent etiologies for diabetes mellitus (DM) in young were T2DM (40%), T1DM (40%), fibrocalculous pancreatic diabetes (FCPD, 15%), MODY (2%), flatbush diabetes (2%), and mitochondrial diabetes (1%).

The exponential increase in T2DM prevalence in India over the past three decades has significantly contributed to the elevated burden of diabetes among young individuals in this region (Anjana et al., 2015). The prevalence of T2DM in India ranges from 8 to 10%, with an additional 15% of the population exhibiting pre-diabetes. T2DM in Indian patients are characterized by lower BMI, increased body fat, elevated clinical and biochemical measures of insulin resistance, and systemic inflammation. This is coupled with one of the highest global rates of pre-diabetes progression to T2DM (14–18, 6, and 2.5% per annum in India, Finland, and USA, respectively), indicating a more aggressive diabetes phenotype in Indians (Dutta and Mukhopadhyay, 2016). The onset of T2DM in Indians occurs nearly two decades earlier than in Western populations. This phenomenon also elucidates the high prevalence of T2DM among young individuals, as documented by Sahoo et al.

Tropical calcific pancreatitis, also referred to as FCPD, is predominantly confined to tropical regions and is characterized by pancreatic intra-ductal calcifications, ketosis-resistant lean diabetes, progressive and irreversible destruction of pancreatic parenchyma, initial positive response to oral diabetes medications, and elevated risk of pancreatic carcinoma in the long term (Goundan et al., 2016). The etiopathogenesis is multifactorial, involving malnutrition, cassava consumption, micronutrient deficiencies, and serine protease inhibitor Kazal type 1 gene variations (Kolly et al., 2017). FCPD contributes significantly to the burden of diabetes in young individuals in this geographical region, as highlighted by Sahoo et al. This observation is noteworthy, as FCPD has conventionally been considered to occur after 30–35 years of age. Further research regarding the prevalence of FCPD in young populations is warranted from other regions of India, particularly West Bengal, Kerala, and Tamil Nadu. MODY is frequently misdiagnosed in young Indian individuals with diabetes, especially those with a strong family history. These patients are often incorrectly diagnosed with T1DM and treated with insulin. Increased utilization of genetic studies would enhance the diagnosis of MODY. The number of MODY subtypes (attributed to specific genes) has increased substantially in recent years from six to more than 13 distinct genes. However, it is probable that MODY would not be as prevalent in India as observed in certain ethnic groups, such as Scandinavians. In the study by Sahoo et al., the reported 2% occurrence of MODY may be an underestimation. Restricting genetic testing for MODY to only those individuals with classical clinical history and pedigree analysis indicative of MODY may account for the lower diagnosis rate of MODY in the current study. It is now well-established that many patients with MODY may present de novo without a strong family history of diabetes (Chapla et al., 2015).

Another form of diabetes, which is prevalent in South Asia, is Flatbush diabetes (Jha et al., 2015). Patients with this condition present with markedly elevated blood glucose levels, varying degrees of ketosis, and one or more characteristics of insulin resistance. These individuals initially demonstrate poor response to oral antidiabetic medications and are effectively managed with insulin in the acute setting. Upon achieving glycemic control within several weeks, insulin therapy can typically be discontinued in these patients, and they subsequently respond well to oral antidiabetic medications for extended periods, similar to individuals with T2DM.

Currently, it is reasonable to assert that the two most prevalent forms of diabetes in young individuals are T1DM and T2DM, each accounting for approximately 40–45% of cases; FCPD and flatbush diabetes contribute to 5–15% of all diabetes cases, while up to 10% are attributed to MODY and other genetic forms of diabetes. The increasing prevalence of childhood obesity is also contributing to the burden of T2DM in young individuals. This distribution contrasts with the situation nearly three decades ago when T1DM was the predominant form of diabetes in young individuals. However, it is important to note that in the general population, the proportion of individuals with T2DM in the 'diabetes with young cohort' is likely to be higher, as the aforementioned prevalence rates have been obtained from hospital-based studies, which are subject to referral bias due to the tendency for individuals with more severe disease to seek medical attention (Dutta and Ghosh, 2019).

Until routine and affordable genetic testing becomes available in India, a more judicious utilization of clinical phenotype would be more pragmatic and cost-effective in determining the medications best suited for establishing the type of diabetes and its management (oral antidiabetes agents vs. early insulin therapy). This approach involves restricting the measurement of diabetes autoantibodies [glutamic acid decarboxylase [GAD] antibody, IA2 antibody, ZnT8 antibodies) and C-peptide (fasting/one hour post-mixed meal) to non-obese patients with diabetes who lack a family history of diabetes or features of the metabolic syndrome (central obesity, increased dorsal pad of fat, skin tags, acanthosis, fatty liver, polycystic ovary syndrome, high triglycerides (TGs) and low HDL cholesterol). Furthermore, a judicious follow-up over 1–2 years often aids in establishing the type of diabetes in a patient (Dutta and Ghosh, 2019).

3.23. Conclusion

The incidence of T2DM in children and adolescence continues to increase, and due to its insidious onset, early diagnosis remains challenging. Screening at-risk patients has facilitated diagnosis; however, preventing complications that affect both patients' morbidity and mortality necessitates more effective treatment modalities. Conducting clinical trials has proven challenging among youth. Numerous studies have stringent inclusion and exclusion criteria, such as specific age ranges of children with T2DM, patients who have not yet initiated treatment, and patients willing to participate for an extended period to adequately assess the long-term effects of the disease (Jalaludin et al., 2020). Moreover, children and adolescents often experience difficulties with adherence to the treatment regimen, whether pharmacologic or lifestyle modifications (Nadeau et al., 2016). This challenge is multifaceted, with unsupportive relationships and social determinants of health serving as significant barriers to care. Novel treatment options for T2DM are urgently required, as the currently approved treatment options—lifestyle modifications, metformin, and insulin—appear to lack long-term efficacy for treating T2DM, a chronic condition (Barr et al., 2019). T2DM in children and adolescents is an emerging public health concern globally that presents with distinct characteristics, demographics, and disease progression in comparison to adult-onset T2DM. It exhibits lower rates of response to oral pharmacotherapy than in adults. Given the relatively recent emergence of T2DM in children and adolescents, the evidence base regarding prevention, optimal treatment approaches, and monitoring of this population is lagging behind the steady increase in cases. The available treatment options to manage youth-onset T2DM and prevent the development of complications are limited. However, two additional GLP-1RAs have already been approved. The trials of oral semaglutide (Pioneer Teens) and tirzepatide (SURPASS-PEDS) in type 2 diabetic children and adolescents are ongoing. It is anticipated that additional therapies will not only facilitate the optimization of glycemic control but also decelerate the progression of disease and reduce long-term co-morbidities and complications. T2DM prevention in youth is another priority. Identification of children and adolescents who are at the highest risk of developing T2DM will facilitate the development of more efficacious interventions to prevent or delay the disease onset. A focus on enhancing knowledge regarding the pathophysiology as well as biology and environment of youth-onset T2DM, determining the optimal approach to working with this population, and utilizing more realistic and effective study designs and interventions suitable to this population is necessary to improve the care of children and adolescents with T2DM globally (Parmanik et al., 2024).

References

1. Akalu, Y., & Belsti, Y. (2020). Hypertension and its associated factors among type 2 diabetes mellitus patients at Debre Tabor General Hospital, Northwest Ethiopia. *Diabetes, Metabolic Syndrome and Obesity: Targets and Therapy, 13*, 1621–1631.

2. Akinci, G., Savelieff, M. G., Gallagher, G., Callaghan, B. C., & Feldman, E. L. (2021). Diabetic neuropathy in children and youth: New and emerging risk factors. *Pediatric Diabetes, 22*, 132–147.

3. Al-Saeed, A. H., Constantino, M. I., Molyneaux, L., D'Souza, M., Limacher-Gisler, F., Luo, C., Wu, T., Twigg, S. M., Yue, D. K., & Wong, J. (2016). An inverse relationship between age of type 2 diabetes onset and complication risk and mortality: The impact of youth-onset type 2 diabetes. *Diabetes Care, 39*, 823–829.

4. Amutha, A., Ranjit, U., Anjana, R. M., Shanthi R., C. S., Rajalakshmi, R., Venkatesan, U., Muthukumar, S., Philips, R., Kayalvizhi, S., Gupta, P. K., Sastry, N. G., & Mohan, V. (2021). Clinical profile and incidence of microvascular complications of childhood and adolescent onset type 1 and type 2 diabetes seen at a tertiary diabetes center in India. *Pediatric Diabetes, 22*, 67–74.

5. Anjana, R. M., Shanthi Rani, C. S., Deepa, M., Pradeepa, R., Sudha, V., Divya Nair, H., et al. (2015). Incidence of diabetes and prediabetes and predictors of progression among Asian Indians: 10-year follow-up of the Chennai Urban Rural Epidemiology Study (CURES). *Diabetes Care, 38*, 1441–1448.

6. Armstrong, S. C., Bolling, C. F., Michalsky, M. P., & Reichard, K. W.; Section on Obesity, Section on Surgery. (2019). Pediatric metabolic and bariatric surgery: Evidence, barriers, and best practices. *Pediatrics, 144*.

7. Arslanian, S. A., El Ghormli, L., Kim, J. Y., Tjaden, A. H., Barengolts, E., Caprio, S., Hannon, T. S., Mather, K. J., Nadeau, K. J., Utzschneider, K. M., Kahn, S. E., & RISE Consortium. (2021). OGTT glucose response curves, insulin sensitivity, and β-cell function in RISE: Comparison between youth and adults at randomization and in response to interventions to preserve β-cell function. *Diabetes Care, 44*, 817–825.

8. Arslanian, S. A., Hannon, T., Zeitler, P., Chao, L. C., Boucher-Berry, C., Barrientos-Pérez, M., Bismuth, E., Dib, S., Cho, J. I., Cox, D.; AWARD-PEDS Investigators. (2022). Once-weekly dulaglutide for the treatment of youths with type 2 diabetes. *New England Journal of Medicine, 387*, 433–443.

9. Arslanian, S., El Ghormli, L., Bacha, F., Caprio, S., Goland, R., Haymond, M. W., Levitsky, L., Nadeau, K. J., White, N. H., Willi, S. M.; TODAY Study Group. (2017). Adiponectin, insulin sensitivity, β-cell function, and racial/ethnic disparity in treatment failure rates in TODAY. *Diabetes Care, 40*, 85–93.

10. Arslanian, S., Kim, J. Y., Nasr, A., Bacha, F., Tfayli, H., Lee, S., & Toledo, F. G. S. (2018). Insulin sensitivity across the lifespan from obese adolescents to obese adults with impaired glucose tolerance: Who is worse off? *Pediatric Diabetes, 19*, 205–211.

11. Bacha, F., Cheng, P., Gal, R. L., Kollman, C., Tamborlane, W. V., Klingensmith, G. J., Manseau, K., Wood, J., & Beck, R. W.; for the Pediatric Diabetes Consortium. (2018). Initial presentation of type 2 diabetes in adolescents predicts durability of successful treatment with metformin

monotherapy: Insights from the Pediatric Diabetes Consortium T2D Registry. *Hormone Research in Pediatrics, 89*, 47–55.

12. Barker, M. M., Davies, M. J., Zaccardi, F., Brady, E. M., Hall, A. P., Henson, J. J., Khunti, K., Lake, A., Redman, E. L., Rowlands, A. V., Speight, J., Yates, T., Sargeant, J. A., & Hadjiconstantinou, M. (2023). Age at diagnosis of type 2 diabetes and depressive symptoms, diabetes-specific distress, and self-compassion. *Diabetes Care, 46*, 579–586.
13. Barr, M. M., Aslibekyan, S., & Ashraf, A. P. (2019). Glycemic control and lipid outcomes in children and adolescents with type 2 diabetes. *PLoS ONE, 14*(7), e0219144.
14. Barrett, J. S., Bucci-Rechtweg, C., Cheung, S. Y. A., Gamalo-Siebers, M., Haertter, S., Karres, J., Marquard, J., Mulugeta, Y., Ollivier, C., Strougo, A., Yanoff, L., Yao, L., & Zeitler, P. (2020). Pediatric extrapolation in type 2 diabetes: Future implications of a workshop. *Clinical Pharmacology & Therapeutics, 108*(1), 29.e–39.e.
15. Barrett, T., Jalaludin, M. Y., Turan, S., Hafez, M., & Shehadeh, N. (2020). Rapid progression of type 2 diabetes and related complications in children and young people—a literature review. *Pediatric Diabetes, 21*(2), 158–172.
16. Bartz, S. K., Caldas, M. C., Tomsa, A., Krishnamurthy, R., & Bacha, F. (2015). Urine albumin-to-creatinine ratio: A marker of early endothelial dysfunction in youth. *The Journal of Clinical Endocrinology & Metabolism, 100*(9), 3393–3399.
17. Berkowitz, R. I., Marcus, M. D., Anderson, B. J., Delahanty, L., Grover, N., Kriska, A., Laffel, L., Syme, A., Venditti, E., Van Buren, D. J., Wilfley, D. E., Yasuda, P., Hirst, K.; TODAY Study Group. (2018). Adherence to a lifestyle program for youth with type 2 diabetes and its association with treatment outcome in the TODAY clinical trial. *Pediatric Diabetes, 19*(2), 191–198.
18. Bjerregaard, L. G., Jensen, B. W., Ängquist, L., Osler, M., Sørensen, T. I. A., & Baker, J. L. (2018). Change in overweight from childhood to early adulthood and risk of type 2 diabetes. *The New England Journal of Medicine, 378*(14), 1302–1312.
19. Buttermore, E., Campanella, V., & Priefer, R. (2021). The increasing trend of type 2 diabetes in youth: An overview. *Diabetes & Metabolic Syndrome: Clinical Research & Reviews, 15*(5), 102253.
20. Campbell, E. G., Alasmar, A., Lawrence, R., Kurpius-Brock, M., DeCamp, M., Kovar, A., Schoen, J., Inge, T., Kelsey, M. M., Boles, R., & Engel, S. (2022). Barriers to metabolic bariatric surgery in adolescents: Results of a qualitative study. *Surgery for Obesity and Related Diseases, 18*(6), 794–802.
21. Centers for Disease Control and Prevention. (2020). Rates of new diagnosed cases of type 1 and type 2 diabetes continue to rise among children, teens.
22. Chapla, A., Mruthyunjaya, M. D., Asha, H. S., Varghese, D., Varshney, M., Vasan, S. K., et al. (2015). Maturity onset diabetes of the young in India—a distinctive mutation pattern identified through targeted next-generation sequencing. *Clinical Endocrinology, 82*(4), 533–542.
23. Christensen, A. A., & Gannon, M. (2019). The beta cell in type 2 diabetes. *Current Diabetes Reports, 19*(9), 81.
24. Cioana, M., Deng, J., Hou, M., Nadarajah, A., Qiu, Y., Chen, S. S. J., Rivas, A., Banfield, L., Chanchlani, R., Dart, A., Wicklow, B., Alfaraidi, H., Alotaibi, A., Thabane, L., & Samaan, M. C. (2021). Prevalence of hypertension and albuminuria in pediatric type 2 diabetes: A systematic review and meta-analysis. *JAMA Network Open, 4*(5), e216069.

25. Cioana, M., Deng, J., Nadarajah, A., Hou, M., Qiu, Y., Chen, S. S. J., Rivas, A., Banfield, L., Toor, P. P., Zhou, F., Guven, A., Alfaraidi, H., Alotaibi, A., Thabane, L., & Samaan, M. C. (2022). The prevalence of obesity among children with type 2 diabetes: A systematic review and meta-analysis. *JAMA Network Open, 5*(8), e2247186.

26. Cioana, M., Deng, J., Nadarajah, A., Hou, M., Qiu, Y., Chen, S. S. J., Rivas, A., Toor, P. P., Banfield, L., Thabane, L., Chaudhary, V., & Samaan, M. C. (2023). Global prevalence of diabetic retinopathy in pediatric type 2 diabetes: A systematic review and meta-analysis. *JAMA Network Open, 6*, e231887.

27. Dabelea, D., Stafford, J. M., Mayer-Davis, E. J., D'Agostino Jr, R., Dolan, L., Imperatore, G., et al. (2017). Association of type 1 diabetes vs type 2 diabetes diagnosed during childhood and adolescence with complications during teenage years and young adulthood. *JAMA, 317*(8), 825–835.

28. Dennis, J. M., Shields, B. M., Henley, W. E., Jones, A. G., & Hattersley, A. T. (2019). Disease progression and treatment response in data-driven subgroups of type 2 diabetes compared with models based on simple clinical features: An analysis using clinical trial data. *The Lancet Diabetes & Endocrinology, 7*(6), 442–451.

29. Donnelly, L. A., Zhou, K., Doney, A. S. F., Jennison, C., Franks, P. W., & Pearson, E. R. (2018). Rates of glycaemic deterioration in a real-world population with type 2 diabetes. *Diabetologia, 61*(3), 607–615.

30. Dutta, D., & Ghosh, S. (2019). Young-onset diabetes: An Indian perspective. *Indian Journal of Medical Research, 149*(4), 441, 442.

31. Dutta, D., & Mukhopadhyay, S. (2016). Intervening at prediabetes stage is critical to controlling the diabetes epidemic among Asian Indians. *Indian Journal of Medical Research, 143*(4), 401–404.

32. ElSayed, N. A., Aleppo, G., Aroda, V. R., Bannuru, R. R., Brown, F. M., Bruemmer, D., et al. (2023). Children and adolescents: Standards of care in diabetes—2023. *Diabetes Care, 46*(Supplement_1), S230–S253.

33. Galderisi, A., Giannini, C., Weiss, R., Kim, G., Shabanova, V., Santoro, N., Pierpont, B., Savoye, M., & Caprio, S. (2018). Trajectories of changes in glucose tolerance in a multiethnic cohort of obese youths: An observational prospective analysis. *The Lancet Child & Adolescent Health, 2*(10), 726–735.

34. Goundan, P., Junqueira, A., Kelleher-Yassen, D., & Steenkamp, D. (2016). Fibro calculous pancreatic diabetes. *Minerva Endocrinological, 41*(1), 70–77.

35. Gow, M. L., Pham-Short, A., Jebeile, H., Varley, B. J., & Craig, M. E. (2021). Current perspectives on the role of very-low-energy diets in the treatment of obesity and type 2 diabetes in youth. *Diabetes, Metabolic Syndrome and Obesity: Targets and Therapy, 14*, 215–225.

36. Gregg, E. W., Hora, I., & Benoit, S. R. (2019). Resurgence in diabetes-related complications. *JAMA, 321*(19), 1867–1868.

37. Huo, L., Magliano, D. J., Rancière, F., Harding, J. L., Nanayakkara, N., Shaw, J. E., & Carstensen, B. (2018). Impact of age at diagnosis and duration of type 2 diabetes on mortality in Australia 1997–2011. *Diabetology, 61*(6), 1055–1063.

38. Inge, T. H., Courcoulas, A. P., Jenkins, T. M., Michalsky, M. P., Brandt, M. L., Xanthakos, S. A., et al. (2019). Five-year outcomes of gastric bypass in adolescents as compared with adults. *The New England Journal of Medicine, 380*(22), 2136–2145.

39. Inge, T. H., Jenkins, T. M., Xanthakos, S. A., Dixon, J. B., Daniels, S. R., Zeller, M. H., & Helmrath, M. A. (2017). Long-term outcomes of bariatric surgery in adolescents with severe obesity (FABS-5+): A prospective follow-up analysis. *The Lancet Diabetes & Endocrinology, 5*(2), 165–173.

40. Jalaludin, M. Y., Barrientos-Pérez, M., Hafez, M., Lynch, J., Shehadeh, N., Turan, S., & Weghuber, D. (2020). Recommendations for improving clinical trial design to facilitate the study of youth-onset type 2 diabetes. *Clinical Trials, 17*(1), 87–98.

41. Jalaludin, M. Y., Deeb, A., Zeitler, P., Garcia, R., Newfield, R. S., Samoilova, Y., Rosario, C. A., Shehadeh, N., Saha, C. K., Zhang, Y., Zilli, M., Scherer, L. W., Lam, R. L. H., Golm, G. T., Engel, S. S., Kaufman, K. D., & Shankar, R. R. (2022). Efficacy and safety of the addition of sitagliptin to treatment of youth with type 2 diabetes and inadequate glycemic control on metformin without or with insulin. *Pediatric Diabetes, 23*(2), 183–193.

42. Janssen, K. C., Phillipson, S., O'Connor, J., & Johns, M. W. (2017). Validation of the Epworth Sleepiness Scale for children and adolescents using Rasch analysis. *Sleep Medicine, 33*, 30–35.

43. Jha, S., Waghdhare, S., Siddiqui, S., Srivastava, K., & Bhargava, A. (2015). First identification of Flatbush diabetes in patients of Indian origin. *Diabetes Care, 38*(6), e164–e165.

44. Kahn, L. G., Philippat, C., Nakayama, S. F., Slama, R., & Trasande, L. (2020). Endocrine-disrupting chemicals: Implications for human health. *The Lancet Diabetes & Endocrinology, 8*(9), 703–718.

45. Karavanaki, K., Paschou, S. A., Tentolouris, N., Karachaliou, F., & Soldatou, A. (2022). Type 2 diabetes in children and adolescents: Distinct characteristics and evidence-based management. *Endocrine, 78*(1), 280–295.

46. Ke, C., Lau, E., Shah, B. R., Stukel, T. A., Ma, R. C., So, W. Y., Kong, A. P., Chow, E., Clarke, P., Goggins, W., Chan, J. C., & Luk, A. (2019). Excess burden of mental illness and hospitalization in young-onset type 2 diabetes: A population-based cohort study. *Annals of Internal Medicine, 170*(2), 145–154.

47. Kelsey, M. M., Braffett, B. H., Geffner, M. E., Levitsky, L. L., Caprio, S., McKay, S. V., Shah, R., Sprague, J. E., Arslanian, S. A.; TODAY Study Group. (2018). Menstrual dysfunction in girls from the Treatment Options for Type 2 Diabetes in Adolescents and Youth (TODAY) study. *The Journal of Clinical Endocrinology & Metabolism, 103*(6), 2309–2318.

48. Kolly, A., Shivaprasad, C., Pulikkal, A. A., Atluri, S., Sarathi, V., Dwarakanath, C. S., et al. (2017). High prevalence of serine protease inhibitor Kazal type 1 gene variations detected by whole gene sequencing in patients with fibro calculous pancreatic diabetes. *Indian Journal of Endocrinology and Metabolism, 21*(4), 510–514.

49. Laffel, L. M., Danne, T., Klingensmith, G. J., Tamborlane, W. V., Willi, S., Zeitler, P., Neubacher, D., Marquard, J.; DINAMO Study Group. (2023). Efficacy and safety of the SGLT2 inhibitor empagliflozin versus placebo and the DPP-4 inhibitor linagliptin versus placebo in young people with type 2 diabetes (DINAMO): A multicenter, randomized, double-blind, parallel group, phase 3 trial. *Lancet Diabetes & Endocrinology, 11*(3), 169–181.

50. Lawrence, J. M., Divers, J., Isom, S., Saydah, S., Imperatore, G., Pihoker, C., Marcovina, S. M., Mayer-Davis, E. J., Hamman, R. F., Dolan, L., Dabelea, D., Pettitt, D. J., Liese, A. D.; SEARCH for Diabetes in Youth Study Group. (2021). Trends in prevalence of type 1 and type 2 diabetes in children and adolescents in the US, 2001–2017. *JAMA, 326*(7), 717–727.

51. Levitt Katz, L., Gidding, S. S., Bacha, F., Hirst, K., McKay, S., Pyle, L., Lima, J. A.; TODAY Study Group. (2015). Alterations in left ventricular, left atrial, and right ventricular structure and function to cardiovascular risk factors in adolescents with type 2 diabetes participating in the TODAY clinical trial. *Pediatric Diabetes, 16*(1), 39–47.

52. Liu, S., Leone, M., Ludvigsson, J. F., Lichtenstein, P., Gudbjörnsdottir, S., Landén, M., Bergen, S. E., Taylor, M. J., Larsson, H., Kuja-Halkola, R., Butwicka, A. (2022). Early-onset type 2 diabetes and mood, anxiety, and stress-related disorders: A genetically informative register-based cohort study. *Diabetes Care, 45*(12), 2950–2956.

53. Lynch, J. L., Barrientos-Pérez, M., Hafez, M., Jalaludin, M. Y., Kovarenko, M., Rao, P. V., & Weghuber, D. (2020). Country-specific prevalence and incidence of youth-onset type 2 diabetes: A narrative literature review. *Annals of Nutrition and Metabolism, 76*(3), 289–296.

54. Maffazioli, G. D., Stanford, F. C., Campoverde Reyes, K. J., Stanley, T. L., Singhal, V., Corey, K. E., Pratt, J. S., Bredella, M. A., & Misra, M. (2016). Comparing outcomes of two types of bariatric surgery in an adolescent obese population: Roux-en-Y gastric bypass vs. sleeve gastrectomy. *Frontiers in Pediatrics, 4*, 78.

55. Marcovecchio, M. L., Chiesa, S. T., Bond, S., Daneman, D., Dawson, S., Donaghue, K. C., Jones, T. W., Mahmud, F. H., Marshall, S. M., Neil, H. A. W., Dalton, R. N., Deanfield, J., Dunger, D. B.; AdDIT Study Group. (2017). ACE inhibitors and statins in adolescents with type 1 diabetes. *The New England Journal of Medicine, 377*(18), 1733–1745.

56. Marcus, M. D., Wilfley, D. E., El Ghormli, L., Zeitler, P., Linder, B., Hirst, K., Ievers-Landis, C. E., van Buren, D. J., Walders-Abramson, N.; TODAY Study Group. (2017). Weight change in the management of youth-onset type 2 diabetes: The TODAY clinical trial experience. *Pediatric Obesity, 12*(4), 337–345.

57. McGavock, J., Dart, A., & Wicklow, B. (2015). Lifestyle therapy for the treatment of youth with type 2 diabetes. *Current Diabetes Reports, 15*(12), 568.

58. Meehan, C., & Silverstein, J. (2016). Treatment options for type 2 diabetes in youth remain limited. *The Journal of Pediatrics, 170*, 20.e1–7.

59. Misra, S., Ke, C., Srinivasan, S., Goyal, A., Nyriyenda, M. J., Florez, J. C., Khunti, K., Magliano, D. J., & Luk, A. (2023). Current insights and emerging trends in early-onset type 2 diabetes. *Lancet Diabetes & Endocrinology, 11*(10), 768–782.

60. Murphy, H. R., Howgate, C., O'Keefe, J., Myers, J., Morgan, M., Coleman, M. A., et al. (2021). Characteristics and outcomes of pregnant women with type 1 or type 2 diabetes: A 5-year national population-based cohort study. *Lancet Diabetes & Endocrinology, 9*(3), 153–164.

61. Nadeau, K. J., Anderson, B. J., Berg, E. G., Chiang, J. L., Chou, H., Copeland, K. C., Hannon, T. S., Huang, T. T., Lynch, J. L., Powell, J., Sellers, E., Tamborlane, W. V., & Zeitler, P. (2016). Youth-onset type 2 diabetes consensus report: Current status, challenges, and priorities. *Diabetes Care, 39*(10), 1635–1642.

62. Narasimhan, S., & Weinstock, R. S. (2014). Youth-onset type 2 diabetes mellitus: Lessons learned from the TODAY study. *Mayo Clinic Proceedings, 89*(6), 806–816.

63. Newton, K. P., Hou, J., Crimmins, N. A., Lavine, J. E., Barlow, S. E., Xanthakos, S. A., et al. (2016). Prevalence of prediabetes and type 2 diabetes in children with nonalcoholic fatty liver disease. *JAMA Pediatrics, 170*(6), e161971.

64. Norris, J. M., Johnson, R. K., & Stene, L. C. (2020). Type 1 diabetes—early life origins and changing epidemiology. *Lancet Diabetes & Endocrinology, 8*(3), 226–238.

65. Patton, S. R., Kahhan, N., Pierce, J. S., Benson, M., Fox, L. A., & Clements, M. A. (2023). Parental diabetes distress is a stronger predictor of child HbA1c than diabetes device uses in school-age children with type 1 diabetes. *BMJ Open Diabetes Research & Care, 11*, e003010.

66. Pramanik, S., Mondal, S., Palui, R., & Ray, S. (2024). Type 2 diabetes in children and adolescents: Exploring the disease heterogeneity and research gaps to optimum management. *World Journal of Clinical Pediatrics, 13*(2), 915–987.

67. Pratt, J. S. A., Browne, A., Browne, N. T., Bruzoni, M., Cohen, M., Desai, A., Inge, T., Linden, B. C., Mattar, S. G., Michalsky, M., Podkameni, D., Reichard, K. W., Stanford, F. C., Zeller, M. H., & Zitsman, J. (2018). ASMBS pediatric metabolic and bariatric surgery guidelines, 2018. *Surgery for Obesity and Related Diseases, 14*(6), 882–901.

68. Protudjer, J. L. P., Dumontet, J., & McGavock, J. M. (2014). My voice: A grounded theory analysis of the lived experience of type 2 diabetes in adolescence. *Canadian Journal of Diabetes, 38*(4), 229–236.

69. Ricci, M., Mancebo-Sevilla, J. J., Cobos Palacios, L., Sanz-Cánovas, J., López-Sampalo, A., Hernández-Negrin, H., Pérez-Velasco, M. A., Pérez-Belmonte, L. M., Bernal-López, M. R., & Gómez-Huelgas, R. (2023). Remission of type 2 diabetes: A critical appraisal. *Frontiers in Endocrinology, 14*, 1125961.

70. Riddle, M. C., Cefalu, W. T., Evans, P. H., Gerstein, H. C., Nauck, M. A., Oh, W. K., Rothberg, A. E., le Roux, C. W., Rubino, F., Schauer, P., Taylor, R., & Twenefour, D. (2021). Consensus report: Definition and interpretation of remission in type 2 diabetes. *Diabetes Care, 44*(11), 2438–2444.

71. RISE Consortium. (2018). Metabolic contrasts between youth and adults with impaired glucose tolerance or recently diagnosed type 2 diabetes: II. Observations using the oral glucose tolerance test. *Diabetes Care, 41*(8), 1707–1716.

72. Rodriquez, I. M., & O'Sullivan, K. L. (2023). Youth-onset type 2 diabetes: Burden of complications and socioeconomic cost. *Current Diabetes Reports, 23*(2), 59–67.

73. Ross, J. A. D., Barron, E., McGough, B., Valabhji, J., Daff, K., Irwin, J., Henley, W. E., & Murray, E. (2022). Uptake and impact of the English National Health Service digital diabetes prevention programmed: Observational study. *BMJ Open Diabetes Research & Care, 10*, e002736.

74. Sahoo, S. K., Zaidi, G., Vipin, V. P., Chapla, A., Thomas, N., Yu, L., et al. (2019). Heterogeneity in the etiology of diabetes mellitus in young adults: A prospective study from North India. *Indian Journal of Medical Research, 149*(4), 479–488.

75. Salama, M., Biggs, B. K., Creo, A., Prissel, R., Al Nofal, A., & Kumar, S. (2023). Adolescents with type 2 diabetes: Overcoming barriers to effective weight management. *Diabetes, Metabolic Syndrome and Obesity: Targets and Therapy, 16*, 693–711.

76. Sam, S., Edelstein, S. L., Arslanian, S. A., Barengolts, E., Buchanan, T. A., Caprio, S., Ehrmann, D. A., Hannon, T. S., Tjaden, A. H., Kahn, S. E., Mather, K. J., Tripputi, M., Utzschneider, K. M., Xiang, A. H., Nadeau, K. J.; RISE Consortium; RISE Consortium Investigators. (2021). Baseline predictors of glycemic worsening in youth and adults with impaired glucose tolerance or recently diagnosed type 2 diabetes in the Restoring Insulin Secretion (RISE) study. *Diabetes Care, 44*(8), 1938–1947.

77. Sattar, N., Rawshani, A., Franzén, S., Svensson, A. M., Rosengren, A., McGuire, D. K., Eliasson, B., & Gudbjörnsdottir, S. (2019). Age at diagnosis of type 2 diabetes mellitus and associations with cardiovascular and mortality risks. *Circulation, 139*(22), 2228–2237.

78. Shah, A. S., Nadeau, K. J., Dabelea, D., & Redondo, M. J. (2022). Spectrum of phenotypes and causes of type 2 diabetes in children. *Annual Review of Medicine, 73*, 501–515.

79. Shah, R. D., Chernausek, S. D., El Ghormli, L., Geffner, M. E., Keady, J., Kelsey, M. M., Farrell, R., Tesfaldet, B., Tryggestad, J. B., Van Name, M., & Isganaitis, E. (2023). Maternal diabetes in youth-onset type 2 diabetes is associated with progressive dysglycemia and risk of complications. *The Journal of Clinical Endocrinology & Metabolism, 108*(3), 1120–1131.

80. Solis-Herrera, C., Triplitt, C. L., & Lynch, J. L. (2014). Nephropathy in youth and young adults with type 2 diabetes. *Current Diabetes Reports, 14*(2), 456.

81. Song, S. H. (2015). Complication characteristics between young-onset type 2 versus type 1 diabetes in a UK population. *BMJ Open Diabetes Research & Care, 3*(1), e000044.

82. Srinivasan, S., Chen, L., Todd, J., Divers, J., Gidding, S., Chernausek, S., et al. (2021). The first genome-wide association study for type 2 diabetes in youth: The Progress in Diabetes Genetics in Youth (ProDiGY) Consortium. *Diabetes, 70*(4), 996–1005.

83. Sun, H., Saeedi, P., Karuranga, S., Pinkepank, M., Ogurtsova, K., Duncan, B. B., Stein, C., Basit, A., Chan, J. C. N., Mbanya, J. C., Pavkov, M. E., Ramachandaran, A., Wild, S. H., James, S., Herman, W. H., Zhang, P., Bommer, C., Kuo, S., Boyko, E. J., & Magliano, D. J. (2022). IDF Diabetes Atlas: Global, regional and country-level diabetes prevalence estimates for 2021 and projections for 2045. *Diabetes Research and Clinical Practice, 183*, 109119.

84. Swei, E. C., & Sullivan, S. A. (2020). Aspiration therapy. *Techniques in Vascular and Interventional Radiology, 23*(4), 100659.

85. Tagi, V. M., Giannini, C., & Chiarelli, F. (2019). Insulin resistance in children. *Frontiers in Endocrinology, 10*, 342.

86. Tamborlane, W. V., Barrientos-Pérez, M., Fainberg, U., Frimer-Larsen, H., Hafez, M., Hale, P. M., et al. (2019). Liraglutide in children and adolescents with type 2 diabetes. *The New England Journal of Medicine, 381*(7), 637–646.

87. Tamborlane, W. V., Bishai, R., Geller, D., Shehadeh, N., Al-Abdulrazzaq, D., Vazquez, E. M., Karoly, E., Troja, T., Doehring, O., Carter, D., Monyak, J., & Sjöström, C. D. (2022). Once-weekly exenatide in youth with type 2 diabetes. *Diabetes Care, 45*(8), 1833–1840.

88. Temneanu, O. R., Trandafir, L. M., & Purcarea, M. R. (2016). Type 2 diabetes mellitus in children and adolescents: A relatively new clinical problem within pediatric practice. *Journal of Medicine and Life, 9*(3), 235–239.

89. TODAY Study Group, Bjornstad, P., Drews, K. L., Caprio, S., Gubitosi-Klug, R., Nathan, D. M., Tesfaldet, B., Tryggestad, J., White, N. H., & Zeitler, P. (2021). Long-term complications in youth-onset type 2 diabetes. *The New England Journal of Medicine, 385*(5), 416–426.

90. TODAY Study Group. (2021). Pregnancy outcomes in young women with youth-onset type 2 diabetes followed in the TODAY study. *Diabetes Care, 45*(5), 1038–1045.

91. Todd, J. N., Srinivasan, S., & Pollin, T. I. (2019). Advances in the genetics of youth-onset type 2 diabetes. *Current Diabetes Reports, 18*(8), 57.

92. Tsai, E., & Lee, T. P. (2018). Diagnosis and evaluation of nonalcoholic fatty liver disease/nonalcoholic steatohepatitis, including noninvasive biomarkers and transient elastography. *Clinical Liver Disease, 22*(1), 73–92.

93. Van Name, M., & Santoro, N. (2013). Type 2 diabetes mellitus in pediatrics: A new challenge. *World Journal of Pediatrics, 9*(4), 293–299.

94. Van Name, M., Klingensmith, G., Nelson, B., Wintergerst, K., Mitchell, J., Norris, K., et al. (2020). Transforming performance of clinical trials in pediatric type 2 diabetes: A consortium model. *Diabetes Technology & Therapeutics, 22*(4), 330–336.

95. Vuorio, A., Kuoppala, J., Kovanen, P. T., Humphries, S. E., Tonstad, S., Wiegman, A., Drogari, E., & Ramaswami, U. (2019). Statins for children with familial hypercholesterolemia. *Cochrane Database of Systematic Reviews, 2019*(9), CD006401.

96. Wagenknecht, L. E., Lawrence, J. M., Isom, S., Jensen, E. T., Dabelea, D., Liese, A. D., et al. (2023). Trends in incidence of youth-onset type 1 and type 2 diabetes in the USA, 2002–18: Results from the population-based SEARCH for Diabetes in Youth study. *The Lancet Diabetes & Endocrinology, 11*(3), 242–250.

97. Wallace, A. S., Wang, D., Shin, J. I., & Selvin, E. (2020). Screening and diagnosis of prediabetes and diabetes in US children and adolescents. *Pediatrics, 146*(3), e2020004317.

98. Wu, H., Patterson, C. C., Zhang, X., Ghani, R. B. A., Magliano, D. J., Boyko, E. J., Ogle, G. D., & Luk, A. O. Y. (2022). Worldwide estimates of incidence of type 2 diabetes in children and adolescents in 2021. *Diabetes Research and Clinical Practice, 185*, 109785.

99. Wu, Z., Gao, Z., Qiao, Y., Chen, F., Guan, B., Wu, L., Cheng, L., Huang, S., & Yang, J. (2023). Long-term results of bariatric surgery in adolescents with at least 5 years of follow-up: A systematic review and meta-analysis. *Obesity Surgery, 33*(5), 1730–1745.

100. Xie, J., Wang, M., Long, Z., Ning, H., Li, J., Cao, Y., Liao, Y., Liu, G., Wang, F., & Pan, A. (2022). Global burden of type 2 diabetes in adolescents and young adults, 1990–2019: Systematic analysis of the Global Burden of Disease Study 2019. *BMJ, 379*, e072385.

101. Zeitler, P., Hirst, K., Copeland, K. C., El Ghormli, L., Levitt Katz, L., Levitsky, L. L., et al. (2015). HbA1c after a short period of monotherapy with metformin identifies durable glycemic control among adolescents with type 2 diabetes. *Diabetes Care, 38*(12), 2285–2292.

102. Zhang, Y., Song, M., Cao, Y., Eliassen, A. H., Wolpin, B. M., Stampfer, M. J., Willett, W. C., Wu, K., Ng, K., Hu, F. B., & Giovannucci, E. L. (2023). Incident early- and later-onset type 2 diabetes and risk of early- and later-onset cancer: Prospective cohort study. *Diabetes Care, 46*(1), 120–129.

103. Zuckerman Levin, N., Cohen, M., Phillip, M., Tenenbaum, A., Koren, I., Tenenbaum-Rakover, Y., Admoni, O., Hershkovitz, E., Haim, A., Mazor Aronovitch, K., Zangen, D., Strich, D., Brener, A., Yeshayahu, Y., Schon, Y., Rachmiel, M., Ben-Ari, T., Levy-Khademi, F., Tibi, R., Weiss, R., Lebenthal, Y., Pinhas-Hamiel, O., & Shehadeh, N. (2022). Youth-onset type 2 diabetes in Israel: A national cohort. *Pediatric Diabetes, 23*(6), 649–659.

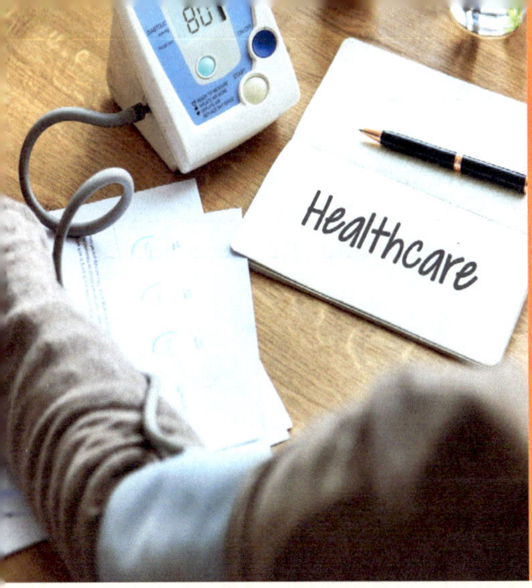

Chapter 4

COMORBIDITIES ASSOCIATED WITH HYPERTENSION: LATEST RESEARCH

Contents

4.1. Introduction

Hypertension, commonly called high blood pressure (BP), is a major global public health concern, affecting over 1 billion individuals (World Health Organization, 2021). It is often termed a "silent killer" because it frequently presents without symptoms but can lead to severe cardiovascular, renal, and cerebrovascular complications. The complexity of hypertension is amplified by its frequent co-occurrence with various comorbid conditions. These comorbidities not only complicate management but also exacerbate morbidity and mortality. Hypertension's comorbidities present diverse challenges that necessitate a multi-pronged approach. Cardiovascular diseases (CVDs) such as coronary artery disease (CAD) and stroke remain the leading causes of death linked to high BP. Moreover, metabolic conditions, including diabetes and dyslipidemia, intertwine with hypertension to form a "syndrome cluster," worsening patient outcomes. Chronic kidney disease (CKD) represents another frequent comorbid condition, where hypertension both contributes to and results from renal dysfunction. Additionally, emerging evidence underscores the role of lifestyle and environmental factors as modulators of hypertensive comorbidities. This chapter delves into the latest research on hypertension-related comorbidities, examining genetic factors, pharmacological interventions, and alternative medicine approaches. The discussion aims to provide insights into current challenges and future opportunities by synthesizing knowledge across these domains. An integrative understanding of these dimensions is essential for improving patient outcomes and reducing the global burden of hypertension. This chapter aims to provide an in-depth analysis of the latest research on comorbidities associated with hypertension. Each section explores a specific category of comorbid conditions, including cardiovascular, renal, neurological, metabolic, pulmonary, and others. It also highlights emerging diagnostic tools, innovative therapies, and integrated care strategies to address the multifaceted challenges posed by hypertension and its associated disorders.

4.1.1. Most Common Comorbidities of Hypertension: Prevalence and Incidence

4.1.1.1. Global Perspective

Hypertension often coexists with several chronic conditions, significantly impacting global health. Among these comorbidities, the most frequently observed include CVDs, diabetes mellitus (DM), CKD, and dyslipidemia. According to a 2020 report by the Global Burden of Disease Study, ischemic heart disease and stroke, which are tightly linked to hypertension, rank as the leading causes of mortality worldwide. Approximately 55% of stroke cases and 47% of ischemic heart disease cases are attributable to hypertension (GBD Collaborators, 2020). The prevalence of DM among hypertensive individuals is alarmingly high, with studies estimating that 30–40% of individuals with hypertension also have diabetes (Sun et al., 2019). Dyslipidemia, another common comorbidity, has a prevalence of approximately 60% among hypertensive patients, contributing to increased cardiovascular risk (Zhou et al., 2018). CKD affects nearly 20% of hypertensive patients globally, underscoring the bidirectional relationship between renal dysfunction and hypertension (Jha et al., 2019). Emerging evidence highlights a rise in the prevalence of mental health disorders, including depression and anxiety, among hypertensive individuals. These conditions not only exacerbate hypertension through mechanisms such as increased sympathetic activity but also complicate its management (Kretchy et al., 2020). The interplay between hypertension and these comorbidities demands an integrated care approach.

4.1.1.2. Indian Context

In India, the burden of hypertension and its associated comorbidities is escalating rapidly, driven by urbanization, dietary changes, and sedentary lifestyles. A nationwide study conducted in 2019 estimated that approximately 30% of adults in India have hypertension, with significant variations across states (Gupta et al., 2020). CVDs remain the most common comorbidity, with hypertension contributing to nearly 28% of all cardiovascular deaths in the country.The prevalence of diabetes among hypertensive individuals in India is strikingly high, ranging from 25% to 40% in different regions (Anjana et al., 2019). CKD, often underdiagnosed, affects an estimated 17% of hypertensive patients in India, highlighting the need for improved screening and management protocols (Singh et al., 2020). Dyslipidemia is another prevalent comorbidity, with nearly 70% of hypertensive patients in urban areas exhibiting abnormal lipid profiles (Joshi et al., 2021). Mental health disorders are also emerging as a significant concern, with studies reporting a prevalence of depression and anxiety ranging from 15% to 30% among hypertensive individuals (Ravindran et al., 2019). Addressing these comorbidities in India requires tailored strategies that account for socio-cultural and economic factors (Figures 4.1 and 4.2).

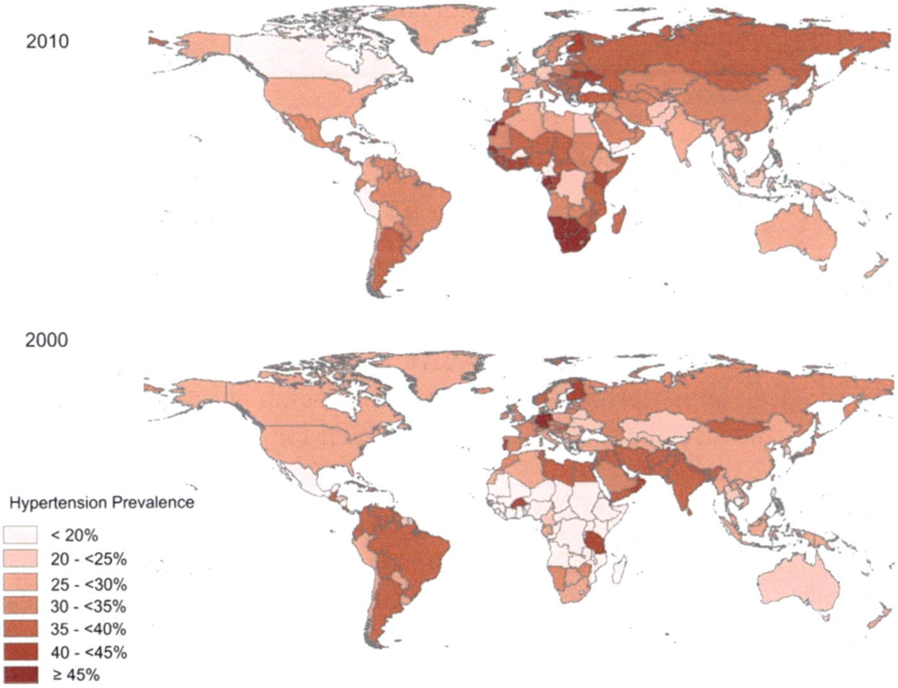

Figure 4.1. Worldwide age- and sex-standardized prevalence of hypertension in adults 20 years and older by country. Top: Country-specific prevalence in 2010. Bottom: Country-specific prevalence in 2000. Maps are shaded according to prevalence, from light (lower prevalence) to dark (higher prevalence).

Source: Katherine, T., Moran, A. E., Forouzanfar, M. H., Roth, G. A., Mensah, G. A., & Murray, C. J. L. (2016). Global disparities of hypertension prevalence and control: A systematic analysis of population-based studies from 90 countries. *Circulation*, *134*(6), 441–450.

Individuals with systolic (SBP) and diastolic (DBP) blood pressure in 2 categories are designated to the higher blood pressure category.

SBP (mmHg)		DBP (mmHg)	JNC 7	ACC/AHA 2017
<120	AND	<80	NORMAL BP	NORMAL BP
120-129	AND	<80	Prehypertension	Elevated BP
130-139	OR	80-89	Prehypertension	Stage 1 Hypertension
140-159	OR	90-99	Stage 1 Hypertension	Stage 2 Hypertension
≥160	OR	≥100	Stage 2 Hypertension	Stage 2 Hypertension

SBP: Systolic blood pressure; DBP: Diastolic blood pressure; JNC 7: Seventh Report of the Joint National Committee on prevention, detection, evaluation, and treatment of high Blood Pressure; ACC/AHA: American College of Cardiology/American Heart Association Task Force on Clinical Practice Guidelines

Figure 4.2. Classification of blood pressure (BP) according to the 2017 ACC/AHA guidelines.

Source: Papaioannou, T. G., Protogerou, A. D., Vrachatis, D. A., Nasothimiou, E. G., Kardara, D., Papamichael, C. M., & Tousoulis, D. (2018). Arterial stiffness and subclinical aortic damage of reclassified subjects as stage 1 hypertension according to the new 2017 ACC/AHA blood pressure guidelines. *Vasa*, *47*(2), 108–115.

4.2. Hypertension and Cardiovascular Comorbidities

- **Background:** Hypertension significantly contributes to CVDs such as CAD, heart failure, and atrial fibrillation. Chronically elevated BP accelerates arterial wall damage, promotes atherosclerosis, and impairs cardiac function. Understanding the genetic, pharmacological, and alternative treatment options for managing hypertension-associated cardiovascular comorbidities is critical for improving patient outcomes (Figure 4.3).
- **Genetics:**
  - **Gene Therapy:** Gene-editing techniques like CRISPR-Cas9 are being explored to modify AGT and ACE genes, which influence hypertension-related cardiac damage (Ehret et al., 2018).
  - **GWAS Insights:** Genome-wide association studies have identified NOS3 and AGTR1 variants that increase susceptibility to CAD in hypertensive populations (Kato et al., 2018).
- **Pharmaceuticals:**
  - **PCSK9 Inhibitors:** Evolocumab significantly reduces LDL cholesterol and cardiovascular risk, particularly in hypertensive patients with CAD (Sabatine et al., 2017).
  - **ARNis:** Sacubitril/valsartan outperforms ACE inhibitors (ACEIs) in reducing heart failure hospitalizations and mortality in hypertensive populations (McMurray et al., 2019).

- **Alternative Medicine:**
  - **Mindfulness-based Stress Reduction (MBSR):** Studies show MBSR reduces BP and improves heart rate variability, benefiting hypertensive CAD patients (Gu et al., 2019).
  - **Hawthorn Extract:** Demonstrates vasodilatory properties and improves coronary perfusion in hypertensive populations (Walker et al., 2020).
- **Recent Advances:**
  - **High-Sensitivity Biomarkers:** Troponins and BNP levels help in early detection of myocardial injury and heart failure in hypertensive patients (Ridker et al., 2018).
  - **Thrombectomy Devices:** Improved mechanical thrombectomy systems enhance stroke treatment outcomes in hypertensive ischemic stroke patients (Goyal et al., 2018).

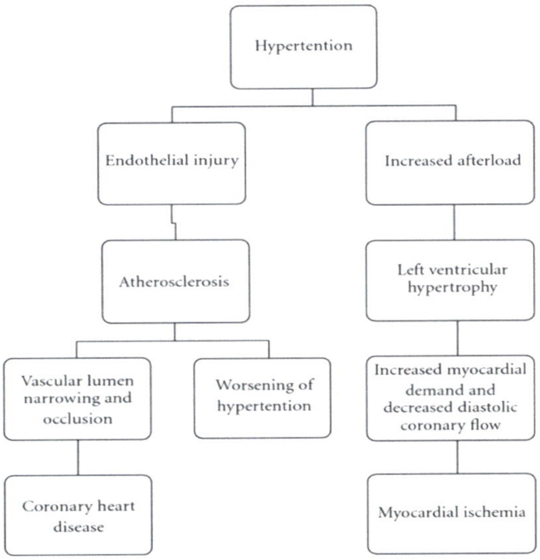

Figure 4.3. The role of hypertension in the pathogenesis of coronary artery disease (CAD).

Source: Oladipupo, O., Ajayi, I. O., & Oyediran, M. A. (2011). Management of hypertension among patients with coronary heart disease. *International Journal of Hypertension*.

4.3. Hypertension and Renal Comorbidities

- **Background:** The relationship between hypertension and renal disorders is bidirectional. Hypertension is both a cause and consequence of CKD, while acute kidney injury (AKI) exacerbates systemic BP dysregulation. Renal dysfunction leads to fluid retention and increases vascular resistance, creating a vicious cycle that worsens hypertension. Addressing this complex interplay requires integrating genetic, pharmaceutical, and lifestyle-based interventions (Figure 4.4).

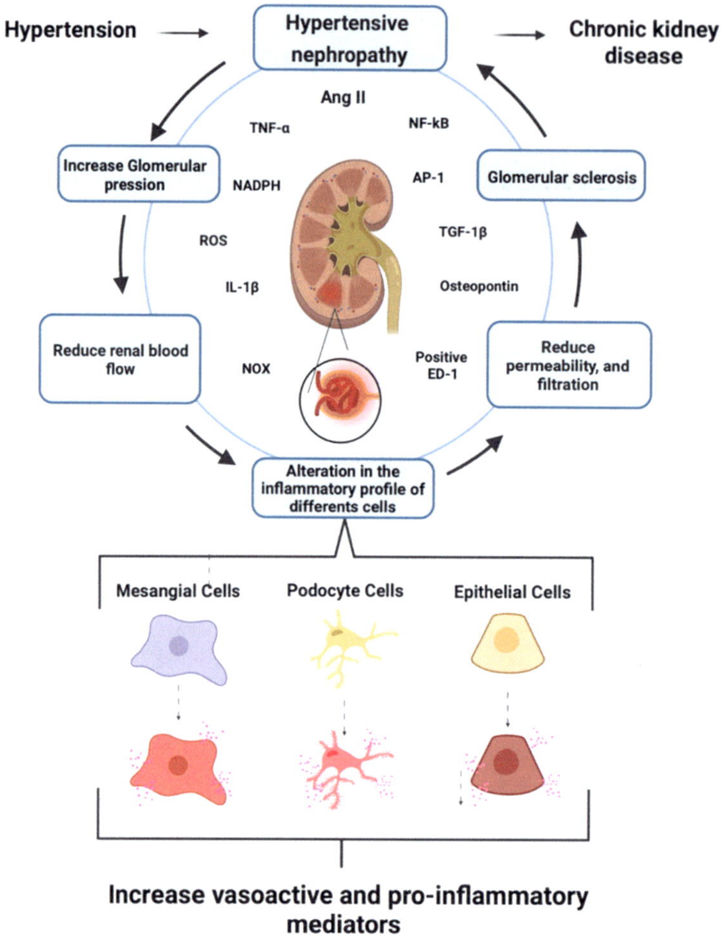

Figure 4.4. Hypertensive nephropathy.

Source: https://encyclopedia.pub/entry/39102.

- **Genetics:**
  - **APOL1 Variants:** Linked to an accelerated progression to kidney failure in hypertensive patients of African ancestry (Friedman et al., 2018).
  - **ACE Polymorphisms:** Variants associated with altered kidney perfusion, influencing personalized antihypertensive strategies (Kuivaniemi et al., 2018).
- **Pharmaceuticals:**
  - **SGLT2 Inhibitors:** Dapagliflozin reduces proteinuria and CKD progression in hypertensive patients, per the DAPA-CKD trial (Heerspink et al., 2020).
  - **Endothelin Receptor Antagonists:** Improve renal hemodynamics in resistant hypertension and hypertensive nephropathy (Kohan et al., 2019).
- **Alternative Medicine:**
  - **Acupuncture:** Reduces proteinuria and improves renal function by regulating blood flow in hypertensive nephropathy (Kim et al., 2018).

- **Dietary Interventions:** The DASH diet lowers systolic BP and improves renal outcomes in hypertensive individuals (Appel et al., 2021).

- **Recent Advances:**
  - **Biomarker Panels:** NGAL and cystatin C allow for early AKI detection in hypertensive patients (Hoste et al., 2020).
  - **Renal Denervation (RDN):** A promising non-pharmacological intervention for resistant hypertension (Kario et al., 2020).

4.4. Hypertension and Neurological Comorbidities

- **Background:** Hypertension is a major risk factor for neurological conditions, including stroke, vascular dementia, and cognitive decline. Persistent high BP leads to small vessel damage, reduced cerebral perfusion, and neuroinflammation. Advances in genetic studies, pharmacological therapies, and alternative medicine approaches offer new opportunities to mitigate these risks and improve neurological outcomes.

- **Genetics:**
  - **APOE Variants:** Linked to increased cognitive decline and Alzheimer's risk in hypertensive populations (Licher et al., 2019).
  - **PICALM Variants:** Associated with vascular dementia in hypertensive individuals (Greenwood et al., 2018).

- **Pharmaceuticals:**
  - **Neuroprotective Agents:** Edaravone mitigates oxidative stress in stroke patients with hypertension (Jiang et al., 2020).
  - **Calcium Channel Blockers (CCBs):** Reduce white matter lesions, preserving cognitive function in hypertensive populations (Guo et al., 2018).

- **Alternative Medicine:**
  - **Meditation:** Decreases BP and enhances cerebral perfusion, reducing stroke and dementia risks (Okonta, 2017).
  - **Ginkgo Biloba:** Shown to improve cognitive function in hypertensive individuals with mild cognitive impairment (Yancheva et al., 2019).

- **Recent Advances:**
  - **Thrombectomy Devices:** New technologies increase stroke recovery success rates in hypertensive patients (Goyal et al., 2018).
  - **Advanced Imaging:** Diffusion tensor imaging improves early detection of small vessel disease in hypertensive populations (Raji et al., 2020).

4.5. Hypertension and Metabolic Disorders

- **Background:** Hypertension frequently coexists with metabolic disorders such as DM, dyslipidemia, and metabolic syndrome. These conditions share common risk factors, including obesity, insulin resistance, and chronic inflammation, which create a synergistic effect, compounding cardiovascular risk. Understanding the pathophysiological connections and addressing them through innovative treatments is crucial for holistic management.

- **Genetics:**
  - **TCF7L2 Variants:** Strongly associated with insulin resistance and hypertension in metabolic syndrome patients (Mahajan et al., 2018).
  - **ADIPOQ Variants:** Linked to reduced adiponectin levels, contributing to obesity and hypertension (Menzaghi et al., 2018).
- **Pharmaceuticals:**
  - **GLP-1 Receptor Agonists:** Liraglutide improves BP, glycemic control, and weight management in hypertensive diabetics (Gerstein et al., 2019).
  - **Fixed-Dose Combination Pills:** Statin-antihypertensive combinations improve adherence and reduce cardiovascular events in metabolic syndrome (Wald et al., 2020).
- **Alternative Medicine:**
  - **Berberine:** Enhances glucose metabolism and reduces BP in hypertensive individuals with metabolic syndrome (Zhang et al., 2018).
  - **Yoga:** Improves insulin sensitivity and lowers BP in hypertensive diabetics (Cramer et al., 2018).
- **Recent Advances:**
  - **Nutritional Genomics:** Research on gene-diet interactions reveals how specific nutrients impact BP regulation in hypertensive metabolic syndrome (Corella et al., 2018).
  - **Continuous Glucose Monitors:** Integrated with AI, these devices improve glycemic and BP control in hypertensive diabetics (Heerspink et al., 2020).

4.6. Hypertension and Pulmonary Comorbidities

- **Background:** Pulmonary hypertension (PH) and obstructive sleep apnea (OSA) are prevalent in hypertensive populations, creating significant morbidity. Systemic hypertension increases pulmonary vascular pressures and promotes hypoxia-induced vascular remodeling. Addressing these pulmonary complications alongside systemic hypertension is key to improving respiratory and cardiovascular outcomes.
- **Genetics:**
  - **BMPR2 Mutations:** Associated with pulmonary arterial hypertension, informing targeted therapeutic strategies (Drake et al., 2020).

- **NOS3 Polymorphisms:** Linked to impaired nitric oxide (NO) production in hypertensive pulmonary conditions (Galiè et al., 2019).

- **Pharmaceuticals:**
  - **Riociguat:** Improves pulmonary pressures and functional capacity in patients with PAH secondary to systemic hypertension (Sitbon et al., 2018).
  - **Macitentan:** Reduces pulmonary vascular resistance and improves exercise tolerance in PAH patients (Sitbon et al., 2018).
- **Alternative Medicine:**
  - **Breathing Exercises:** Techniques like pranayama enhance oxygenation and reduce pulmonary pressures (Kaushik et al., 2019).
  - **Boswellia Serrata:** Anti-inflammatory properties benefit hypertensive pulmonary disorders (Gupta et al., 2018).
- **Recent Advances:**
  - **Combination Therapy:** Upfront use of macitentan and riociguat improves outcomes in high-risk PH patients (Humbert et al., 2019).
  - **Wearable Pulse Oximeters:** Real-time oxygen saturation monitoring aids in managing PH in hypertensive patients (Galiè et al., 2019).

4.7. Hypertension and Vascular Disorders

- **Background:** Hypertension exacerbates vascular conditions such as peripheral arterial disease (PAD) and aortic aneurysms or dissections. Chronic high BP accelerates endothelial dysfunction and arterial stiffening, leading to life-threatening complications. An integrated approach involving genetic, pharmaceutical, and lifestyle interventions is vital for managing these vascular comorbidities.
- **Genetics:**
  - **COL3A1 Mutations:** Associated with aortic dissection and vascular fragility in hypertensive patients (Kuivaniemi et al., 2018).
  - **ELN Polymorphisms:** Linked to arterial stiffness, influencing PAD severity in hypertensive populations (Shen et al., 2019).
- **Pharmaceuticals:**
  - **Beta-Blockers:** Essential for reducing aneurysm progression and preventing rupture in hypertensive patients (Milewicz et al., 2019).
  - **Drug-Eluting Stents:** Minimize restenosis in hypertensive PAD patients by releasing antiproliferative agents (Kabra et al., 2019).
- **Alternative Medicine:**
  - **Horse Chestnut Extract:** Improves circulation and reduces symptoms of PAD-

related claudication (Umar et al., 2019).

  - **Tai Chi:** Enhances vascular elasticity and reduces arterial stiffness in hypertensive individuals (Zeng et al., 2019).

- **Recent Advances:**
  - **Advanced Imaging:** 4D flow MRI offers insights into aneurysm wall stress and rupture risk in hypertensive patients (Roth et al., 2019).
  - **Angiogenic Therapies:** Research into growth factor delivery for PAD shows promise in restoring blood flow in ischemic limbs (Shen et al., 2019).

4.8. Hypertension and Autoimmune/Inflammatory Conditions

- **Background:** Autoimmune and inflammatory conditions, including rheumatoid arthritis (RA), systemic lupus erythematosus (SLE), and psoriasis, frequently coexist with hypertension. Chronic systemic inflammation promotes vascular dysfunction and accelerates the progression of hypertension. Novel therapeutic strategies targeting inflammatory pathways are emerging as effective approaches to address this intersection.
- **Genetics:**
  - **HLA Variants:** Linked to increased hypertension risk in autoimmune conditions like lupus (Agca et al., 2018).
  - **IL6R Polymorphisms:** Associated with elevated cytokine levels and hypertension in RA patients (Kitas et al., 2019).
- **Pharmaceuticals:**
  - **IL-6 Inhibitors:** Tocilizumab reduces inflammation and improves BP control in hypertensive RA patients (Kitas et al., 2019).
  - **TNF-α Blockers:** Etanercept demonstrates cardiovascular protective effects in hypertensive autoimmune populations (Madhok et al., 2019).
- **Alternative Medicine:**
  - **Omega-3 Fatty Acids:** Anti-inflammatory properties improve endothelial function and BP in autoimmune conditions (Calder et al., 2019).
  - **Curcumin:** Reduces cytokine levels and enhances vascular health in hypertensive patients (Gupta et al., 2018).
- **Recent Advances:**
  - **Biologic Therapies:** Advances in targeted biologics like IL-23 inhibitors demonstrate efficacy in managing both BP and inflammation (Madhok et al., 2019).
  - **Epigenetic Research:** DNA methylation studies reveal potential for reversing inflammation-induced hypertension (Agca et al., 2018).

4.9. Hypertension and Cancer

- **Background:** Hypertension often complicates cancer management, particularly in patients undergoing anti-angiogenic therapies that inhibit vascular endothelial growth factor (VEGF). These treatments exacerbate BP dysregulation, increasing cardiovascular risk. Addressing hypertension in cancer patients requires an integrated approach that balances oncological and cardiovascular care.
- **Genetics:**
  - **VEGF Polymorphisms:** Associated with increased susceptibility to therapy-induced hypertension during anti-angiogenic cancer treatments (Drake et al., 2020).
  - **BRCA1 Variants:** Linked to hypertension in cancer survivors receiving certain chemotherapy agents (Ghosh et al., 2018).
- **Pharmaceuticals:**
  - **VEGF Inhibitor Combinations:** Antihypertensives like amlodipine combined with VEGF inhibitors manage therapy-induced hypertension effectively (Choueiri et al., 2018).
  - **ACE Inhibitors (ACEIs):** Provide cardioprotective effects during chemotherapy, reducing hypertension and associated risks (Moudgil et al., 2019).
- **Alternative Medicine:**
  - **Green Tea Extract:** Antioxidant-rich extract reduces vascular inflammation in cancer patients undergoing chemotherapy (Basu et al., 2018).
  - **Ashwagandha:** Mitigates stress-induced BP elevations in cancer survivors (Gupta et al., 2018).
- **Recent Advances:**
  - **Cardio-Oncology:** Multidisciplinary management of cancer therapy-induced hypertension improves outcomes and therapy adherence (Tini et al., 2019).
  - **Biomarker Monitoring:** Circulating endothelial cells are being explored for early detection of VEGF inhibitor-induced vascular damage (Choueiri et al., 2018).

4.10. Hypertension and Psychosocial Comorbidities

- **Background:** Psychosocial factors such as stress, anxiety, and depression significantly influence the development and progression of hypertension. Chronic stress activates the hypothalamic-pituitary-adrenal (HPA) axis, increasing sympathetic activity and systemic BP. Behavioral and pharmacological interventions targeting these factors are essential for comprehensive hypertension management.

- **Genetics:**
  - **SLC6A4 Variants:** Associated with serotonin transport and increased stress-related hypertension in vulnerable populations (Esler et al., 2018).
  - **COMT Polymorphisms:** Influence stress reactivity and BP regulation, particularly in hypertensive individuals with anxiety (Lichtman et al., 2018).
- **Pharmaceuticals:**
  - **SSRIs:** Antidepressants like sertraline improve mood without significantly raising BP in hypertensive patients (Lichtman et al., 2018).
  - **Beta-Blockers:** Manage anxiety symptoms and hypertension simultaneously (Esler et al., 2018).
- **Alternative Medicine:**
  - **Biofeedback Therapy:** Proven to reduce BP through autonomic nervous system modulation (McGrady et al., 2019).
  - **Chamomile Tea:** Offers anxiolytic properties, reducing BP in hypertensive patients with mild anxiety (Amsterdam et al., 2018).
- **Recent Advances:**
  - **Digital Mental Health Tools:** CBT-based apps show promise in reducing stress and BP in hypertensive patients (McGrady et al., 2019).
  - **Stress Biomarkers:** Salivary cortisol and α-amylase levels are under study for monitoring stress-induced BP fluctuations (Esler et al., 2018).

4.11. Gender and Age-Related Considerations

- **Background:** Gender and age significantly influence hypertension pathophysiology and management. Women face unique challenges during pregnancy, menopause, and postmenopause, while elderly patients often exhibit isolated systolic hypertension due to arterial stiffening. Tailored approaches are essential to address these demographic-specific needs effectively.
- **Genetics:**
  - **ESR1 Variants:** Linked to estrogen's protective role in BP regulation, particularly in premenopausal women (Barton and Meyer, 2019).
  - ACE Polymorphisms: Contribute to isolated systolic hypertension in elderly hypertensive populations (Benetos et al., 2019).
- **Pharmaceuticals:**
  - **Diuretics for the Elderly:** Thiazide diuretics remain effective and safe for older hypertensive individuals (Whelton et al., 2019).
  - **HRT Options:** Transdermal estrogen formulations are associated with neutral or reduced BP effects in postmenopausal women (Barton and Meyer, 2019).
- **Alternative Medicine:**
  - **Soy Isoflavones:** Improve arterial elasticity and BP,

particularly in postmenopausal hypertensive women (Wu et al., 2018).

- **Resistance Training:** Reduces arterial stiffness and improves vascular health in elderly hypertensive individuals (Zouhal et al., 2019).

- **Recent Advances:**
  - **Sarcopenia Management:** Addressing muscle loss in elderly hypertensive individuals enhances BP regulation through improved vascular function (Benetos et al., 2019).
  - **Menopause-Related Research:** Studies emphasize the role of hormone replacement therapies in managing menopause-induced hypertension (Barton and Meyer, 2019).

4.12. Emerging Biomarkers and Predictive Tools

- **Background:** Advances in genomics, proteomics, and artificial intelligence (AI) have revolutionized hypertension management. Emerging biomarkers provide insights into disease progression and therapy response, while predictive tools enable early detection and personalized interventions. These developments are paving the way for precision medicine in hypertension care.

- **Genetics:**
  - **Polygenic Risk Scores (PRS):** Combine genetic variants to predict hypertension risk and guide prevention strategies (Ehret et al., 2018).
  - **Epigenetic Biomarkers:** DNA methylation studies reveal insights into hypertension pathogenesis and therapy responses (Kato et al., 2018).

- **Pharmaceuticals:**
  - **RNA-based Therapies:** Emerging treatments target specific genetic pathways, offering precision management for hypertension (Murray et al., 2019).
  - **Omics-Driven Drug Development:** Multi-omics data guide the development of drugs targeting specific molecular pathways in hypertensive patients (Corella et al., 2018).

- **Alternative Medicine:**
  - **Traditional Chinese Medicine (TCM):** Herbal formulations like astragalus and ginseng show potential for BP regulation (Zhang et al., 2018).
  - **Acupressure:** Demonstrates efficacy as a complementary therapy in managing hypertension (Kim et al., 2018).

- **Recent Advances:**
  - **Wearable Technology:** Devices combining BP monitoring with AI analytics enable real-time feedback and risk stratification (Whelton et al., 2019).

- **AI-Powered Predictive Models:** Algorithms integrating EHR data with biomarkers improve hypertension risk assessment (Ehret et al., 2018).

4.13. Conclusion

Hypertension is a multifaceted condition intricately linked to various comorbidities, including cardiovascular, renal, neurological, metabolic, pulmonary, vascular, and psychosocial disorders. Each of these comorbidities significantly impacts the progression, management, and outcomes of hypertension, creating a need for integrated and personalized care. Recent advances in genomics, pharmacotherapy, and alternative medicine offer promising avenues for improved management. Developments in predictive tools and AI have revolutionized hypertension care, providing early detection and precision medicine capabilities. Furthermore, lifestyle interventions and holistic care approaches play an essential role in addressing the broader determinants of health in hypertensive patients. A multidisciplinary approach, combining state-of-the-art technology with evidence-based interventions, is pivotal in mitigating the global burden of hypertension. Future research must focus on bridging gaps in care, addressing health disparities, and leveraging emerging technologies to deliver patient-centered outcomes.

References

1. Aburto, N. J., et al. (2020). Effect of increased potassium intake on cardiovascular risk factors and disease. *Cochrane Database of Systematic Reviews, 2020*(6), CD010048.
2. Agca, R., et al. (2018). Inflammation in hypertension: Role of genetics and epigenetics. *Journal of Clinical Hypertension, 20*(8), 1226–1234.
3. Amsterdam, J. D., et al. (2018). Chamomile (*Matricaria recutita*) as a treatment for generalized anxiety disorder. *Journal of Clinical Psychopharmacology, 38*(6), 615–620.
4. Barton, M., & Meyer, M. R. (2019). Postmenopausal hypertension: Mechanisms and therapy. *Hypertension, 74*(3), 705–712.
5. Benetos, A., Petrovic, M., & Strandberg, T. (2019). Hypertension management in older and frail older patients. *Circulation Research, 124*(7), 972–992.
6. Bhatnagar, V., et al. (2019). Pharmacogenetics of antihypertensive therapy. *Frontiers in Cardiovascular Medicine, 6*, 68.
7. Calder, P. C., et al. (2019). Omega-3 fatty acids and inflammation in hypertension. *Hypertension Research, 42*(5), 543–554.
8. Carey, R. M., et al. (2018). Resistant hypertension: Detection, evaluation, and management. *Circulation, 138*(16), e426–e493.
9. Choueiri, T. K., et al. (2018). VEGF-targeted therapies and cardiovascular side effects. *Journal of Clinical Oncology, 36*(10), 905–913.
10. Cramer, H., et al. (2018). Yoga for managing hypertension in metabolic syndrome. *Journal of Hypertension, 36*(3), 577–583.
11. Drake, K. M., et al. (2020). BMPR2 mutations and pulmonary hypertension. *American Journal of Respiratory and Critical Care Medicine, 202*(1), 110–119.
12. Ehret, G. B., & Caulfield, M. J. (2018). Genomic insights into hypertension. *Nature Reviews Cardiology, 15*(7), 375–386.
13. Filippini, T., et al. (2020). Potassium intake and blood pressure. *Nutrients, 12*(5), 1264.
14. Friedman, D. J., & Pollak, M. R. (2018). APOL1 kidney disease risk variants. *Journal of the American Society of Nephrology, 29*(9), 2495–2508.
15. Friedman, D. J., et al. (2017). APOL1 nephropathy: From genetics to clinical applications. *Clinical Journal of the American Society of Nephrology, 12*(8), 1203–1213.
16. Gencer, B., et al. (2020). PCSK9 inhibitors in lipid management. *European Heart Journal, 41*(24), 2363–2372.
17. Gerstein, H. C., et al. (2019). Cardiovascular and renal outcomes with GLP-1 receptor agonists. *New England Journal of Medicine, 381*(4), 322–333.
18. Gupta, S. K., et al. (2018). Anti-inflammatory effects of curcumin in hypertension. *Hypertension Research, 41*(3), 253–259.
19. Heerspink, H. J. L., et al. (2020). Dapagliflozin in patients with CKD. *New England Journal of Medicine, 383*(15), 1436–1446.

20. Heerspink, H. J. L., et al. (2020). SGLT2 inhibitors and kidney protection in T2DM. *Lancet Diabetes & Endocrinology, 8*(8), 653–663.
21. Huang, Y., et al. (2019). Mindfulness-based interventions and hypertension: A meta-analysis. *Journal of Hypertension, 37*(3), 432–440.
22. Kitas, G. D., et al. (2019). Tocilizumab in hypertensive rheumatoid arthritis patients. *The Lancet Rheumatology, 1*(2), e78–e89.
23. Lichtman, J. H., et al. (2018). Depression, anxiety, and cardiovascular risk in hypertension. *Circulation, 138*(24), 2631–2640.
24. Mahajan, A., et al. (2018). Genetic insights into diabetes and hypertension risk. *Nature Genetics, 50*(11), 1505–1513.
25. Martinez-Zapata, M. J., et al. (2020). Coenzyme Q10 for the treatment of hypertension. *Cochrane Database of Systematic Reviews, 2020*(4), CD007435.
26. McGrady, A., et al. (2019). Biofeedback and hypertension management. *Journal of Clinical Psychology in Medical Settings, 26*(3), 229–241.
27. McMurray, J. J. V., et al. (2019). Sacubitril/valsartan in heart failure: A review. *The Lancet, 394*(10206), 1313–1323.
28. Natarajan, P., et al. (2018). Epigenetics and cardiovascular disease. *Nature Reviews Cardiology, 15*(7), 398–408.
29. Navarese, E. P., et al. (2018). Meta-analysis of PCSK9 inhibitors effects on cardiovascular outcomes. *European Heart Journal, 39*(17), 1360–1371.
30. Omboni, S., et al. (2020). Telemedicine in hypertension management. *Current Hypertension Reports, 22*(11), 1–9.
31. Sabatine, M. S., et al. (2017). Evolocumab and cardiovascular outcomes. *New England Journal of Medicine, 376*(18), 1713–1722.
32. Shen, J., et al. (2019). Arterial stiffness and ELN polymorphisms in hypertension. *Hypertension Research, 42*(7), 574–581.
33. Sitbon, O., et al. (2018). Macitentan in pulmonary arterial hypertension. *The Lancet Respiratory Medicine, 6*(7), 523–534.
34. Tini, G., et al. (2019). Cardio-oncology advances in cancer therapy-induced hypertension. *Cardio-Oncology, 5*(1), 5–14.
35. Wald, N. J., et al. (2020). Fixed-dose combination therapy for hypertension management. *Journal of the American Medical Association, 323*(4), 356–364.
36. Whelton, P. K., Carey, R. M., & Aronow, W. S. (2019). 2017 guideline for the management of hypertension in adults. *Hypertension, 71*(6), e13–e115.

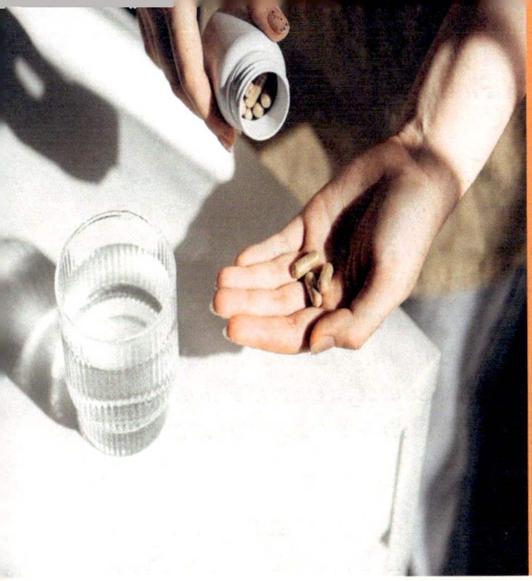

Chapter 5

SUPPORT AND ALTERNATIVE TREATMENTS FOR DIABETES

Contents

"When you are inspired by some great purpose, some extraordinary project, all your thoughts break their bonds: Your mind transcends limitations, your consciousness expands in every direction, and you find yourself in a new, great, and wonderful world. Dormant forces, faculties, and talents become alive, and you discover yourself to be a greater person by far than you ever dreamed yourself to be."

—*Patanjali (Yoga Sutras)*

5.1. "Apps" for Diabetes

According to Healy et al. (2013), the readmission to hospitals in diabetic patients was significantly lower when they received inpatient diabetes education (IDE). This further bolsters the concept of *self-management* in diabetes. The widespread use of mobiles/apps in our lives can be corroborated in the ICT Facts and Figures (2015) datasheet:

"Over the past 15 years the ICT revolution has driven global development in an unprecedented way. Technological progress, infrastructure deployment, and falling prices have brought unexpected growth in ICT access and connectivity to billions of people around the world. In 2015 there are more than 7 billion mobile cellular subscriptions worldwide, up from less than 1 billion in 2000. Globally 3.2 billion people are using the Internet of which 2 billion are from developing countries. ICTs will play an even more significant role in the post 2015 development agenda and in achieving future sustainable development goals as the world moves faster and faster towards a digital society. Our mission is to connect everyone and to create a truly inclusive information society, for which we need comparable and high-quality data and statistics to measure progress."

—Brahima Sanou, Director of the ITU Telecommunication Development Bureau

This section summarizes research findings on how apps and smartphones have found use in managing diabetes. Mobile health or m-health is defined as a '*medical and public health practice supported by mobile devices, such as mobile phones, patient monitoring devices, personal digital assistants (PDAs), and other wireless devices*' (Istepanian, 2022). Figure 5.1 shows the concept of m-Health.

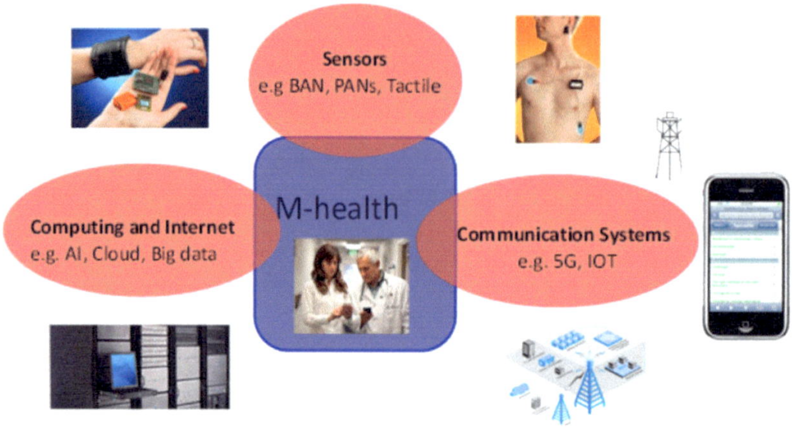

Figure 5.1. The concept of m-Health.

Source: Istepanian, R. S. H. (2022). Mobile health (m-Health) in retrospect: The known unknowns. *International Journal of Environmental Research and Public Health*, *19*(7), 3747. https://doi.org/10.3390/ijerph19073747 (accessed on 29th May 2025). Licensee MDPI, Basel, Switzerland. This article is an open access article distributed under the terms and conditions of the Creative Commons Attribution (CC BY) license (https://creativecommons.org/licenses/by/4.0/) (accessed on 29th May 2025).

According to R2G mHealth Economics 2017 – Current Status and Future Trends in Mobile Health Berlin (2017), diabetes was considered the best market for digital health innovation. For example, a two-arm (usual care and intervention) randomized controlled trial (RCT) was reported by Kirwan et al. (2013) assessing the utility of a free smartphone app along with text-message feedback from a certified diabetes educator (CDE) to improve glycemic control and diabetes-related outcomes in type 1 diabetes patients (Australian New Zealand Clinical Trials Registry: ACTRN12612000132842).

The app was the freely available "Glucose Buddy" developed by SkyHealth LLC for self-managing diabetes. Figure 5.2 shows screenshots of the app for diabetes management and reminder (Table 5.1).

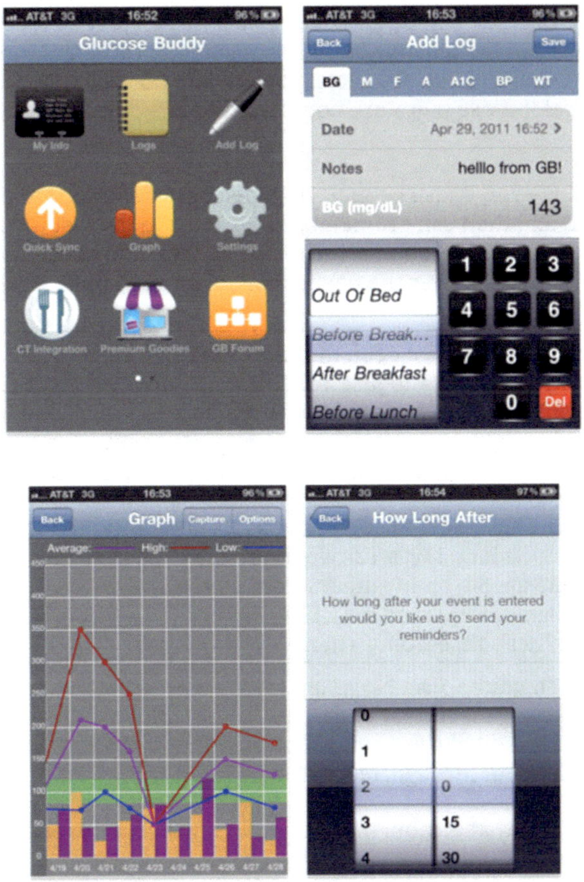

Figure 5.2. Glucose Buddy.

Source: Kirwan, M., Vandelanotte, C., Fenning, A., & Duncan, M. J. (2013). [Full article title not provided]. *Journal of Medical Internet Research*. Retrieved from http://www.jmir.org/ (accessed on 29th May 2025). This is an open-access article distributed under the terms of the Creative Commons Attribution License (http://creativecommons.org/licenses/by/2.0/) (accessed on 29th May 2025), which permits unrestricted use, distribution, and reproduction in any medium, provided the original work, first published in the *Journal of Medical Internet Research*, is properly cited. The complete bibliographic information, a link to the original publication on http://www.jmir.org/, as well as this copyright and license information must be included.

Table 5.1. Examples and Statistics of Interactions with the Certified Diabetes Educator (CDE) in the Trial by Kirwan et al. (2013)

Themes	Examples
Feedback on logs (blood glucose, insulin, diet)	Hi <patient name> – Another pretty good week – just a bit concerned about some odd higher levels in the morning. Looks like some of these are forgotten doses – would that be right? Otherwise, all are getting better and no real hypos. Be aware you may need to tweak basal if those highs are not related to forgotten doses. Your thoughts? [Sent from CDE] Hi Veronica – Yes, I have been having my breakfast later after I arrive at work. I get distracted and then can't remember if I have had my insulin or not. I think I will just have a piece of fruit and insulin before I leave for work to prevent the high. I think the basal is OK, but I will check over the next couple of days. Thanks for your help. [Response from Patient]
Diabetes questions	Hi <patient name> – I've been thinking about your CHO ratio. Have you ever done a basal check – which is simply to just have basal insulin overnight and on waking up, have no CHO and omit fast-acting insulin for breakfast or lunch, and just check how your levels go? If basal is right, you should stay pretty constant. It's a good place to start – if basal is right, we can start on CHO ratio with *Novo*? [Sent from CDE] Hi Veronica, I have never heard of a basal check, but I did this as you said, and you can see on my download I was 12 two hours after tea (before bed) and went down to 8 when I woke up. So, I now understand, as you say, I need to adjust my CHO ratio with the evening meals, so my after-tea BSL is lower. Will adjust and let you have a look at levels next week. [Response from Patient]
Educational tips	Hi <patient name> – Great logging this week – just a few Xmas tips: don't forget to give extra fast-acting insulin for extra treats. Remember, extra alcohol will make you low, so eat carbs if you drink! Today I will be standing by to answer Xmas queries, so please feel free to send them through. Merry Xmas! [Sent from CDE] I didn't realize that alcohol made my BSL lower. That explains a lot – I have had some bad hypos in the morning after a big night out. I usually give myself extra insulin for each beer I drink. Should I give any fast-acting insulin for alcohol at all, or just eat extra CHO serves? [Response from Patient]
Positive reinforcement	Hi <patient name> – Great logging this week – WOW, I'm thrilled with your HbA1c and your positive comment about it being the best in six years. It is a testament to you because you are keeping such good track of your own adjustments and control. Looks like another great week again! [Sent from CDE] Thanks. After I was first diagnosed, I kept a log, but then I didn't bother to keep track of anything because I just always felt out of control. By getting direct feedback, I have understood more about the finer details of insulin/carbs/exercise and alcohol, which has made me less reactive and think more about my adjustments. [Response from Patient]

Source: Kirwan, M., Vandelanotte, C., Fenning, A., & Duncan, M. J. (2013). The effectiveness of a web-based computer-tailored physical activity intervention using Fitbit activity trackers: Randomized trial. *Journal of Medical Internet Research*, *15*(2), e38. Retrieved from http://www.jmir.org/ (accessed on 29th May 2025).

the original work, first published in the *Journal of Medical Internet Research*, is properly cited. The complete bibliographic information, a link to the original publication on http://www.jmir.org/, as well as this copyright and license information must be included.

Of the 53 participants who completed the study (28 controls and 25 interventions), the glycemic control (measured by glycosylated hemoglobin or HbA1c levels) documented an improvement in those who used the app: baseline (mean 9.08%, SD 1.18) to 9-month follow-up (mean 7.80%, SD 0.75) than the control group (baseline: mean 8.47%, SD 0.86, follow-up: mean 8.58%, SD 1.16) (Table 5.2).

Table 5.2. The Results Obtained by Kirwan et al. (2013) in Using "Glucose Buddy" for Diabetes Management*

	Overall[a]	Control[b]	Intervention[c]	Overall *F* statistic (*df* = 1246)		
	Mean (SD)	Mean (SD)	Mean (SD)	Time	Group	Time x Group
HbA1c (%)						
Baseline	8.78 (1.07)	8.47 (0.86)	9.08 (1.18)[d]	–	–	–
3-month	8.27 (0.86)	8.23 (0.89)	8.32 (0.84)	28.79[e]	10.55[d]	20.07[e]
6-month	8.22 (0.91)	8.43 (1.00)	7.97 (0.73)	–	–	–
9-month	8.21 (1.05)	8.58 (1.16)	7.80 (0.75)	–	–	–
SDSCA[f]						
General Diet						
Baseline	3.81 (2.06)	4.19 (1.88)	3.42 (2.19)	–	–	–
3-month	4.10 (2.00)	3.97 (2.13)	4.23 (1.86)	5.30[d]	1.92	3.40
6-month	4.36 (1.86)	4.16 (1.98)	4.59 (1.73)	–	–	–
9-month	4.37 (1.83)	4.14 (1.85)	4.62 (1.80)	–	–	–
Specific Diet						
Baseline	3.08 (1.89)	2.60 (1.98)	3.56 (1.70)[d]	–	–	–
3-month	3.10 (1.63)	3.00 (1.76)	3.22 (1.48)	0.52	6.90[d]	3.36

6-month	3.68 (1.63)	3.56 (1.66)	3.80 (1.60)	–	–	–
9-month	3.93 (1.61)	4.05 (1.43)	3.80 (1.82)	–	–	–
Exercise						
Baseline	2.74 (2.09)	2.92 (2.12)	2.57 (2.08)	–	–	–
3-month	2.45 (2.12)	2.53 (2.31)	2.36 (1.91)	1.44	2.22	0.93
6-month	2.83 (1.95)	3.06 (1.97)	2.55 (1.92)	–	–	–
9-month	2.96 (1.79)	2.82 (1.75)	3.12 (1.86)	–	–	–
Glucose Testing						
Baseline	5.46 (2.04)	5.51 (2.08)	5.40 (2.03)	–	–	–
3-month	5.88 (1.64)	5.75 (1.65)	6.02 (1.64)	3.65	1.42	1.86
6-month	6.10 (1.56)	6.02 (1.67)	6.20 (1.46)	–	–	–
9-month	5.92 (1.62)	5.61 (1.95)	6.28 (1.06)	–	–	–
DES-SF[g]						
Baseline	3.62 (0.77)	3.62 (0.65)	3.62 (0.89)	–	–	–
3-month	3.78 (0.64)	3.70 (0.65)	3.88 (0.61)	0.01	0.16	0.001
6-month	3.73 (0.77)	3.64 (0.81)	3.82 (0.73)	–	–	–
9-month	3.61 (0.72)	3.62 (0.74)	3.60 (0.71)	–	–	–
DQOL[h]						
Satisfaction						
Baseline	3.14 (0.61)	3.09 (0.55)	3.20 (0.66)	–	–	–
3-month	3.22 (0.61)	3.11 (0.54)	3.35 (0.67)	0.55	1.42	0.01
6-month	3.32 (0.60)	3.23 (0.62)	3.43 (0.58)	–	–	–

9-month	3.35 (0.66)	3.29 (0.65)	3.42 (0.68)	–	–	–
Impact						
Baseline	3.70 (0.53)	3.66 (0.54)	3.75 (0.52)	–	–	–
3-month	3.81 (0.57)	3.75 (0.56)	3.89 (0.58)	0.58	0.71	0.07
6-month	3.83 (0.61)	3.74 (0.61)	3.94 (0.62)	–	–	–
9-month	3.85 (0.53)	3.77 (0.55)	3.93 (0.52)	–	–	–
Worry						
Baseline	3.98 (0.66)	3.90 (0.78)	4.06 (0.52)	–	–	–
3-month	4.10 (0.70)	4.01 (0.77)	4.19 (0.61)	1.77	1.26	0.70
6-month	4.16 (0.70)	3.99 (0.82)	4.35 (0.46)	–	–	–
9-month	4.15 (0.63)	3.99 (0.76)	4.34 (0.36)	–	–	–

[a]Number of participants included in both groups at each time point is baseline n = 72, 3-month n = 68, 6-month n = 60, 9-month n = 53.

[b]Number of participants included in the Intervention group at each time point is baseline n = 36, 3-month n = 32, 6-month n = 28, 9-month n = 25.

*Results of linear mixed model analysis for diabetes glycemic control, self-efficacy, self-care, and quality of life measures.

Source: Kirwan, M., Vandelanotte, C., Fenning, A., & Duncan, M. J. (2013). The physical activity status, preferences and experiences of culturally and linguistically diverse (CALD) women living in Australia: A qualitative study. *Journal of Medical Internet Research*, *15*(2), e196. Retrieved from http://www.jmir.org/ (accessed on 29th May 2025).

A pilot study (9 months) by Roca et al. (2021) reported the development of a virtual assistant to improve medicine adherence in patients with T2DM and depression (comorbidity). The virtual assistant had messaging layers with the artificial intelligence markup language (AIML) being employed between the assistant and the user. An example of the interaction and details are shown in Figure 5.3 and Table 5.3.

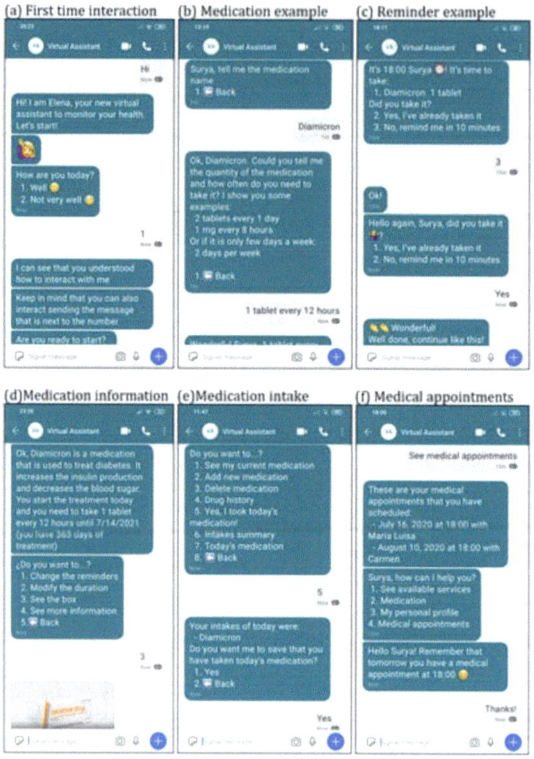

Figure 5.3. Virtual assistant interactions.

Source: Roca, S., Surya, S., Lozano, M. L., García, J., & Alesanco, Á. (2021). Validation of a virtual assistant for improving medication adherence in patients with comorbid type 2 diabetes mellitus and depressive disorder. *International Journal of Environmental Research and Public Health*, *18*(22), 12056. https://doi.org/10.3390/ijerph182212056 (accessed on 29th May 2025). © 2021 by the authors. Licensee MDPI, Basel, Switzerland. This article is an open access article distributed under the terms and conditions of the Creative Commons Attribution (CC BY) license (https://creativecommons.org/licenses/by/4.0/) (accessed on 29th May 2025).

The study from May 2019 to February 2020 included 5 healthcare professionals and 13 patients with type 2 diabetes mellitus (T2DM) and depressive disorder. Interestingly, the patient acceptance was reported as satisfactory with 9/13 expressing their opinion of continuing the assistant use after the study. Further, an increase in medicine adherence with a lowering of the HbA1c level (glycemic control) and patient health questionnaire (PHQ-9) scores (depression). Table 5.4 summarizes these results.

Table 5.3. Virtual Assistant Functions in the Study by Roca et al. (2021)

Functionality	**Tasks**
Reminders	· Sends a message at the reminder time · Sends three reminders, one every 10 min · Provides the medication box image if selected

Medication	• Shows the current medication • Adds new medication • Deletes medication • Shows the drug history • Informs the virtual assistant that the patient has taken the day's medication • Shows the medication intake summary • Shows the remaining medication to be taken during the day • Sets the reminders for taking the medication • Shows the medication information (box, information pamphlet, etc.)
Suggestions	• Receives feedback from users
Medical appointments	• Shows the medical appointments • Adds new medical appointments • Modifies medical appointments • Deletes medical appointments • Sets notifications of the appointments
Tutorials	• Lists the tutorials available on YouTube

Source: Roca, S., Surya, S., Lozano, M. L., García, J., & Alesanco, Á. (2021). Validation of a virtual assistant for improving medication adherence in patients with comorbid type 2 diabetes mellitus and depressive disorder. *International Journal of Environmental Research and Public Health, 18*(22), 12056. https://doi.org/10.3390/ijerph182212056 (accessed on 29th May 2025).

Table 5.4. Glycosylated Hemoglobin and PHQ-9 for Each Patient Before and After Using the Virtual Assistant (Roca et al., 2021)

Patient	**HbA1c Values (%) (p = 0.02)**		**PHQ-9 Score (p = 0.002)**	
	Before	**After**	**Before**	**After**
1*	7.6	7.4	11	9
2	7.4	6.9	5	4
3	7.5	7.2	18	10
4	6.9	6.2	6	4

5	7.8	7.6	9	5
6	7.8	6.9	22	12
7*	7.9	7.9	14	8
8	9.3	9.2	5	5
9	6.9	6.9	16	7
10	7.9	6.9	20	14
11*	7.8	8.0	21	15
12	6.7	6.8	13	10
13	7.5	7.2	12	9

*Patients who had uninstalled Signal: results calculated using the period they had Signal installed.

Source: Roca, S., Surya, S., Lozano, M. L., García, J., & Alesanco, Á. (2021). Validation of a virtual assistant for improving medication adherence in patients with comorbid type 2 diabetes mellitus and depressive disorder. *International Journal of Environmental Research and Public Health, 18*(22), 12056. https://doi.org/10.3390/ijerph182212056 (accessed on 29th May 2025).

While these results are encouraging, the researchers reported a few hitches that needed addressing, such as the occasional failure of the assistant and the "boring" weather forecasts. Table 5.5 summarizes the feedback of the patients and medical professionals.

Table 5.5. Feedback from Patients and Healthcare Professionals Regarding the Virtual Assistant for Medication Adherence in Diabetes

Patients		
Question	**Yes, % (*n*)** **(*N* = 13)**	**No, % (*n*)** **(*N* = 13)**
Do you ever forget to take medications to treat your disease?	23.1 (n = 3)	76.9 (n = 10)
When you are well, do you stop taking your medication?	0.0	100.0
If you ever feel bad, do you stop taking it?	15.4 (n = 2)	84.6 (n = 11)
Did you find it easy to use the virtual assistant?	92.3 (n = 12)	7.7 (n = 1)
Do you think it is useful for you?	92.3 (n = 12)	7.7 (n = 1)
Do you think the virtual assistant improves your medication adherence?	92.3 (n = 12)	7.7 (n = 1)
Do you think you will continue using the virtual assistant after the project?	69.2 (n = 9)	30.8 (n = 4)
From a certain moment, the virtual assistant began to give the weather forecast. Has this helped you use it more often?	100.0	0.0

Healthcare Professionals		
Question	**Yes, % (*n*) (*N* = 5)**	**No, % (*n*) (*N* = 5)**
Did you find the virtual assistant easy to use?	80.0 ($n = 4$)	20.0 ($n = 1$)
Do you think it is useful for you?	80.0 ($n = 4$)	20.0 ($n = 1$)
Do you think it is useful for the patients?	100.0	0.0
Do you think the virtual assistant improves the medication adherence of the patients?	100.0	0.0
Did you use the functionalities to monitor the medication intakes of your patients?	60.0 ($n = 3$)	40.0 ($n = 2$)
Do you think you will continue using the virtual assistant after the project?	80.0 ($n = 4$)	20.0 ($n = 1$)

Question	**Mean (SD)**
In the medical appointment, did you observe motivation in using the virtual assistant by patients?	4.2 (1.3)
In the medical appointment, did you observe dissatisfaction with the virtual assistant by patients?	1.8 (0.8)
In the medical appointment, did you observe an improvement in the patients' medication intake?	4.2 (0.8)

Source: Roca, S., Surya, S., Lozano, M. L., García, J., & Alesanco, Á. (2021). Validation of a virtual assistant for improving medication adherence in patients with comorbid type 2 diabetes mellitus and depressive disorder. *International Journal of Environmental Research and Public Health*, *18*(22), 12056. https://doi.org/10.3390/ijerph182212056 (accessed on 29th May 2025).

A systematic review was reported by Dening et al. (2020) as *"the first to demonstrate the potential for web-based interventions to achieve significant improvements in dietary behavior in people with T2DM."* The study entailed analyzing five studies ($n = 1056$) scoring changes in diet from RCTs of web-based interventions in adults with T2DM (Table 5.6).

Table 5.6. Studies on Diet Management in T2DM Patients Using Web-based Interventions Reviewed by Dening et al. (2020)

Author/Date	Study Design	Sample Size, *N*	Population Characteristics	Theory/Model	Intervention Participants, *N*, Program Name, Digital Intervention Characteristics	Type of Diets Prescribed	Intervention/ Follow-Up Period
Ramadas et al. (2018)	RCT[a]	128	Adults with T2DM[b], mean age 50.5 years, most with a family history of T2DM. Malaysia	Transtheoretical Model Stages of Change, user-centered design	*N* = 62, *myDIDeA*[c], received personalized intensive dietary intervention via website + standard care	IG[d]: standard dietary guidelines CG[e]: no prescribed diet	6-month intervention, 12-month follow-up
Hansel et al. (2017)	RCT	120	Adults with abdominal obesity and T2DM, mean age 57 years. Paris	No theory reported	*N* = 60, *ANODE*[f], fully automated web-based nutritional support program	IG: National Nutrition and Health Program guidelines CG: received general diet advice	16-week intervention
Saslow et al. (2017)	Pilot RCT	25	Overweight adults with T2DM, mean age 55.6 years. California	No theory reported	*N* = 12, dietary instruction provided via email lessons including mindfulness training and lifestyle advice	IG: *VLCKD*[g] (20–50 g/carbs per day) CG: *ADA*[h] "create your plate" diet	16-week intervention, 32-week follow-up
Glasgow et al. (2003)	RCT	320	Adults with T2DM, mean age 59 years. Colorado	Self-efficacy theory, social support theory	*N* = *N/A*[i], *D-Net*[j], two intervention arms: tailored self-management training, peer support	All groups received general healthy eating advice to decrease fat and increase fruit and vegetable intake	3-month intervention, 10-month follow-up
Glasgow et al. (2012)	RCT	463	Adults with T2DM, mean age 58.4 years. Colorado	Social-ecological theory, social cognitive theory, and the "5 As" self-management model	*N* = 189, two intervention arms: *CASM*[k]: self-administered computer-assisted self-management; *N* = 182, *CASM+*[l] with enhanced social support	All groups received general advice to decrease fat and eat a healthy diet	4-month intervention, 12-month follow-up

[a] RCT: randomized controlled trial.

[b] T2DM: type 2 diabetes mellitus.

[c] *myDIDeA:* Malaysian Dietary Intervention for People with Type 2 Diabetes: An e-Approach.

[d] IG: intervention group.

[e] CG: control group.

[f] ANODE*:* Accompagnement Nutritionnel de l'Obésité et du Diabète par E-coaching.

[g] VLCKD*:* very low carbohydrate ketogenic diet.

[h] ADA*:* American Diabetes Association.

[i] N/A: not applicable.

[j] D-Net: Diabetes Network.

[k] CASM: computer-assisted self-management.

[l] CASM+: computer-assisted self-management plus social support.

Source: Dening, J., Islam, S. M. S., George, E. S., & Maddison, R. (2020). mHealth for non-communicable diseases in low and middle-income countries: A systematic review of reviews. *Journal of Medical Internet Research*, *22*(3), e14309. Retrieved from http://www.jmir.org/ (accessed on 29th May 2025).

Dietary patterns were significantly improved in four of these studies (seen as lowered saturated fat, sodium, added sugar, and eating habits) and improved awareness. Further, average reductions were reported in three studies in terms of fasting blood glucose, hemoglobin A1c (HbA1c), etc. These results as presented by the authors are given in Table 5.7.

Table 5.7. Results of Diet Management Analyses in T2DM Patients Using Web-based Interventions Reviewed by Dening et al. (2020)

Dietary Assessment	Baseline Dietary Assessment Results	Postintervention Dietary Changes	References
DKAB[a] score, DSOC[b]	IG[c]: DKAB 34.2 (5.2), DSOC 193.3 (14.6) CG[d]: DKAB 33.7 (5.5), DSOC 191.2 (16.2)	IG: DKAB 54.0 (8.7), DSOC 199.7 (18.2) CG: DKAB 41.3 (7.7), DSOC 191.5 (15.1) DKAB score significantly improved in both groups, with greater improvement in the IG (difference of 12.2 points). No group difference in DSOC at 6 months. IG showed improved DSOC at 12-month follow-up; no change in CG.	Ramadas et al. (2018)
DQI-I[e]	IG: DQI-I 54.0 CG: DQI-I 52.8	IG: Significant increase in DQI-I score by 4.55 (total = 58.55) CG: Decrease in DQI-I score by −1.68 (total = 51.12) Dietary changes toward healthier foods in IG, especially saturated fat ($P = 0.02$) and sodium ($P < 0.001$).	Hansel et al. (2017)
Self-reported dietary intake (*MyFitnessPal*) and self-reported subjective experience	IG: Nonfiber carbohydrates (g): 163.6 (86.7), Fat (g): 77.1 (41.4), Protein (g): 83.3 (18.0), Sugar (g): 50.6 (33.8) CG: Nonfiber carbohydrates (g): 152.0 (58.9), Fat (g): 81.3 (27.3), Protein (g): 74.5 (17.2), Sugar (g): 44.9 (23.8)	IG consumed fewer grams of nonfiber carbohydrates and sugar than CG. No difference in protein and fat intake. IG's mean carbohydrate intake dropped from 39.6% to 15.5% of total calories. IG rated themselves less likely to cheat, with a large effect size (Cohen $d = -1.0$).	Saslow et al. (2017)
FFB[f] and the NCI[g] Fat Screener	Not reported	Trending improvements in FFB in both IGs but no significant differences between groups.	Glasgow et al. (2003)
"Starting the Conversation" scale and NCI[g] Fat Screener	IG: Eating habits 2.18 (0.2), Fat intake 34.86 (28) CG: Eating habits 2.13 (0.3), Fat intake 35.18 (40)	IG: Eating habits 2.32 (0.2), Fat intake 33.22 (24) CG: Eating habits 2.23 (0.3), Fat intake 33.91 (37) The combined IG CASM[h]/CASM+[i] significantly improved eating habits and fat intake over 12 months ($\chi^2 = 9.01$, $\chi^2 = 6.01$). Clinical outcomes were statistically significant for intervention groups ($P < 0.05$).	Glasgow et al. (2012)

Significant clinical outcomes for dietary intervention groups. Data were considered statistically significant if $P < 0.05$.

Author/Date/ Reported Mean and Outcomes Measured	Baseline	Timepoint	Outcome	Within-Group Changes (*P* Value)	Between-Group Changes (*P* Value)
Ramadas et al. (2018), Mean (SD)					
HbA1c[a] (%)	9.1 (2.0)	6 months = 8.7 (1.9)	12 months = 8.5 (1.8)	0.004	–[b]
Fasting blood glucose (mmol/L)	8.9 (3.9)	6 months = 8.1 (2.7)	12 months = 7.9 (2.5)	0.015	–
Hansel et al. (2017), Mean (SD)					
HbA1c (%)	7.16 (0.78)	–	6.86 (0.94)	–	<0.001
Weight (kg)	93.3 (16.2)	–	91 (3.0)	–	0.01
Waist circumference (cm)	110 (10)	–	109.1 (4.7)	–	0.01
Saslow et al. (2017), Mean (SD) and Mean (EMM[c])					
HbA1c (%)	7.1 (0.4)	16 weeks = 6.2 (−1.1, −0.6)	32 weeks = 6.3 (−1.1, −0.6)	–	0.002
Weight (kg)	109 (24.9)	16 weeks = 100.5 (−11.9, −5.2)	32 weeks = 96.3 (−7.3, 1.3)	–	<0.001
Triglycerides (mg/dL)	183 (135)	16 weeks = 147.5 (−65.7, −5.2 EMM)	32 weeks = 122.9 (−46.0, 33.6 EMM)	–	0.01

[a] DKAB: Dietary knowledge, attitude, and behavior.

[b] DSOC: Dietary stages of change.

[c] IG: Intervention group.

[d] CG: Control group.

[e] DQI-I: International diet quality index.

[f] FFB: Kristal fat and fiber behavior scale.

[g] NCI: National Cancer Institute.

[h] CASM: Computer-assisted self-management.

[i] CASM+: Computer-assisted self-management plus social support.

[a] HbA1c: Hemoglobin A1c

[b] Not applicable

[c] EMM: Estimated marginal means.

Source: Dening, J., Islam, S. M. S., George, E. S., & Maddison, R. (2020). mHealth for noncommunicable disease prevention and management in low and middle-income countries: A systematic review of

A systematic review by Islam et al. (2022) reported 8 high-quality apps freely and publicly available in the Apple App Store and Google Play. Of 249 apps in Google Play and 209 apps in the Apple App Store, these were selected based on the mean app-specific score (MASS): the average of six dimensions, including awareness, knowledge, attitudes, intention to change, help-seeking, and behavior change. The features of these apps are summarized in Figure 5.4.

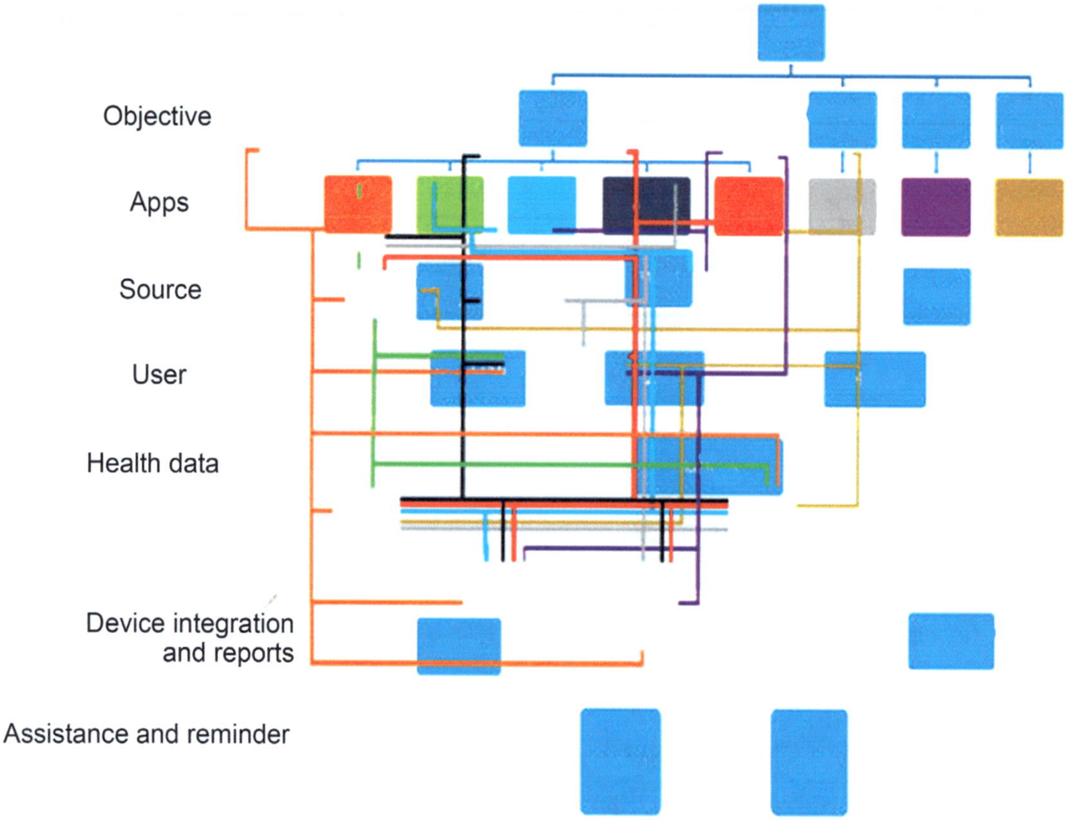

Figure 5.4. Features of apps selected for diabetes management (Islam et al., 2022).

Abbreviations: CGM: Continuous glucose monitoring; DM: diabetes mellitus; T1DM: type 1 diabetes mellitus; and T2DM: type 2 diabetes mellitus.

Further, 50% of these apps supported low adherence to medications while 25% (2 apps) facilitated high adherence and 25% (2 apps) allowed moderate adherence. Table 5.8 summarizes the findings.

Table 5.8. Diabetes Medication Adherence and Apps – An Analysis by Islam et al. (2022)

App	**Primary Factors**						**App Features**					
	Blood Glucose	**Food**	**Physical Activity**	**Medi cation**	**Vital Signs**	**Score**	**Over view**	**Rem inder**	**Notifi cation**	**Assis tance**	**Motiv ation**	**Sco re**
Diabetes:M	Yes	Yes	Yes	Yes	No	4	Yes	Yes	Yes	Yes	No	4
mySugr – Diabetes Tracker Log	Yes	Yes	No	Yes	No	3	Yes	No	No	No	Yes	2
Health2Sync	Yes	No	No	No	Yes	2	Yes	Yes	Yes	Yes	Yes	5
MyTherapy Pill Reminder	Yes	No	No	No	Yes	2		Yes	No	Yes	Yes	3
One Drop: Transform Your Life	Yes	Yes	Yes	Yes	Yes	5	Yes	Yes	No	No	Yes	3
Glucose Buddy Diabetes Tracker	Yes	No	No	Yes	Yes	3	Yes	No	No	Yes	No	2
OneTouch Reveal	Yes	Yes	Yes	Yes	No	4	Yes	Yes	Yes	Yes	Yes	5
Sugarmate	Yes	Yes	No	Yes	Yes	4	Yes	No	Yes	No	Yes	3

Source: Islam, S. M. S., Mishra, V., Siddiqui, M. U., Moses, J. C., Adibi, S., Nguyen, L., & Wickramasinghe, N. (2022). Smartphone apps for diabetes medication adherence: Systematic review. *JMIR Diabetes*, 7(2), e33264. Retrieved from https://diabetes.jmir.org/ (accessed on 29th May 2025).

Overall, the authors reported that close to 50% of the free/public apps facilitated moderate to high adherence while the remaining half did not provide medication adherence. The way ahead is the standardization to boost the development of only those apps that provide optimal diabetes management.

"We believe consumer health technologies—apps, wearables, self-diagnosis tools—have the potential to strengthen the patient-physician connection and improve health outcomes."

—Dr. Glen Stream, Chairman, Family Medicine for America's Health

5.2. Herbs and Ethnobotany

"There are no incurable diseases—only the lack of will. There are no worthless herbs—only the lack of knowledge."

—Avicenna

According to the National Institutes of Health Office of Dietary Supplements, "A botanical is a plant or plant part valued for its medicinal or therapeutic properties, flavor, and/or scent. Herbs are a subset of botanicals. Products made from botanicals that are used to maintain or improve health are sometimes called herbal products, botanical products, or phytomedicines." A 2017-published article described that more than one-third of respondents analyzed (the source was the 2015 National Consumer Survey on the Medication Experience and Pharmacist Role or NCSME-PR) used herbal medicines. Interestingly, this usage was more with higher education, older age, and chronic conditions (Rashrash et al., 2017). This section presents research findings from the use of herbal medicines for diabetes.

Modak et al. (2007) compiled a list of Indian medicinal plants and their formulations used for managing diabetes. Tables 5.9 and 5.10 highlight these lists.

Table 5.9. Indian Medicinal Plants with Anti-Diabetic Effects

Plant Name	Ayurvedic/Common Name/Herbal Formulation	Antidiabetic and Other Beneficial Effects in Traditional Medicine
Annona squamosa	Sugar apple	Hypoglycemic and antihyperglycemic activities of ethanolic leaf extract; increased plasma insulin level
Artemisia pallens	Davana	Hypoglycemic; increases peripheral glucose utilization or inhibits glucose reabsorption
Areca catechu	Supari	Hypoglycemic
Beta vulgaris	Chukkander	Increases glucose tolerance in OGTT
Boerhavia diffusa	Punarnava	Increases hexokinase activity; decreases glucose-6-phosphatase (G6PC) and fructose bisphosphatase activity; increases plasma insulin level; antioxidant
Bombax ceiba	Semul	Hypoglycemic
Butea monosperma	Palasa	Antihyperglycemic
Camellia sinensis	Tea	Antihyperglycemic activity; antioxidant
Capparis decidua	Karir or Pinju	Hypoglycemic; antioxidant; hypolipidemic
Caesalpinia bonducella	Sagarghota, Fevernut	Hypoglycemic; insulin secretagogue; hypolipidemic

Coccinia indica	Bimb or Kanturi	Hypoglycemic
Emblica officinalis	Amla, Dhatriphala; a constituent of the herbal formulation "Triphala"	Decreases lipid peroxidation; antioxidant; hypoglycemic
Eugenia uniflora	Pitanga	Hypoglycemic; inhibits lipase activity
Enicostema littorale	Krimihrita	Increases hexokinase activity; decreases G6PC and fructose 1,6-bisphosphatase activity; dose-dependent hypoglycemic activity
Ficus benghalensis	Bur	Hypoglycemic; antioxidant
Gymnema sylvestre	Gudmar or Merasingi	Antihyperglycemic effect; hypolipidemic
Hemidesmus indicus	Anantamul	Anti-snake venom activity; anti-inflammatory
Hibiscus rosa-sinensis	Gudhal or Jasson	Initiates insulin release from pancreatic beta cells
Ipomoea batatas	Sakkargand	Reduces insulin resistance
Momordica cymbalaria	Kadavanchi	Hypoglycemic; hypolipidemic
Murraya koenigii	Curry patta	Hypoglycemic; increases glycogenesis and decreases gluconeogenesis and glycogenolysis
Musa sapientum	Banana	Antihyperglycemic; antioxidant
Phaseolus vulgaris	Hulga, white kidney bean	Hypoglycemic; hypolipidemic; inhibits α-amylase activity; antioxidant; alters insulin receptor and GLUT-4 mRNA levels in skeletal muscle
Punica granatum	Anar	Antioxidant; antihyperglycemic effect
Salacia reticulata	Vairi	Inhibitory activity against sucrase; α-glucosidase inhibitor
Scoparia dulcis	Sweet broomweed	Insulin secretagogue activity; antihyperlipidemic; hypoglycemic; antioxidant
Swertia chirayita	Chirata	Stimulates insulin release from islets
Syzygium alternifolium	Shahajire	Hypoglycemic; antihyperglycemic
Terminalia bellirica	Behada; a constituent of "Triphala"	Antibacterial; hypoglycemic
Terminalia chebula	Hirda	Antibacterial; hypoglycemic
Tinospora crispa	–	Antihyperglycemic; stimulates insulin release from islets
Vinca rosea	Sadabahar	Antihyperglycemic
Withania somnifera	Ashvagandha, winter cherry	Hypoglycemic; diuretic; hypocholesterolemic

Source: Modak, M., Dixit, P., Londhe, J., Ghaskadbi, S., & Devasagayam, T. P. (2007). Indian herbs and herbal drugs used for the treatment of diabetes. *Journal of Clinical Biochemistry and Nutrition*, *40*(3), 163–173. https://doi.org/10.3164/jcbn.40.163 (accessed on 29th May 2025).

Table 5.10. Formulations for Diabetes Used in India

Drug	Company	Ingredients
Diabecon	Himalaya	*Gymnema sylvestre, Pterocarpus marsupium, Glycyrrhiza glabra, Casearia esculenta, Syzygium cumini, Asparagus racemosus, Boerhavia diffusa, Sphaeranthus indicus, Tinospora cordifolia, Swertia chirata, Tribulus terrestris, Phyllanthus amarus, Gmelina arborea, Gossypium herbaceum, Berberis aristata, Aloe vera,* Triphala, *Commiphora wightii,* shilajeet, *Momordica charantia, Piper nigrum, Ocimum sanctum, Abutilon indicum, Curcuma longa, Rumex maritimus*
Diasulin	–	*Cassia auriculata, Coccinia indica, Curcuma longa, Emblica officinalis, Gymnema sylvestre, Momordica charantia, Scoparia dulcis, Syzygium cumini, Tinospora cordifolia, Trigonella foenum-graecum*
Pancreatic Tonic 180 cp	Ayurvedic herbal supplement	*Pterocarpus marsupium, Gymnema sylvestre, Momordica charantia, Syzygium cumini, Trigonella foenum-graecum, Azadirachta indica, Ficus racemosa, Aegle marmelos, Cinnamomum tamala*
Ayurveda Alternative Herbal Formula to Diabetes	Chakrapani Ayurveda	Gurmar (*Gymnema sylvestre*), Karela (*Momordica charantia*), Pushkarmool (*Inula racemosa*), Jamun Gutli (*Syzygium cumini*), Neem (*Azadirachta indica*), Methika (*Trigonella foenum-graecum*), Guduchi (*Tinospora cordifolia*)
Bitter Gourd Powder	Garry and Sun Natural Remedies	Bitter gourd (*Momordica charantia*)
Dia-care	Admark Herbals Limited	Sanjeevan Mool; Himej, Jambu beej, Kadu, Namejav, Neem chal
Diabetes-Daily Care	Nature's Health Supply	Alpha lipoic acid, cinnamon 4% extract, Chromax, vanadium, fenugreek 50% extract, *Gymnema sylvestre* 25% extract, *Momordica* 7% extract, licorice root 20% extract
Gurmar Powder	Garry and Sun Natural Remedies	Gurmar (*Gymnema sylvestre*)
Epinsulin	Swastik Formulations	Vijaysar (*Pterocarpus marsupium*)
Diabecure	Nature Beaute Santé	*Juglans regia, Berberis vulgaris, Erythraea centaurium, Millefolium, Taraxacum*
Diabeta	Ayurvedic Cure Ayurvedic Herbal Health Products	*Gymnema sylvestre, Vinca rosea* (Periwinkle), *Curcuma longa* (Turmeric), *Azadirachta indica* (Neem), *Pterocarpus marsupium* (Kino Tree), *Momordica charantia* (Bitter Gourd), *Syzygium cumini* (Black Plum), *Acacia arabica* (Black Babhul), *Tinospora cordifolia, Zingiber officinale* (Ginger)
Syndrex	Plethico Laboratories	Germinated fenugreek seed extract

Source: Modak, M., Dixit, P., Londhe, J., Ghaskadbi, S., & Devasagayam, T. P. (2007). Indian herbs and herbal drugs used for the treatment of diabetes. *Journal of Clinical Biochemistry and Nutrition, 40*(3), 163–173. https://doi.org/10.3164/jcbn.40.163 (accessed on 29th May 2025).

In a 2016-published work, Baharvand-Ahmadi et al. conducted interviews with 25 herbalists to outline herbs employed to treat diabetes in Shiraz, Iran. The results are presented in Tables 5.11 and 5.12.

Table 5.11. Medicinal Plants Used in Shiraz for Diabetes

Scientific Name	Family	Persian Names	Usable Part of Plant	How to Use	Traditional Use in Shiraz
Juglans regia L.	Juglandaceae	Gerdoo	Leaves	Oral	Diabetes
Cinnamomum verum	Lauraceae	Darchin	Bark	Oral	Diabetes
Ficus johannis Boiss.	Moraceae	Anjir-Vahshi-Daraki	Leaves	Oral	Diabetes
Lamium amplexicaule L.	Lamiaceae	Gazaneh Say	Aerial parts	Decoction	Diabetes
Trigonella monspeliaca L.	Papilionaceae	Shanbalileh	Aerial parts	Decoction	Diabetes
Phaseolus vulgaris L.	Leguminosae	Loobia	Aerial parts	Decoction	Diabetes
Arctium lappa	Compositae	Baba-adam	Aerial parts	Decoction	Diabetes
Urtica dioica L.	Urticaceae	Gazaneh	Aerial parts	Decoction	Diabetes
Olea europaea	Oleaceae	Zeitoon	Leaves	Oral	Diabetes
Amygdalus scoparia Spach.	Rosaceae	Badam-Koohi-Arzhan	Leaves	Decoction	Diabetes
Salvia officinalis	Lamiaceae	Maryam-Goli	Aerial parts	Decoction	Diabetes
Anethum graveolens Dhi	Apiaceae	Shevid	Leaves	Decoction	Diabetes
Achillea millefolium L.	Compositae	Boomadaran-Sefid	Aerial parts	Decoction	Diabetes
Cotoneaster persica Pojark.	Rosaceae	Shirkhesht	Aerial parts	Decoction	Diabetes
Ixilirion tataricum (Pall.) Roem et Schult.	Amaryllidaceae	Khiarak	Leaves	Decoction	Diabetes
Securigera securidaca	Fabaceae	Adas-almolk	Leaves and fruits	Decoction	Diabetes
Citrullus colocynthis	Cucurbitaceae	Hendavaneh-Aboojahl	Fruit	Fresh fruit, decoction	Diabetes
Allium sativum	Alliaceae	Sir	Bulb	Oral	Diabetes
Lagenaria vulgaris	Cucurbitaceae	Kedoo	Fruit	Oral	Diabetes
Curcuma longa	Zingiberaceae	Zardchooveh	Bark	Decoction	Diabetes
Gundelia tournefortii	Compositae	Kangar	Leaves	Oral	Diabetes
Zataria multiflora	Lamiaceae	Avishan-Shirazi	Leaves	Decoction	Diabetes

Berberis vulgaris	Berberidaceae	Zereshk	Fruit	Decoction	Diabetes
Mespilus germanica	Rosaceae	Azgil	Fruit	Decoction	Diabetes

Source: Baharvand-Ahmadi, B., Bahmani, M., Tajeddini, P., Naghdi, N., & Rafieian-Kopaei, M. (2016). An ethno-medicinal study of medicinal plants used for the treatment of diabetes. *Journal of Nephropathology*, *5*(1), [page range not specified]. Published by Society of Diabetic Nephropathy Prevention.

Zanzabil et al. (2022) compiled several studies conducted on the potential of herbs in managing diabetes that has been presented in Table 5.12.

Table 5.12. Select Studies on Research on Herbs and Diabetes Control

Scientific Name	Common Name	Family	Parts Used	Model Organism	Solvent	Dosage	Reference Drug	Result
Ficus racemosa	Cluster fig, Dumur	Moraceae	Leaves	STZ-induced diabetic rats	Petroleum ether	200 mg/kg and 400 mg/kg body weight	Glibenclamide	Reduction in blood glucose levels ($p < 0.001$)
Asparagus racemosus	Satamuli	Liliaceae	Whole plant	STZ-induced diabetic Wistar rats	Ethanol	200 and 400 mg/kg body weight	Glibenclamide (10 mg/kg)	Decreased blood glucose level ($p < 0.05$)
Bombax ceiba	Shimul, red silk-cotton tree	Bomba caceae	Bark	STZ-induced diabetic rats	Ethyl acetate	600 mg/kg body weight	Glibenclamide (10 mg/kg)	Displayed significant hypoglycemic activity ($p < 0.001$)
Cajanus cajan	Arhar, pigeon pea	Fabaceae	Root	Alloxan-induced diabetic mice	Methanol	200 mg/kg or 400 mg/kg body weight	Metformin (50 mg/kg)	Significantly lowered fasting serum glucose and blood glucose levels ($p < 0.001$)
Coccinia cordifolia	Telakucha, Ivy gourd	Cucurbit aceae	Leaves	STZ-induced diabetic rats	Petroleum ether, ethyl acetate	150 mg/kg body weight	Metformin HCl (150 mg/kg)	Reduced blood glucose by 50.39% and 50% at 10th and 24th hours, respectively ($p < 0.001$)
Momordica charantia	Korola, bitter gourd	Cucurb itaceae	Seed	STZ-induced diabetic rats	Water	150 mg/kg body weight	Glibenclamide (600 µg/kg)	Significantly reduced plasma glucose ($p < 0.05$)
Syzygium cumini	Kalojam, Java plum	Myrtaceae	Whole fruit; Leaves	STZ-induced diabetic albino Wistar rats; STZ-induced diabetic rats	Ethanol	200 mg/kg; 250 mg/kg body weight	Glibenclamide (200 mg/kg)	Decreased blood glucose levels ($p < 0.01$); increased muscle glycogen ($p < 0.001$)
Neolamarckia cadamba	Burflower tree, Kodom	Rubiaceae	Leaves	Glucose-loaded hyperglycemic mice	Methanol	200 mg/kg and 400 mg/kg body weight	Glibenclamide (10 mg/kg)	Reduced elevated blood glucose ($p < 0.05$)
Mangifera indica	Mango, Aam	Anacar diaceae	Leaves	Alloxan-induced diabetic rats	Water	200 mg/kg and 400 mg/kg body weight	Gliclazide (2 mg/kg and 4 mg/kg)	Significantly lowered fasting blood glucose ($p < 0.0001$)

Cocos nucifera	Coconut	Arecaceae	Spadix	STZ-induced diabetic rats	Hydrom ethanol	250 mg/kg and 500 mg/kg body weight	Glibenclamide (0.5 mg/kg)	Significantly lowered fasting blood glucose ($p < 0.001$)
Tamarindus indica	Tamarind	Fabaceae	Seed	STZ-induced diabetic Long–Evans rats	–	1.25 g/kg	Glibenclamide (5 mg/kg)	Demonstrated anti-hyperglycemic properties ($p < 0.03$)
Punica granatum	Pomegranate	Lythraceae	Leaves; Fruit	STZ-induced type 2 diabetic rats; Alloxan-induced diabetic rats	Methanol; Water	100–600 mg/kg; 100–350 mg/kg body weight	Glibenclamide (1 mg/kg); –	Demonstrated anti-diabetic activity ($p < 0.05$); reduced fasting blood glucose ($p < 0.001$)
Azadirachta indica	Neem	Meliaceae	Leaves	STZ-induced diabetic rats	Ethanol	200 mg/kg body weight	Glibenclamide (0.25 mg/kg)	Normalized glucose levels after STZ-induced hyperglycemia ($p < 0.05$)
Costus speciosus	Crepe ginger	Costaceae	Rhizome; root	Alloxan-induced diabetic rats	Ethanol	200 mg/kg; 300 and 450 mg/kg body weight	Glibenclamide (2.5 mg/kg); Glibenclamide (600 μg/kg)	Enhanced insulin secretion; lowered blood glucose; decreased gluconeogenesis; increased glycogenesis
Moringa oleifera	Drumstick tree	Moringaceae	Leaves	STZ-induced Sprague-Dawley rats	Ethyl acetate	200 mg/kg body weight	Glibenclamide (5 mg/kg)	Reversed STZ effects on glucose and insulin; demonstrated anti-diabetic activity ($p < 0.05$)
Andrographis paniculata	Green chiretta	Acanthaceae	Leaves	Alloxan-induced diabetic Wistar rats	Ethanol	1000 mg/kg body weight	Glimepiride (4 mg/kg)	Significantly reduced blood glucose ($p < 0.01$)
Ficus benghalensis	Banyan	Moraceae	Leaves; bark	Alloxan-induced diabetic rats; STZ-induced rats	Ethanol	200, 400 mg/kg; 150, 300, 500 mg/kg body weight	Glibenclamide (5 mg/kg); Glibenclamide (0.5 mg/kg)	Reduced triglycerides, cholesterol, and glucose; stimulated insulin secretion ($p < 0.01$)
Anacardium occidentale	Cashew nut, kaju badam	Sumac	Leaves	STZ-induced diabetic Wistar rats	Methanol	300 mg/kg body weight	Insulin (1 IU/kg)	Significantly reduced blood glucose ($p < 0.05$)
Annona squamosa	Custard apple	Annon aceae	Leaves	STZ-induced rats	Water and ethanol	200 mg/kg, 400 mg/kg body weight	Metformin (300 mg/kg)	Reduced blood glucose ($p < 0.05$)
Boerhaavia diffusa	Hogweed	Nyctagin aceae	Leaves	STZ-induced diabetic rats	Chloroform	50, 100, 200 mg/kg body weight	Glibenclamide (25 μg/kg)	Reduced blood glucose, possibly via pancreatic β-cell regeneration
Catharanthus roseus	Nayantara	Apocynaceae	Leaf	Alloxan-induced diabetic rat	Juice	0.5, 0.75, 1.0 mL/kg body weight	Glibenclamide (40 μg/kg)	Lowered blood glucose ($p < 0.01$)
Cocculus hirsutus	Broom creeper, Daikhali, Jalajmani	Menispe rmaceae	Leaf	Alloxan-induced diabetic rat	Water	250, 500, 1000 mg/kg body weight	Glyburide (10 mg/kg)	Reduced serum glucose level ($p < 0.01$)

Ficus hispida	Hairy fig	Moraceae	Bark	Alloxan-induced diabetic albino rat	Ethanol	1.25 g/kg body weight	Glibenclamide (0.5 mg/kg)	Reduced blood glucose ($p < 0.001$)
Terminalia chebula	Myrobalan	Comb retaceae	Fruit	STZ-induced diabetic rats	Ethanol	200 mg/kg body weight	Glibenclamide (600 µg/kg)	Stimulated insulin; lowered blood glucose ($p < 0.05$)
Terminalia catappa	Bangla badam	Combre taceae	Leaf	Alloxan-induced diabetic Wistar albino rats	Water; Cold extract	43 mg/kg (aqueous), 46 mg/kg (cold extract)	Glibenclamide (10 mg/kg)	Regenerated pancreas
Amaranthus tricolor	Edible amaranth	Amara nthaceae	Leaf	Alloxan-induced diabetic male albino rats	Water	400 mg/kg body weight	–	Reduced serum glucose levels ($p < 0.001$)
Blumea lacera	Lettuce leaf blumea	Asteraceae	Leaf	Swiss albino mice	Methanol	50–400 mg/kg body weight	Glibenclamide (10 mg/kg)	Reduced blood glucose ($p < 0.0001$)
Piper betle	Betel leaf	Piperaceae	Leaf	STZ-induced diabetic rats	Ethanol	100, 200, 300, 1500 mg/kg body weight	Tolbutamide (22.5 mg/kg)	Reduced blood glucose significantly ($p < 0.050$)
Achyranthes aspera	Devil's horsewhip	Amara nthaceae	Seed	STZ-induced diabetic rat	Ethanol	300, 600 mg/kg body weight for 24 days	Glibenclamide (5 mg/kg)	Reduced blood glucose level ($p < 0.001$)
Kalanchoe pinnata	Cathedral bells, life plant	Crassu laceae	Leaf	Alloxan-induced diabetic rats	Ethanol	5.8, 11.6, and 33.2 mg/kg body weight	Glibenclamide (1.35 mg/kg), Acarbose (13.5 mg/kg)	Reduced fasting blood glucose ($p < 0.05$); increased pancreatic β-cells
Nelumbo nucifera	Indian lotus	Nymp haeaceae	Flower	STZ-induced diabetic male Wistar rat	Ethanol	250 mg/kg body weight	Glibenclamide (0.25 mg/kg)	Lowered fasting blood glucose
Mikania cordata	Bitter vine	Asteraceae	Leaf	Alloxan-induced diabetic rat	Ethanol	200 mg/kg, 400 mg/kg body weight	Metformin hydrochloride (100 mg/kg)	Reduced blood glucose ($p < 0.05$, $p < 0.01$)
Wedelia chinensis	Wedelia	Asteraceae	Leaf	Alloxan-induced diabetic Swiss albino mice	Methanol	100 mg/kg, 200 mg/kg body weight	Glibenclamide (5 mg/kg)	Reduced blood glucose levels ($p < 0.01$)
Murraya koenigii	Curry tree	Rutaceae	Leaf	STZ- and nicotinamide-induced hyperglycemic rats	Ethanol (corrected from "Ethaol")	200 mg/kg, 400 mg/kg body weight	Glibenclamide (1 mg/kg)	Decreased blood glucose ($p < 0.01$)
Aloe barbadensis	Aloe	Asphode laceae	Gel	Alloxan-induced diabetic rat	Methanol	300 mg/kg body weight	Glibenclamide (0.25 mg/kg)	Reduced blood glucose level ($p < 0.05$)
Bryophyllum pinnatum	Goethe	Crassu laceae	Leaf	Alloxan-induced diabetic rat	Ethanol	200 mg/kg, 400 mg/kg body weight	Glibenclamide (2.5 mg/kg)	Reduced blood glucose level ($p < 0.05$)
Argemone mexicana	Mexican prickly poppy, Sialkanta	Papave raceae	Aerial parts	Alloxan-induced diabetic rat	Ethanol, Water	200 mg/kg, 400 mg/kg body weight	Glibenclamide (5 mg/kg)	Demonstrated significant anti-diabetic effect ($p < 0.05$)

Source: Zanzabil, K., Zohura, K., Hossain, M. S., & Hasan, M. K. (2023). Diabetes mellitus management: An extensive review of 37 medicinal plants. *Diabetology*, *4*(2), 186–234. https://doi.org/10.3390/diabetology4020019 (accessed on 29th May 2025).

An evaluation of clinical trials of herbs was published in 2023 by Elmi et al. Tables 5.13 and 5.14 summarizes these results.

Table 5.13. Clinical Trials of Herb Combinations in Diabetics

Combined Product	Plants	Administered Form	Participants	Intervention	Treatment Period	Results	References
Combined herbal capsule	*Galega officinalis* leaves, *Cinnamomum zeylanicum*, *Trigonella foenum-graecum* seeds, *Berberis vulgaris* fruit, and *Vaccinium bracteatum* thumb leaves	500 mg capsule	80	Combined herbal and placebo capsules were administered twice a day before meals to intervention and placebo groups, respectively	3 months	HbA1c, fasting blood sugar, and 2-hour postprandial were reduced significantly. Also, there were decreased serum lipids in patients with T2DM.	Ghafarzadegan et al. (2021)
Plantabetics capsule of fenugreek, Indian gooseberry, turmeric, and grape seed	*Curcuma longa*, *Trigonella foenum-graecum*, *Emblica officinalis*, and *Vitis vinifera*	350 mg capsule	50	One capsule two times daily was given alongside their diabetes medication	84 days	Reduced HbA1c and postprandial blood and fasting blood sugar	Banerji and Banerjee (2016)
Viabet capsule	*Cinnamomum cassia*, *Urtica dioica*, *Trigonella foenum-graecum*, *Stevia rebaudiana*, and *Cyamopsis tetragonoloba*	500 mg capsule	30	Viabet capsules of 500 mg and a placebo were given randomly to participants three times a day	3 months	HbA1c and body weight reduced significantly in the treatment group with no effects on fasting blood sugar	Tanzidi et al. (2023)

Source: Elmi, G. R., Anum, K., Saleem, K., Fareed, R., Noreen, S., Wei, H., Chen, Y., Chakraborty, A., Rehman, M. U., Liyuan, S., Abbas, M., & Duan, Y. (2023). Evaluation of clinical trials of ethnomedicine used for the treatment of diabetes: A systematic review. *Frontiers in Pharmacology, 14*, 1176618. https://doi.org/10.3389/fphar.2023.1176618 (accessed on 29th May 2025).

Table 5.14. Clinical Trials of Herbs in Diabetics*

Name	Botanical Name	Adminis tered Form	Partici pants	Intervention	Treatment Period	Results	References
Aloe	*Aloe vera*	300 mg dry gel capsule	240	Group A: Metformin + Glimepiride + rosuvastatin + 300 mg *Aloe vera* capsule twice daily	84 days	Reduced blood sugar, triglyceride, and cholesterol in Group A	Shoaib et al. (2022)
				Group B: Metformin + Glimepiride + rosuvastatin			
American ginseng	*Panax quinquefolius*	Extract capsules	38	3 g/day (1 capsule t.i.d.) taken 40 minutes before meals, along with lifestyle modification and pharmacotherapy; Corn starch (3 g/day) as control	8 weeks	↓ HbA1c and fasting glucose; ↓ blood lipids and systolic BP; ↑ nitric oxide (NO) due to improved endothelial function	Vuksan et al. (2019)
American ginseng + konjac fiber	*Panax quinquefolius* + konjac	Dried roots	39	6 g/day fiber (KGB) + 3 g/day ginseng along with standard care; corn starch (3 g/day) given to controls	12 weeks	Significantly reduced HbA1c and lipid levels	Jenkins et al. (2018)
Korean red + American ginseng	*Panax ginseng, P. quinquefolius*	Dried roots	80	AG + Rg3-KRG (2.25 g/day); wheat bran used as placebo	12 weeks	Greater reduction in HbA1c and serum lipids; no toxicity	Jovanovski et al. (2021)
Bilberry	*Vaccinium myrtillus*	Fruit	47	Group A: 200 g purée + 40 g dried bilberry/day	8 weeks	↑ Serum hippuric acid only in Group A, leading to ↓ fasting glucose and ↑ insulin secretion	DeMello et al. (2017)
				Group B: 100 g fresh strawberries, raspberries, cloudberries			
				Control: berry-restricted diet			

Bitter melon	*Momordica charantia*	500 mg dried fruit pulp capsules	24	500 mg capsules 4× daily; calcined magnesia as placebo	3 months	↓ Glucose AUC, HbA1c, 2-h glucose, weight, BMI, and fat %; ↑ insulin AUC and total insulin output	Cortez et al. (2018)
Cinnamon	*Cinnamomum cassia*	500 mg stem bark capsules	99	500 mg cinnamon capsule or placebo daily (randomized)	60 days	↓ Plasma glucose, HbA1c, triglycerides, and BP; ↑ HDL-C and eGFR	Sengsuk et al. (2016)
Ceylon cinnamon	*Cinnamomum zeylanicum*	Stem bark supplement capsule	30	85 mg (Month 1), 250 mg (Month 2), 500 mg (Month 3) daily	3 months	Anti-hyperlipidemic and BP-lowering effects in healthy adults; no hepatotoxicity or anti-coagulation toxicity observed	Ranasinghe et al. (2017a)
Fenugreek	*Trigonella foenum-graecum*	500 mg seed extract (Fenfuro)	154	500 mg Fenfuro twice daily	90 days	↓ Fasting sugar, HbA1c, and postprandial sugar; reduced need for anti-diabetic meds in 48.8% of patients	Verma et al. (2016)
Gymnema	*Gymnema sylvestre*	300 mg leaf powder capsules	30	300 mg Gymnema b.i.d. before meals; placebo to control group	12 weeks	↓ 2-h OGTT, HbA1c, and serum lipids; ↑ insulin sensitivity; reduced medication dosage in 48.8% of patients	Gaytán et al. (2021)
Garlic	*Allium sativum*	Aged garlic extract	26	1200 mg/day garlic extract or placebo for 4 weeks + 4-week washout	4 weeks	No significant improvement in vascular inflammation, oxidative stress, insulin resistance, or endothelial function	Atkin et al. (2016)

Ginger	*Zingiber officinale*	Root powder	45	2 g ginger powder (intervention) vs. 2 g wheat flour (placebo)	10 weeks	↓ ADMA serum concentration; minor ↓ in sICAM-1 in treatment group	Zarezadeh et al. (2019)
Jamun	*Syzygium cumini*	5 g/day seed powder	99	5 g twice daily before meals (treatment); placebo to control group	90 days	Significantly ↓ HbA1c, fasting, and postprandial glucose in treatment group	Sidana et al. (2017)
Psyllium	*Plantago ovata*	Psyllium seed husk	51	10 g psyllium in cookies twice daily vs. placebo cookies	12 weeks	↓ Body weight, HbA1c, fasting glucose, cholesterol, triglycerides; relieved constipation symptoms in T2DM	Noureddin et al. (2018)
Turmeric	*Curcuma longa*	700 mg rhizome powder capsules	80	700 mg capsule t.i.d. after meals; cornstarch flour to placebo group	8 weeks	↓ Body weight and lipids in hyperlipidemic T2DM patients	Adab et al. (2019)

*Interested Readers can access the back references in the reference column in the cited reference.

Source: Elmi, G. R., Anum, K., Saleem, K., Fareed, R., Noreen, S., Wei, H., Chen, Y., Chakraborty, A., Rehman, M. U., Liyuan, S., Abbas, M., & Duan, Y. (2023). Evaluation of clinical trials of ethnomedicine used for the treatment of diabetes: A systematic review. *Frontiers in Pharmacology, 14,* 1176618. https://doi.org/10.3389/fphar.2023.1176618 (accessed on 29th May 2025).

While the use of herbs shows potential, their approval for use is limited. Further research incorporating larger sample sizes and understanding mechanisms of dose-relation and phytochemical identification can pave the way for successful approval.

"Everything on the earth has a purpose, every disease and herb to cure it, and every person a mission. This is the Indian theory of existence."

—Mourning Dove (1994). "Mourning Dove: A Salishan Autobiography," p.69, U of Nebraska Press

5.3. Ayurveda, Traditional Chinese Medicine (TCM), and Other Approaches: What Does Research Say?

"Ayurveda is the science of life that teaches us how to live in harmony with nature and the world around us."

—***Dr. Robert Svoboda.***

Chattopadhyay et al. (2022) conducted a search of publications from inception to 16 January 2021 on the use of ayurvedic medicines for diabetes management. Analyses were done of 219 articles (from 32,519) with 98 medicines representing 199 RCTs (21,191 participants). The promise of ayurvedic medicines was highlighted, and serious adverse effects were not detected (apart from mild gastrointestinal issues). The levels of glycated hemoglobin were lowered with the use of *Aegle marmelos* (L.) Corrêa (MD −1.6%; 95% CI −3 to −0.3), *Nigella sativa* L. (−0.4; −0.6 to −0.1), *Momordica charantia* L. (−0.3; −0.4 to −0.1), *Tinospora cordifolia* (Willd.) Hook.f. & Thomson (−0.5; −0.6 to −0.5), etc. (Table 5.15).

Table 5.15. A Few of the Summarized Findings of Chattopadhyay et al. (2022) on the Potential of Ayurveda in Diabetes Management

***Cinnamomum aromaticum* Nees compared to comparator for T2DM management**

Patient or population: T2DM management
Intervention: *Cinnamomum aromaticum*
Comparison: comparator (i.e., no medicine, no additional medicine, or placebo)

Outcomes	Absolute effect (95% CI)	№ of participants (studies)	Certainty of the evidence (GRADE)	Comments
HbA1c	**MD 0.2 % lower** (0.5 lower to 0.1 higher)	794 (10 RCTs)	⊕⊕⊕◯ MODERATE [a]	
FBG	**MD 1 mg/dL higher** (6 lower to 9 higher)	692 (9 RCTs)	⊕⊕⊕⊕ HIGH	
HRQoL - not reported	-	-	-	
Adverse events	3 studies reported 0 adverse event (this includes 1 study which reported 0 adverse event in the intervention arm). 2 studies reported gastrointestinal tract and skin related adverse events (this includes 1 study which reported 0 adverse event in the intervention arm and 1 study which reported 0 adverse event in the comparator arm).	(5 RCTs)	⊕⊕⊕◯ MODERATE [b]	

CI: Confidence interval; **MD:** Mean difference

GRADE Working Group grades of evidence
High certainty: We are very confident that the true effect lies close to that of the estimate of the effect
Moderate certainty: We are moderately confident in the effect estimate: The true effect is likely to be close to the estimate of the effect, but there is a possibility that it is substantially different
Low certainty: Our confidence in the effect estimate is limited: The true effect may be substantially different from the estimate of the effect
Very low certainty: We have very little confidence in the effect estimate: The true effect is likely to be substantially different from the estimate of effect

Explanations
a. Publication bias detected in the funnel plot.
b. Selective outcome reporting.

Summary of Findings

***Aegle marmelos* (L.) Corrêa compared to comparator for T2DM management**

Patient or population: T2DM management
Intervention: *Aegle marmelos*
Comparison: comparator (i.e., no medicine, no additional medicine, or placebo)

Outcomes	Absolute effect (95% CI)	№ of participants (studies)	Certainty of the evidence (GRADE)	Comments
HbA1c	**MD 1.6 % lower** (3 lower to 0.3 lower)	210 (2 RCTs)	⊕⊕⊕◯ MODERATE [a]	
FBG	**MD 56 mg/dL lower** (104 lower to 9 lower)	228 (3 RCTs)	⊕◯◯◯ VERY LOW [a,b,c]	
HRQoL - not reported	-	-	-	
Adverse events	1 study reported 0 adverse event. Exact details were not provided in the other 2 studies.	(3 RCTs)	⊕⊕◯◯ LOW [a,d]	

CI: Confidence interval; **MD:** Mean difference

GRADE Working Group grades of evidence
High certainty: We are very confident that the true effect lies close to that of the estimate of the effect
Moderate certainty: We are moderately confident in the effect estimate: The true effect is likely to be close to the estimate of the effect, but there is a possibility that it is substantially different
Low certainty: Our confidence in the effect estimate is limited: The true effect may be substantially different from the estimate of the effect
Very low certainty: We have very little confidence in the effect estimate: The true effect is likely to be substantially different from the estimate of effect

Explanations
a. Small sample size.
b. Attrition bias.
c. Statistical heterogeneity.
d. Selective outcome reporting.

***Boswellia serrata* Roxb. compared to comparator for T2DM management**

Patient or population: T2DM management
Intervention: *Boswellia serrata*
Comparison: comparator (i.e., no medicine, no additional medicine, or placebo)

Outcomes	Absolute effect (95% CI)	№ of participants (studies)	Certainty of the evidence (GRADE)	Comments
HbA1c	**MD 0.5 % lower** (0.7 lower to 0.4 lower)	127 (2 RCTs)	⊕⊕⊕◯ MODERATE [a]	
FBG	**MD 24 mg/dL lower** (28 lower to 21 lower)	127 (2 RCTs)	⊕⊕⊕◯ MODERATE [a]	
HRQoL - not reported	-	-	-	
Adverse events	2 studies reported 0 adverse event (this includes 1 study which reported 0 adverse event in the intervention arm).	(2 RCTs)	⊕⊕◯◯ LOW [a,b]	

CI: Confidence interval; **MD:** Mean difference

GRADE Working Group grades of evidence
High certainty: We are very confident that the true effect lies close to that of the estimate of the effect
Moderate certainty: We are moderately confident in the effect estimate: The true effect is likely to be close to the estimate of the effect, but there is a possibility that it is substantially different
Low certainty: Our confidence in the effect estimate is limited: The true effect may be substantially different from the estimate of the effect
Very low certainty: We have very little confidence in the effect estimate: The true effect is likely to be substantially different from the estimate of effect

Explanations
a. Small sample size.
b. Selective outcome reporting.

***Tinospora cordifolia* (Willd.) Hook.f. & Thomson compared to comparator for T2DM management**

Patient or population: T2DM management
Intervention: *Tinospora cordifolia*
Comparison: comparator (i.e., no medicine, no additional medicine, or placebo)

Outcomes	Absolute effect (95% CI)	№ of participants (studies)	Certainty of the evidence (GRADE)	Comments
HbA1c	MD **0.5 % lower** (0.6 lower to 0.5 lower)	159 (2 RCTs)	⊕⊕⊕◯ MODERATE [a]	
FBG	MD **4 mg/dL lower** (6 lower to 3 lower)	140 (2 RCTs)	⊕⊕⊕◯ MODERATE [a]	
HRQoL - not reported	-	-	-	
Adverse events	2 studies reported 0 adverse event (this includes 1 study which reported 0 adverse event in the intervention arm).	(2 RCTs)	⊕⊕⊕◯ MODERATE [a]	

CI: Confidence interval; **MD:** Mean difference

GRADE Working Group grades of evidence
High certainty: We are very confident that the true effect lies close to that of the estimate of the effect
Moderate certainty: We are moderately confident in the effect estimate: The true effect is likely to be close to the estimate of the effect, but there is a possibility that it is substantially different
Low certainty: Our confidence in the effect estimate is limited: The true effect may be substantially different from the estimate of the effect
Very low certainty: We have very little confidence in the effect estimate: The true effect is likely to be substantially different from the estimate of effect

Explanations
a. Small sample size.

***Nigella sativa* L. compared to comparator for T2DM management**

Patient or population: T2DM management
Intervention: *Nigella sativa*
Comparison: comparator (i.e., no medicine, no additional medicine, or placebo)

Outcomes	Absolute effect (95% CI)	№ of participants (studies)	Certainty of the evidence (GRADE)	Comments
HbA1c	MD **0.4 % lower** (0.6 lower to 0.1 lower)	325 (4 RCTs)	⊕⊕⊕◯ MODERATE [a]	
FBG	MD **15 mg/dL lower** (30 lower to 0)	458 (7 RCTs)	⊕⊕⊕◯ MODERATE [b]	
HRQoL - not reported	-	-	-	
Adverse events	3 studies reported 0 adverse event (this includes 1 study which reported 0 adverse event in the intervention arm). 2 studies reported gastrointestinal tract related adverse events (this includes 1 study which reported 0 adverse event in the comparator arm and exact details were not provided in the other study).	(5 RCTs)	⊕⊕◯◯ LOW [a,c]	

CI: Confidence interval; **MD:** Mean difference

GRADE Working Group grades of evidence
High certainty: We are very confident that the true effect lies close to that of the estimate of the effect
Moderate certainty: We are moderately confident in the effect estimate: The true effect is likely to be close to the estimate of the effect, but there is a possibility that it is substantially different
Low certainty: Our confidence in the effect estimate is limited: The true effect may be substantially different from the estimate of the effect
Very low certainty: We have very little confidence in the effect estimate: The true effect is likely to be substantially different from the estimate of effect

Explanations
a. Small sample size.
b. Statistical heterogeneity.
c. Selective outcome reporting.

***Elettaria cardamomum* (L.) Maton compared to comparator for T2DM management**

Patient or population: T2DM management
Intervention: *Elettaria cardamomum*
Comparison: comparator (i.e., no medicine, no additional medicine, or placebo)

Outcomes	Absolute effect (95% CI)	№ of participants (studies)	Certainty of the evidence (GRADE)	Comments
HbA1c	MD **0.2 % higher** (0.2 lower to 0.5 higher)	164 (2 RCTs)	⊕⊕⊕◯ MODERATE [a]	
FBG	MD **1 mg/dL higher** (9 lower to 12 higher)	164 (2 RCTs)	⊕⊕⊕◯ MODERATE [a]	
HRQoL - not reported	-	-	-	
Adverse events	1 study reported 0 adverse event in the intervention arm. The other study reported adverse events (this study reported 0 adverse event in the comparator arm).	(2 RCTs)	⊕⊕⊕◯ MODERATE [a]	

CI: Confidence interval; **MD**: Mean difference

GRADE Working Group grades of evidence
High certainty: We are very confident that the true effect lies close to that of the estimate of the effect
Moderate certainty: We are moderately confident in the effect estimate: The true effect is likely to be close to the estimate of the effect, but there is a possibility that it is substantially different
Low certainty: Our confidence in the effect estimate is limited: The true effect may be substantially different from the estimate of the effect
Very low certainty: We have very little confidence in the effect estimate: The true effect is likely to be substantially different from the estimate of effect

Explanations
a. Small sample size

***Trigonella foenum-graecum* L. compared to comparator for T2DM management**

Patient or population: T2DM management
Intervention: *Trigonella foenum-graecum*
Comparison: comparator (i.e., no medicine, no additional medicine, or placebo)

Outcomes	Absolute effect (95% CI)	№ of participants (studies)	Certainty of the evidence (GRADE)	Comments
HbA1c	MD **0.6 % lower** (0.9 lower to 0.4 lower)	1095 (12 RCTs)	⊕⊕⊕◯ MODERATE [a]	
FBG	MD **14 mg/dL lower** (22 lower to 5 lower)	1069 (13 RCTs)	⊕⊕⊕◯ MODERATE [a,b]	
HRQoL - not reported	-	-	-	
Adverse events	5 studies reported 0 adverse event (this includes 2 studies which reported 0 adverse event in the intervention arm). 5 studies reported different body systems related adverse events but mainly gastrointestinal tract related and hypoglycemia (this includes 1 study which reported 0 adverse event in the comparator arm). Exact details were not provided in 1 study.	(11 RCTs)	⊕⊕⊕◯ MODERATE [c]	

CI: Confidence interval; **MD**: Mean difference

GRADE Working Group grades of evidence
High certainty: We are very confident that the true effect lies close to that of the estimate of the effect
Moderate certainty: We are moderately confident in the effect estimate: The true effect is likely to be close to the estimate of the effect, but there is a possibility that it is substantially different
Low certainty: Our confidence in the effect estimate is limited: The true effect may be substantially different from the estimate of the effect
Very low certainty: We have very little confidence in the effect estimate: The true effect is likely to be substantially different from the estimate of effect

Explanations
a. Publication bias.
b. Statistical heterogeneity.
c. Selective outcome reporting.

Source: Chattopadhyay, K., Wang, H., Kaur, J., Nalbant, G., Almaqhawi, A., Kundakci, B., Panniyammakal, J., Heinrich, M., Lewis, S. A., Greenfield, S. M., Tandon, N., Biswas, T. K., Kinra, S., & Leonardi-Bee, J. (2022). Effectiveness and safety of Ayurvedic medicines in type 2 diabetes mellitus management: A systematic review and meta-analysis. *Frontiers in Pharmacology*, *13*, 821810. https://doi.org/10.3389/fphar.2022.821810 (accessed on 29th May 2025).

Murudkar et al. (2022) presented antidiabetic formulations employed in Ayurvedic, traditional Chinese, and Unani systems. Their results are presented in Figure 5.5 and Table 5.16.

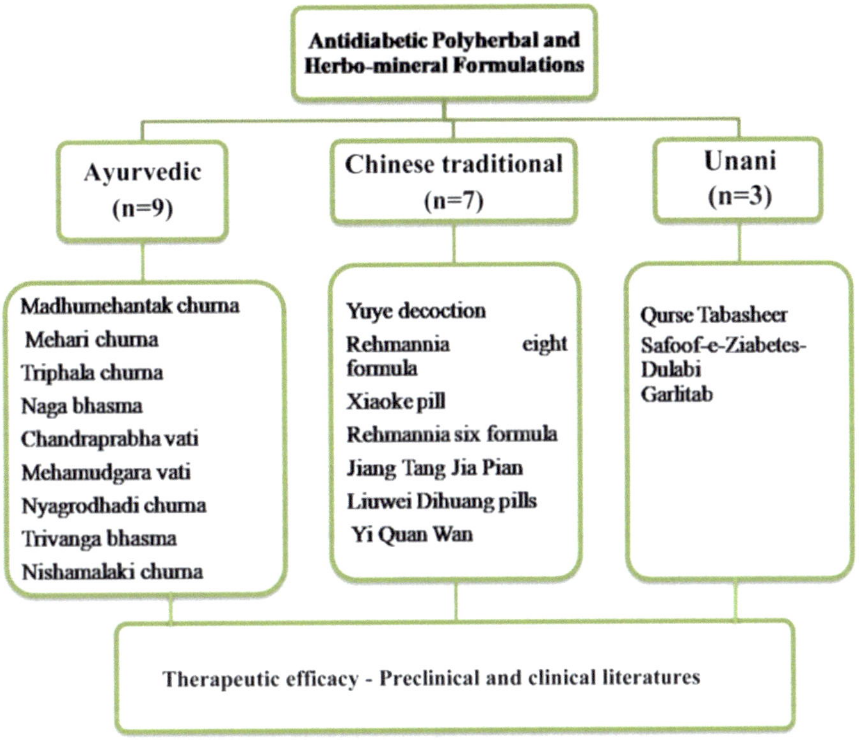

Figure 5.5. Review of antidiabetic formulations employed in Ayurvedic, traditional Chinese, and Unani systems.

Source: Murudkar, P. H., Tambe, M. S., Chandrasekar, S. B., Boddeda, B., & Pawar, A. T. (2022). Common Ayurvedic, Chinese traditional and Unani antidiabetic formulations – A review. *Frontiers in Pharmacology*, *13*, 991083. https://doi.org/10.3389/fphar.2022.991083 (accessed on 29th May 2025).

Table 5.16. Antidiabetic Formulations Employed in Ayurvedic, Traditional Chinese, and Unani Systems*

Formulation	Type of Study	Dose and Mode of Administration	Outcome Parameter	Improvement in Diabetes	References
Madhumehantak churna	*In vivo* (clinical trial)	4 g thrice daily, 30 min before food	Blood glucose level and HbA1c	Yes	Bhattacharya and Reddy (2016)
Mehari churna	*In vivo* (clinical trial)	1 to 2 teaspoonfuls with warm water	Blood glucose level and HbA1c	Yes	Kandalkar and Bhajipale (2016)
Triphala churna	*In vivo* (pre-clinical trial)	250, 500, and 1000 mg/kg	Urine parameters, plasma proteins, albumin, creatinine, blood urea nitrogen levels, and oxidative stress in the kidney	Yes	Ganeshpurkar et al. (2015); Suryavanshi et al. (2020)
Naga bhasma	*In vivo* (pre-clinical study)	100 and 200 mg/kg	Weight deviation and glucose tolerance test	Yes	Deshmukh et al. (2013)
Chandraprabha vati	*In vivo* (pre-clinical study)	50, 100, and 200 mg/kg	Fasting glucose levels, glucose tolerance test, cholesterol, and triglycerides	Yes	Wanjari et al. (2016)
Mehamudgara vati	*In vivo* (clinical trial)	Three tablets thrice a day	Fasting blood sugar, postprandial blood sugar in blood and urine, serum cholesterol, triglyceride, and high-density lipoprotein	Yes	Tanna et al. (2011)

Nyagrodhadi churna	*In vivo* (clinical trial)	Two tablets thrice daily with lukewarm water	Fasting and postprandial blood sugar, serum cholesterol, triglyceride, HDL, LDL, VLDL, fasting serum insulin, blood urea, and serum creatinine	Yes	Kumari et al. (2010)
Trivanga bhasma	*In vivo* (clinical trial)	200 mg/kg in water 200 mg/kg in honey	Various blood parameters; fasting blood sugar	Yes	Das et al. (2018)
Nishamalaki churna	*In vivo* (pre-clinical study)	900 and 1800 mg/kg	Blood glucose level	Yes	Dawane et al. (2016)
Yuye decoction	*In vivo* (pre-clinical study)	6.4, 12.7, and 25.4 g/kg	Fasting blood glucose, OGTT, ALT, AST, creatinine, BUN, LDL, total cholesterol, triglyceride, HDL, number and volume of islet cells	Yes	Liu et al. (2021)
Rehmannia Eight Formula	*In vivo* (pre-clinical study)	12 pills each time, three times daily	Blood glucose levels and lipid profile	Yes	Zhang et al. (2004)
Xiaoke Pill	*In vivo* (clinical trial)	Five pills per day	Blood glucose levels, HbA1c	Yes	Zhang et al. (2017)
Rehmannia Six Formula	*In vivo*	27 g/day	Frantic fever and spontaneous perspiration, total cholesterol, systolic BP, waist circumference, phosphatidylcholines, and Yin deficiencies	Yes	Poon et al. (2011); Wietmarschen et al. (2009)
Jiang Tang Jia Pian	*In vivo* (clinical trial)	40 mg tablets thrice a day	Glucose tolerance	76.3%	Grant et al. (2009)

Liuwei Dihuang pills	*In vivo* (pre-clinical study)	2.4 g/kg	Diabetic nephropathy, fasting blood glucose, total cholesterol, triglycerides, LDL-C, HbA1c, urine volume, urine sugar, and HDL-C	Yes	Lin et al. (2016); Wang et al. (2018)
Yu Quan Wan	*In vivo*	–	Proinflammatory cytokines, blood glucose levels, and glucose tolerance	Yes	Grant et al. (2009)
Qurse Tabasheer	–	–	–	–	Shaikh et al. (2016)
Safoof-e-Ziabetes-Dulabi	*In vivo* (pre-clinical study)	200 and 400 mg/kg	Serum alkaline phosphatase, total bilirubin, SGPT, and SGOT	Yes	Syed Hussain et al. (2020)
Garlitab	*In vivo* (pre-clinical study)	1.25 mg/kg once daily	Blood glucose level	Yes	Hossain (2015)

*The references have been included as presented-they can be accessed in Murudkar et al. (2022).

Source: Murudkar, P. H., Tambe, M. S., Chandrasekar, S. B., Boddeda, B., & Pawar, A. T. (2022). Common Ayurvedic, Chinese traditional and Unani antidiabetic formulations – A review. *Frontiers in Pharmacology, 13*, 991083. https://doi.org/10.3389/fphar.2022.991083 (accessed on 29th May 2025).

"Life (ayu) is the combination (samyoga) of body, senses, mind, and reincarnating soul. Ayurveda is the most sacred science of life, beneficial to humans both in this world and the world beyond."

—Charaka

In an interesting article by Bablis et al. (2024), a new approach entailing neuro-emotional technique (NET) was employed in a male with Type 2 Diabetes (46 years). The NET approach is a mind-body intervention (MBI) entailing 15 steps to locate and address Neuro-Emotional Complexes or stress patterns. The patient had glucose levels in the range of 10–15 mmol/L (the regular range is 4–10 mmol/L) had anxiety/stress (ACE-Q or Adverse Childhood Experiences Questionnaire score of 4) and was on insulin injections. The recommended approach was 8 sessions of NET over 4 weeks and the glucose levels were measured, along with psychometric tests at baseline and at the end.

The baseline glucose levels were above the "normal" range: after the treatment, the levels were in the normal range (as measured by "FreeStyle Libre 2": a continuous glucose monitoring (CGM) sensor). Further, mental health also documented an improvement as evidenced by the DASS-21 (depression, anxiety, and stress scale) Questionnaire, DRAM (distress and risk assessment method), and short form McGill pain questionnaire (SF-MPQ) (Figure 5.6).

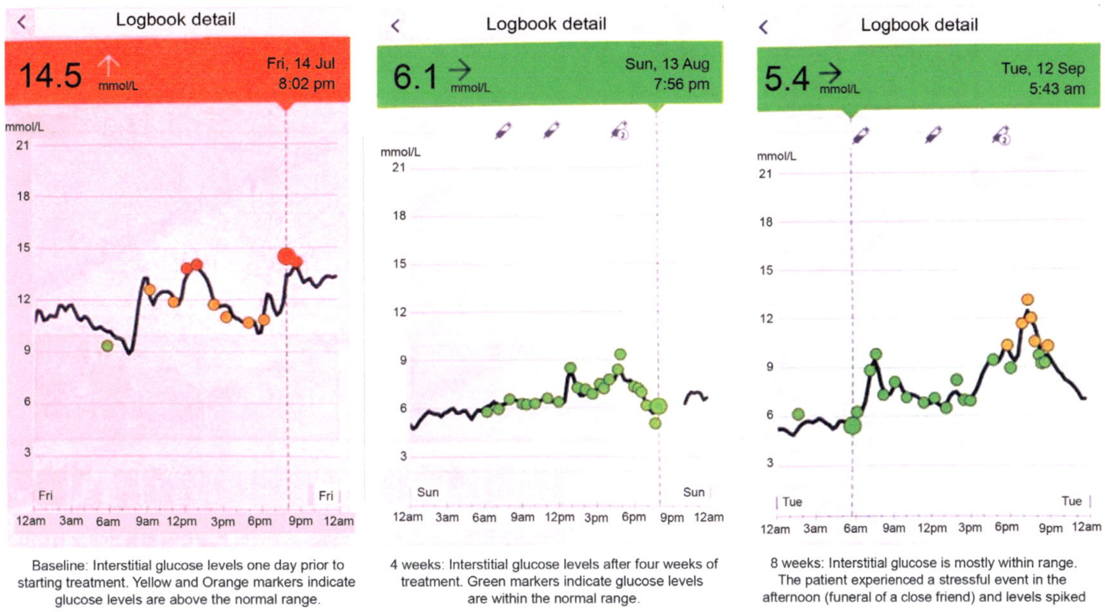

Figure 5.6. The effect of neuro-emotional technique (NET) on glucose levels in a 46-year-old male with type 2 diabetes.

Source: Bablis, P., Day, R. R., & Pollard, H. (2024). Treatment of type 2 diabetes and stress using neuro-emotional technique: Case report. *Frontiers in Endocrinology (Lausanne)*, *15*, 1382757. https://doi.org/10.3389/fendo.2024.1382757 (accessed on 29th May 2025).

Given the promise of this approach, the use of MBI techniques can be recommended as supplementary therapy. Further studies can support these findings.

Rodríguez et al. (2023) reviewed patents filed for natural products/isolated substances to highlight the potential of such alternative approaches to manage diabetes. Notwithstanding the promise, the stringent checking of safety profiles and rigorous tests can pave the way for natural product-based management (Table 5.17).

Table 5.17. Natural Product Patents for Diabetes in the European Patent Office (EPO): 2016–2022

Year	Country	Registration Number	Species	Part of the Plant	Secondary Metabolites	Mechanism of Action	Formulation	Safety Asses sments	Efficacy Tests
2020	WO	WO202 0115767 (A1)	*Premna herbacea*	Leaves	Isoverbascoside	Improved insulin signaling via the AKT/AMPK pathway	ND	A single dose of 2000 mg/ kg of *P. herbacea* methanol extract was reported as safe in Swiss ICR male mice (acute toxicity test).	*In vitro*: (a) Uptake of glucose in L6 cells; (b) Lipid accumulation in HepG2 cells by Oil Red O staining. *In vivo*: ND Clinical studies: ND
2020	US	US1100 7237 (B2); US2020147160 (A1)	*Pinus* spp.	Resin	ND	α-Glucosidase inhibition	Syrup, tablets, capsules, granules, powders	ND	*In vitro*: (a) Suppression of α-glucosidase activity; (b) Glucose uptake potential. Clinical studies: ND
2020	WO	WO2020 012299 (A1)	*Curcuma longa*, *Phyllanthus emblica*	ND	ND	Insulin sensitization and antihyper glycemic action	ND	Non-cytotoxic doses confir med by cytot oxicity assay and PPARγ expression in fibr oblasts using MTT assay.	*In vitro*: PPARγ expression in fibroblasts. *In vivo*: STZ-induced insulin resistance in rats. Clinical studies: ND

2019	SG	SG11201 908574T (A)	*Curcuma longa, Emblica officinalis, Vernonia anthelmintica, Tinospora cordifolia, Trigonella foenum-graecum, Ixora coccinea, Syzygium cumini*	ND	Tannins, organic acids, curcuminoids	ND	Powders, pastes, granules, capsules, tablets, emulsions, suspensions, syrup, elixir, oral drops, nutraceuticals	Safe after acute toxicity test in Swiss ICR mice (male and female).	*In vitro*: Glucose uptake in L6 rat skeletal muscle cells. *In vivo*: ND Clinical studies: ND
2019	WO	WO2019 205943 (A1)	*Polygonatum* spp., *Poria cocos, Lycium barbarum, Pueraria, Panax ginseng, Lentinula edodes* (shiitake), *Cordyceps, Ganoderma lucidum, Hericium erinaceus, Tremella, Dendrobium officinale*	ND	Flavonoids and oligosacc harides (inulin, fructooligosa ccharides)	Reduced Firmicutes/ Bacteroides ratio in the gut microbiota	ND	Prepa ration reported as safe (method not detailed).	*In vitro*: ND *In vivo*: Oral glucose tolerance test in mice Clinical studies: ND
2019	WO	WO2019 186579 (A1)	*Trigonella foenum-graecum, Solanum lycopersicum, Lagenaria siceraria* (dudhi bhopla), *Vitis vinifera, Medicago sativa*	Roots, stems, leaves, buds, flowers, fruits, seeds	Osmotin	Adiponectin mimetic; AMPK pathway activation	Tablets, syrup, granules, transmucosal film	ND	*In vitro*: ND *In vivo*: ND Clinical studies: ND

2019	US	US1096 7025 (B2); US20192 09634 (A1)	*Moringa oleifera*, *Origanum vulgare*, *Shilajit*, *Phyllanthus emblica*, *Piper nigrum*, *Salvia rosmarinus*, *Punica granatum*, *Trigonella foenum-graecum*, *Curcuma longa*, blue-green algae	Leaves, fruits, seeds	Polyphenols, carvacrol, phycocyanin	Antioxidant, anti-inflammatory (COX-1 inhibition)	Capsules	ND	*In vitro*: (a) ROS scavenging; (b) DPPH assay; (c) LDL oxidation; (d) Insulin release in rat islets; (e) COX-1 enzyme inhibition. *In vivo*: ND Clinical studies: ND
2019	WO	WO2019 088958 (A2); WO2019 088958 (A3)	*Paliurus spina-christi*	Fruits	Naringenin	Regulates ALT, AST, insulin secretion, glucose, antioxidant levels, and magnesium absorption	ND	ND	*In vitro*: ND *In vivo*: STZ-induced diabetic rats Clinical studies: ND
2019	MX	MX2018 004489 (A)	*Agavaceae* spp.	Leaves, rhizomes, mead	Steroidal saponins and sapogenins (e.g., kammogenin, manogenin)	Improves glucose and lipid metabolism, energy expenditure, oxidative capacity, thermogenesis (via PGC-1α, UCP1, AMPK)	Pills, capsules	ND	*In vitro*: ND *In vivo*: ND Clinical studies: ND
2019	US	US10640 480 (B2); US2019 031635 (A1)	*Gnetum gnemon*	Fruits	Gnetin C	Antioxidant, antibacterial, inhibition of lipase, α-glucosidase, α-amylase	Powders, granules, tablets, capsules	ND	*In vitro*: ND *In vivo*: ND Clinical studies: ND

2019	AU	AU2018 278958 (A1); AU2018 278958 (B2)	*Cichorium endivia*, *Lactuca sativa* (var. *latifolia*, *longifolia*), *Asteraceae*, *Lamiaceae*, *Brassicaceae*, *Amaranthaceae* spp.	Fruits, leaves, stems, roots	ND	IRS2 pathway activation	ND	ND	*In vitro*: ND *In vivo*: ND Clinical studies: ND
2019	US	US105 76117 (B2); US2019 125816 (A1)	*Salacia chinensis*, *Gymnema sylvestre*, *Emblica officinalis*, *Eugenia jambolana*, *Curcuma longa*, *Commiphora mukul*, *Tinospora cordifolia*, *Withania somnifera*, *Terminalia chebula*, *Andrographis paniculata*, etc.	Roots, fruits, bark, leaves, flowers, seeds, gum, stems	ND	Hypogl ycemic, hypolip idemic, pancreatic regeneration, tissue enzyme modulation, FBS, PPBS, HbA1c reduction	Tablets, granules, capsules, solution, suspension, emulsion	OECD-compliant safety in rodents (tests 423, 407, 408, 452).	*In vitro*: ND *In vivo*: Alloxan-diabetic Wistar rats Clinical studies: Phase III, open-label, non-randomized study at Muniyal Ayurvedic Hospital, Manipal, India
2017	US	US106681 22 (B2); US20172 52393 (A1)	*Toona sinensis*	Leaves	Monoterpenes, diterpenes, triterpenes, sesquiterpenes, saturated and unsaturated fatty acids	Improves glucose absorption, lipid degradation, and metabolic syndrome prevention	ND	ND	*In vitro*: (a) 24-h glucose consumption in 3T3-L1 cells; (b) Adipogenesis inhibition by TSL-SCF; (c) Antidiabetic effects of polar TSL components. *In vivo*: ND Clinical studies: ND

2017	US	US10111923 (B2); US2017173103 (A1)	*Cyclocarya paliurus*, *Puerariae lobatae* radix, *Polygonatum odoratum* rhizome	ND	ND	ND	Pills, capsules, granules, powders, tea	ND	*In vitro*: ND *In vivo*: STZ-induced diabetic rats Clinical studies: ND
2017	NZ	NZ630125 (A)	*Calophyllum inophyllum*	Cortex	ND	Inhibits DGAT-1 and SCD-1 activity	Tablets, capsules, powders, elixir, syrup	ND	*In vitro*: DGAT-1, SCD-1 assays, triglyceride synthesis in HepG2 cells. *In vivo*: STZ-induced diabetic rats on high-fat diet. Clinical studies: ND
2016	US	US2016361341 (A1); US9828442 (B2)	*Hirsutella sinensis*	ND	Polysaccharides	Reduces hyperglycemia and improves insulin sensitivity	ND	ND	*In vitro*: ND *In vivo*: STZ-induced diabetic rats on high-fat diet Clinical studies: ND
2016	US	US10028930 (B2); US2016228400 (A1)	*Ephedra sinica* and brown algae concentrate	ND	Fucoxanthin, caffeine, ephedrine	Thermogenic potentiation	Extended-release tablets, transdermal patches	ND	*In vitro*: ND *In vivo*: ND Clinical studies: ND

2016	US	US10799547 (B2); US2016067294 (A1)	*Suaeda japonica*	Leaves, seeds	ND	The cytoprotective activity of pancreatic β-cells, hypoglycemic action, insulin secretion increase, improvement of glucose tolerance, and increase of adiponectin content in the blood.	Pills, powders, granules, capsules	ND	*In vitro*: ND *In vivo*: Overfed diabetic OLETF mice Clinical studies: ND
2016	UA	UA104161 (U)	*Equisetum arvense*, *Sambucus* spp., *Hypericum perforatum*, *Tilia* spp., *Polygonum aviculare*, *Urtica* spp., *Inula helenium*, *Vaccinium myrtillus*	Flowers, leaves, rhizomes, roots	Ascorbic acid, tannins, flavonoids, organic and hydroxycinnamic acids	GLP-1 related hypoglycemia, ↑ insulin, improved carbohydrate and lipid metabolism	ND	ND	*In vitro*: ND *In vivo*: Alloxan-induced diabetic female rats Clinical studies: ND

Abbreviations: WO: World Intellectual Property Organization (WIPO); xUS: United States; SG: Singapore; MX: Mexico; AU: Australia; NZ: New Zealand; UA: Ukraine; AKT/AMPK: Protein kinase B or AKT / AMP-activated protein kinase; ICR: Cancer Research Institute; PPARγ: Peroxisome proliferator-activated receptor gamma; COX-1: Cyclooxygenase-1; ROS: Reactive oxygen species; DPPH: 2,2-Diphenyl-1-picrylhydrazyl; LDL: Low-density lipoproteins; ALT: Alanine aminotransferase; AST: Aspartate aminotransferase; PGC-1α: Peroxisome proliferator-activated receptor gamma coactivator 1-alpha; UCP1: Uncoupling protein 1 or thermogenin; IRS2: Insulin receptor substrate 2; FBS: Fasting blood sugar; PPBS: Postprandial blood sugar; HbA1c: Glycosylated hemoglobin; TS-SCF: *T. sinensis*–supercritical carbon dioxide fluid; TSL-SCF: Hojas de *T. sinensis*–supercritical carbon dioxide fluid; DGAT-1: Diacylglycerol O-acyltransferase 1; Human hDGAT-1: Human diacylglycerol acyltransferase-1; SCD-1: Stearoyl-CoA desaturase-1.

Source: Rodríguez, I. A., Serafini, M., Alves, I. A., Lang, K. L., Silva, F. R. M. B., & Aragón, D. M. (2023). Natural products as outstanding alternatives in diabetes mellitus: A patent review. *Pharmaceutics*, *15*(1), 85. https://doi.org/10.3390/pharmaceutics15010085 (accessed on 29th May 2025).

When looking at acupuncture, the effects of acupuncture in handling diabetic neuropathy were summarized by Chu et al. (2021). Among the studies that predominantly employed ST36, BL13, BL20, SP6, and SP9 points, the potential of acupuncture was outlined (only minor side effects like numbness were reported) (Table 5.18).

Table 5.18. Studies Employing Acupuncture for Diabetes in Humans

Author	**Characteristics of Patients**	**Acupuncture Treatment** ① **Acupuncture Types** ② **Acupoints** ③ **Retention Time** ④ **Treatment Duration (Sessions)** ⑤ **Conventional Treatment** ⑥ **Control to Acupuncture** **Patients-Related Outcomes**		**Outcomes** **Nerve-Function Outcomes**	
Abuaisha et al. (1998)	Participants: $n = 44$	①	Manual acupuncture	Improvement in primary (74.9 ± 2.4 to 44.5 ± 4.3) and secondary (70.3 ± 2.9 to 43.5 ± 4.2) symptoms was observed in 34/44 patients (77%) Complete symptom relief after treatment was observed in 7 out of 34 patients (21%). No significant change in NDS (7.3 ± 0.5 to 7.2 ± 0.7).	No significant change in VPT (30.4 ± 1.9 to 31.1 ± 2.2 volts)
		②	*LI3, SP6, SP9, ST36*		
		③	20 min (first week: 5 min)		
		④	10 weeks (6)		
		⑤	Analgesics, tricyclic drugs, anticonvulsants (63%)		
		⑥	–		

Jiang et al. (2006)	Participants: n = 90 Wrist-ankle acupuncture: n = 30 Body acupuncture: n = 30 Control: n = 30	①	Manual acupuncture	Wrist-ankle acupuncture: 56.67% markedly relieved, 36.67% improved. Body acupuncture: 56.67% markedly relieved, 33.33% improved. Control: 23.33% markedly relieved, 40.00% improved.	Wrist-ankle acupuncture: Improved CV of median (42.12 ± 3.80 → 46.87 ± 5.57 m/s) and common peroneal nerve (41.42 ± 4.47 → 45.45 ± 4.82 m/s). Body acupuncture: Improved CV of median (42.17 ± 4.51 → 45.48 ± 4.92 m/s) and common peroneal nerve (42.12 ± 4.63 → 45.37 ± 4.90 m/s) Control: No change in CV of median (42.22 ± 4.90 → 43.15 ± 5.24 m/s) and common peroneal nerve (42.04 ± 4.53 → 43.91 ± 5.51 m/s)
		②	Wrist-ankle acupuncture: upper 2 and lower 2 Body acupuncture: SP6, SP10, KI3, LI11, GB34 Additional acupoints according to symptoms were applied to both groups		
		③	15–30 min		
		④	25 days (21)		
		⑤	–		
		⑥	VB_1 and VB_{12}, i.m.		
Zhang et al. (2010)	Participants: n = 65 Acupuncture: *n* = 32 Control: *n* = 33	①	Manual acupuncture	Acupuncture: 16 markedly relieved, 12 improved, 4 failed Control: 7 markedly relieved, 14 improved, 12 failed	–
		②	BL18, BL20, BL23, BL58, ST36, SP6, SP3, CV6, CV4, ST40, GB34, Ex-B3 + acupoints according to symptoms		
		③	25 min		
		④	3 months (70)		
		⑤	–		
		⑥	Inositol, p.o., 2 g/day		

Tong et al. (2010)	Participants: $n = 63$ Acupuncture: $n = 42$ Control: $n = 21$	①	Manual acupuncture	Improved numbness of lower extremities Improved spontaneous pain of lower extremities. Improved rigidity in upper extremities Improved alterations in temperature perception in lower extremities	Improved F-wave minimum latency in tibial nerve (52.6 ± 0.5 → 53.0 ± 0.3 m/s) Improved MNCV in tibial nerve (39.5 ± 0.5 → 40.2 ± 3.9 m/s) Improved FCV in median nerve (55.6 ± 0.4 → 56.5 ± 0.5 m/s) Improved SNCV of forearm (47.8 ± 0.5 → 48.3 ± 0.7 m/s) Improved VPT (8.05 ± 3.22 → 8.56 ± 3.43 s)
		②	LI4, ST40, LI11, ST36, SP6		
		③	30 min		
		④	15 days (15)		
		⑤	–		
		⑥	0.3 cm (vs. 1.2–2.3 cm) needle insertion without stimulation		
Garrow et al. (2014)	Participants: $n = 45$ Acupuncture: $n = 24$ Control: $n = 21$	①	Manual acupuncture	Improved LANSS score (14.3 ± 6.4 → 13.6 ± 7.2) Improved VAS pain intensity (73 ± 24 → 58 ± 26) Improved MYMOP score (4.3 ± 1.2 → 3.4 ± 1.3) Improved SF-36 physical component score (40.7 ± 13.2 → 39.2 ± 14.0) No change in SF-36 bodily pain score (37.7 ± 27.4 → 40.2 ± 20.2)	–
		②	*LR3, KI3, SP6, ST36*		
		③	30 min		
		④	10 weeks (10)		
		⑤	–		
		⑥	Sham acupuncture (blunt and slides into the handle)		
Jeon et al. (2015)	Participants: $n = 9$	①	Manual acupuncture	No significant change in TSS score (7.99 ± 3.55 → 4.95 ± 4.41) No significant change in MNSI score (6.33 ± 1.31 → 4.33 ± 3.00)	–
		②	Ex-LE10, LR3, GB34, GB39, GB41, ST36, SP6, SP9		
		③	21–28 min		
		④	4 weeks (12)		
		⑤	–		
		⑥	–		

Bailey et al. (2017)	Participants: $n = 25$	①	Manual acupuncture	Improved NTSS-6 scores: aching pain (2.4 ± 0.6 → 1.6 ± 0.5), burning pain (1.7 ± 0.7 → 1.0 ± 0.6), tingling and prickling (2.2 ± 0.5 → 1.2 ± 0.6), numbness (1.7 ± 0.6 → 1.0 ± 0.6), allodynia (1.9 ± 0.6 → 1.2 ± 0.7) No significant difference in NTSS-6 scores: lancinating pain (2.0 ± 0.6 → 1.6 ± 0.6) NDS (5.2 ± 3.6 → 4.9 ± 3.4)	–
		②	Ex-LE10, ST32, ST37, ST42, SP7, SP9, KI1, KI3, KI9, LR4, LR7, GB34, GB37		
		③	30 min		
		④	10 weeks (10)		
		⑤	–		
		⑥	–		
Shin et al. (2018)	Participants: $n = 126$ Acupuncture: $n = 63$ Control: $n = 63$	①	EA (2/120 Hz)	Improved PI-NRS scores (−0.67 [95% CI −1.29 to −0.06] vs. control) at week 9 Improved short-form McGill Pain Questionnaire, sleep interference scores, and EuroQol-5 Dimensions at week 9	No significant difference in nerve conduction velocity
		②	ST36, GB39, SP9, SP6, LR3, GB41 + additional acupoints according to symptoms (Ex-LE10)		
		③	–		
		④	8 weeks (16)		
		⑤	Anti-diabetes and rescue medication allowed (acetaminophen 500 mg, max 3000 mg/day)		
		⑥	No EA treatment		
Chao et al. (2019)	Participants: $n = 40$ Acupuncture (1/week): $n = 14$ Acupuncture (2/week): $n = 12$ Control: $n = 14$	①	Manual acupuncture	Improved NRS score (between-group differences): Average pain intensity (−1.86 [week 6], −2.06 [week 12]) Worst pain intensity (−1.88 [week 6], −2.34 [week 12]) Least pain intensity (−1.24 [week 6], −1.46 [week 12])	–
		②	Jing-well and shu-stream acupoints + acupoints according to symptoms (8–12 acupoints)		
		③	20–40 min.		
		④	12 weeks (12 and 24)		
		⑤	Antidepressants, opiates, and anticonvulsants		
		⑥	No acupuncture treatment		

Meyer-Hamme et al. (2020)	Participants: *n* = 120 Acupuncture: *n* = 60 Laser acupuncture: *n* = 60 Control: *n* = 60	①	Manual and laser acupuncture	Improved 12/12 items of patient-related outcomes in acupuncture group Improved 11/12 items of patient-related outcomes (exclusion: hyperesthesia) in laser acupuncture group Improved 9/12 items of patient-related outcomes (exclusions: hyperesthesia, heat sensation, muscle cramps) in control	Improved sural SNAP (μV) in all three groups Improved sural SNCV (m/s) in manual and laser acupuncture groups Improved tibial MNCV (m/s) in manual acupuncture group No significant difference in tibial MNAP (mV) in any group
		②	Ex-LE10, Ex-LE12, ST34		
		③	20 min		
		④	10 weeks (10)		
		⑤	–		
		⑥	Laser acupuncture without laser		

Abbreviations: Ach: Acetylcholine; CV: Conduction velocity; FCV: F-wave conduction velocity; HbA1c: Glycosylated hemoglobin; LANSS: Leeds Assessment of Neuropathic Symptoms and Signs; LDF: Laser Doppler fluxmetry; LDS: Neuropathy Disability Score; MNAP: Motor nerve action potential; MNCV: Motor nerve conduction velocity; MNSI: Michigan Neuropathy Screening Instrument; MYMOP: Measure Yourself Medical Outcome Profile; NDS: Neuropathy Disability Score; NRS: Numerical rating scale; NS: Non-significant; NTSS: Neuropathy Total Symptom Scale; PI-NRS: Pain Intensity Numerical Rating Scale; SF-36: Short Form 36; SNAP: Sensory nerve action potential; SNCV: Sensory nerve conduction velocity; SNP: Sodium nitroprusside; SPS: Sleep Problem Scale; TSS: Total Symptom Score; VAS: Visual analog scale; VB: Vitamin B; VPT: Vibration perception threshold.

Source: Cho, E., & Kim, W. (2021). Effect of acupuncture on diabetic neuropathy: A narrative review. *International Journal of Molecular Sciences, 22*(16), 8575. https://doi.org/10.3390/ijms22168575 (accessed on 29th May 2025).

Chapman et al. (2015) reviewed 45 RCTs assessing the efficacy of psychological therapy (cognitive behavioral therapy [CBT] and motivational interviewing [MI]) in Chinse patients with T2DM or non-insulin-dependent diabetes mellitus (NIDDM). Interestingly, they noted lowered levels of glycated hemoglobin due to (CBT: –0.97 [95% CI –1.37 to –0.57]; MI: –0.71 [95% CI –1.00 to –0.43]). Notwithstanding the promise of these mindfulness interventions, the issues of bias and heterogeneity would need to be addressed (Table 5.19).

Table 5.19. The Role of Psychological Therapy (Cognitive Behavioral Therapy [CBT] and Motivational Interviewing [MI]) in Chinese Patients with T2DM or Non-Insulin-Dependent Diabetes Mellitus

Number of Participants Recruited/ at Follow-Up	Mean Age ± SD (or Range) (Years)	Clinical Subgroup	Mean Duration of Diabetes ± SD (or Range) (Years)	Setting	Model and Duration of Therapy in Intervention Group	Regimen in Intervention Group and Specialty of Therapist	Model and Duration of Therapy in Control Group	Regimen in Control Group and Specialty of Therapist	Follow-Up (Months from Baseline)	Outcome Measures of Relevance
60/60	72.9 ± 9.6	Depression	8.6 ± 3.0	Hospital (I)	Individual CBT[a] for 2 months	CBT sessions consisting of relaxation training, music relaxation therapy, emotional adjustment, and psychological support by nurse (number of sessions and manualization not specified)	UC for 2 months	Usual nutrition and medication for DM and depression by doctor and nurse (regimen not specified)	2	FBG and HAM-D
100/95	NS	General	NS	Community health	Individual MI for 12 months	31 MI sessions (therapist and manualization NS)	UC for 12 months	UC (regimen and therapist NS)	12	WHOQoL-BREF
105/105	NS	General	NS	Hospital (I and O)	Individual CBT[a] for 2 months	8 CBT sessions consisting of *Morita* therapy, emotional adjustment, and psychological support (therapist and manualization NS)	UC for 2 months	Usual medication (regimen and therapist NS)	2	QOL-I
80/80	47.7 ± 10.8	Depression and anxiety	NS	Hospital (I)	Individual CBT[a] and family therapy for 2 weeks	CBT sessions consisting of emotional adjustment, music relaxation therapy, psychological support, and family therapy by doctor and nurse (number of sessions and manualization NS)	UC for 2 weeks	UC consisting of nutrition, medication, education, and supportive psychological nursing by nurse (regimen NS)	0.5	SAS, SDS
72/72	66.0 ± 17.4	General	6.8 ± 14.9	Hospital (I)	Individual CBT[a] for 2 months	20 CBT sessions consisting of rational emotive therapy and relaxation training (therapist and manualization NS)	UC for 2 months	UC and education by doctor and nurse (regimen NS)	2	SAS, SDS

60/60	41.5 ± 8.1	General	2.3 ± 0.2	NS	Individual MI and exercise therapy for 6 months	6 MI sessions and 72 sessions of moderate-intensity exercise training, all by nurse (manualization NS)	Exercise therapy and education for 6 months	72 sessions of moderate-intensity exercise training (therapist NS); 6 education sessions consisting of the benefits of exercise and exercise-related knowledge (therapist NS)	6	HbA1c, FBG, and DQoL
60/60	53.0 ± 10.6	Depression and anxiety	6.4 ± 3.1	Hospital (I and O)	Individual CBT and group education for 1 month	8 CBT sessions consisting of behavior modification, planning, stress management, and psychological support (therapist NS); group education (number of sessions, therapist, and manualization NS)	UC for 1 month	Usual nutrition, exercise, and medication (regimen and therapist NS)	1	HbA1c, FBG, SAS, and SDS
132/132	49.6 ± 12.0	General	6.1 ± 3.1	Hospital (I)	Individual CBT for 1 month	8 CBT sessions consisting of behavior modification, relaxation training, music relaxation therapy, psychological support, and family therapy by psychologist (manualization NS)	UC for 1 month	Usual medication/ insulin treatment (regimen and therapist NS)	1	HbA1c, FBG, SAS, and SDS
62/62	58.6 ± 7.5	Depression	6.1 ± 2.6	Community health	Individual and group CBT for 3 months	14 CBT sessions by doctor and endocrinologist (manualization NS)	UC for 3 months	UC (regimen and therapist NS)	5	HbA1c, FBG, and SDS
598/598	56.4 ± 11.6	General	4.8 ± 3.9	Hospital (O)	Individual CBT[a] and individual and group education for 7 months	CBT consisting of behavior modification and planning (number of sessions, therapist, and manualization NS), and individual and group education sessions (number of sessions and therapist NS)	UC for 7 months	UC and usual medication (regimen and therapist NS)	7	HbA1c and FBG

120/105	57.0 ± 8.5	General	5.3 ± 2.2	Hospital (I and O)	Individual CCT[a] and health education for 6 months	12 non-directive counseling sessions with an emphasis on positive thinking by therapist; education sessions by doctor and therapist (number of sessions and manualization NS)	UC for 6 months	UC (regimen and therapist NS)	6	HbA1c and FBG
87/87	51.6 ± 8.0	General	5.3 ± 4.4	Hospital (I)	Individual CBT[a], family therapy, and group education for 3 months	12–24 CBT sessions consisting of behavior modification, exercise therapy, psychological support, and family therapy; 12 education sessions by psychiatric attending physician (manualization NS)	UC for 3 months	UC and usual medication (regimen and therapist NS)	3	HbA1c, FBG, SAS, and SDS
108/108	50.9 ± 11.1	Depression	4.6 ± 3.4	Hospital (I and O)	Individual CBT for 6 weeks	CBT sessions consisting of relaxation training, music relaxation therapy, planning, and psychological support (number of sessions, therapist, and manualization NS)	UC for 6 weeks	UC (regimen and therapist NS)	1.5	HbA1c, FBG, and HAM-D
86/86	53.0 ± 8.2	General	6.3 ± 2.2	Hospital (I)	Individual CBT for 1 month	8 CBT sessions consisting of stress management, behavior modification, planning, and psychological support by psychologist (manualization NS)	UC for 1 month	Usual nutrition, exercise, and medication (regimen and therapist NS)	1	SDS
94/94	53.1 ± 7.4	Nephro pathy	NS	Hospital (I)	Individual and group CBT for 6 months	24 CBT sessions by psychologist (manualization NS)	UC for 6 months	UC consisting of education, glucose monitoring, nutrition, exercise, and monitoring of blood glucose, BP, and lipids (regimen and therapist NS)	6	HbA1c, FBG, SAS, and SDS
438/438	51.6 ± NS	General	NS	Hospital (I)	Individual CBT for 1 month	CBT sessions by DM health professional (number of sessions and manualization NS)	UC for 1 month	Usual medication (regimen and therapist NS)	1	HbA1c, FBG, SAS, and SDS

82/80	56.8 ± 13.2	General	5.5 ± 4.7	Hospital (I and O)	Individual CBT[a] for 1 month	8 CBT sessions consisting of relaxation training and psychological support (therapist and manualization NS)	UC for 1 month	UC (regimen and therapist NS)	1	HbA1c, FBG, and SCL-90
60/60	51.2 ± 11.7	General	3.3 ± 3.7	Hospital (I)	Individual CBT[a] for 1 month	10 CBT sessions consisting of rational emotive therapy by diabetes specialist nurse (manualization NS)	UC and education for 1 month	UC and education (regimen and therapist NS)	1	SCL-90
118/118	NS (40–80)	Depression	6.0 ± 7.0	Hospital (I)	Individual CBT for 1 month	3–4 CBT sessions consisting of cognitive restructuring, relaxation training, and psychological support (therapist and manualization NS)	UC for 1 month	UC (regimen and therapist NS)	1	HbA1c, FBG, SAS, and SDS
72/72	53.1 ± 11.0	General	NS	Hospital (I)	Individual and group CBT and family therapy for 6 months	CBT sessions and family therapy by psychiatrist (number of sessions, therapist, and manualization NS)	UC for 6 months	Usual medication (regimen and therapist NS)	6	SCL-90 and DSQoL
63/63	63.1 (60–79)	Elderly (60+)	NS	Hospital (Military Psychiatric Hospital) (I)	Individual CBT[a] and group education for 2 weeks	10 sessions of *Qigong* relaxation training, 10 sessions of music relaxation therapy, and 4 group education sessions all by doctor (manualization NS)	UC for 2 weeks	UC (regimen and therapist NS)	0.5	HAM-A and SCL-90
96/96	56.8 ± 3.9	General	7.5 (3–12)	Hospital (I)	Individual CCT[a] and individual and group education for 3 months	Non-directive counseling sessions with an emphasis on improvement of self-esteem and positive thinking by psychologist (number of sessions and manualization NS); education sessions by DM specialist and nurse (number of sessions NS)	UC for 3 months	UC (regimen and therapist NS)	3	HbA1c, FBG, and SDS
67/67	44.5 ± 11.0	Depression and anxiety	4.6 ± 3.4	Hospital (I and O)	Individual and group CBT[a] for 6 weeks	6 CBT sessions consisting of relaxation training, behavior modification, and psychological support by psychiatric attending physician (manualization NS)	UC for 6 weeks	Usual medication (regimen and therapist NS)	1.5	HbA1c, FBG, SAS, and SDS

70/70	60.5 ± 10.2	Depression	NS	Hospital (I)	Individual and group CBT[a] for 2 months	8 CBT sessions (individual and group) consisting of relaxation training, emotional adjustment, and psychological support (therapist and manualization NS)	UC and education for 2 months	Usual nutrition, exercise, and medication (regimen and therapist NS); 8 education sessions; and DM hotline by DM specialist nurse (regimen NS)	2	HbA1c, FBG, HAM-D, and DSQoL
93/93	53.6 ± 8.3	General	5.7 ± 3.7	Hospital (I)	Individual CBT[a] and group education for 1 month	CBT consisting of emotional adjustment, relaxation training, and exercise therapy (number of sessions and manualization NS); 8 group education sessions by multidisciplinary team (endocrinologist, nurse, and dietitian)	UC for 1 month	Usual nutrition, exercise, and medication (regimen and therapist NS)	1	FBG, SAS, and SDS
300/300	NS (41–79)	General	6.0 ± NS	Hospital (I)	Individual CBT[a] for 6 months	48 CBT sessions consisting of relaxation training, exercise therapy, emotional adjustment, behavior modification, and psychological support (therapist and manualization NS)	UC for 6 months	Usual medication by doctor (regimen NS)	6	HbA1c, FBG, and SCL-90
80/80	40.8 (22–60)	General	NS	Hospital (I)	Individual and group CBT[a] for 3 months	12 CBT sessions consisting of *Morita* therapy (individual and group), relaxation training, music relaxation therapy, and psychological support by doctor and nurse (manualization NS); and education sessions by doctor and nurse (number of sessions NS)	UC for 3 months	UC consisting of clinical treatment and nursing care (regimen and therapist NS)	3	HbA1c, FBG, SAS, SDS, and DQoL
59/59	54.9 ± 8.4	General	NS (0.5–12)	Hospital (I)	Individual CBT[a] and group education for 1 month	30 CBT sessions consisting of music relaxation therapy (therapist and manualization NS) and 2 group education sessions (therapist NS)	UC for 1 month	UC (regimen and therapist NS)	1	HbA1c, FBG, SAS, and SDS

300/300	52.6 ± 17.6	General	5.0 ± 3.6	Hospital (O)	Individual CBT[a] and group education for 6 months	CBT sessions consisting of relaxation training and exercise therapy (number of sessions, therapist, and manualization NS), and education (number of sessions and therapist NS)	UC for 6 months	Usual medication (regimen and therapist NS)	6	HbA1c, FBG, SCL-90, and A-DQoL
80/80	54.8 ± 16.2	Low income	8.3 ± 6.7	Hospital (O)	Individual CBT for 3 months	12 CBT sessions consisting of *Morita* therapy, emotional adjustment, and psychological support (therapist and manualization NS)	UC for 3 months	Usual nutrition, exercise, medication, and glucose monitoring (regimen and therapist NS)	3	HbA1c, FBG, and SDS
100/100	NS (20–70)	General	NS	Hospital (I)	Individual CBT[a] for 1 month	8 CBT sessions consisting of behavior modification, relaxation training, cognitive restructuring, and psychological support by psychologist (manualization NS)	UC for 1 month	UC (regimen and therapist NS)	1	FBG, HAM-A, and HAM-D
68/68	58.0 ± 6.5	Depression	NS (3–5)	Hospital (I)	Individual CBT[a] for 1 month	CBT sessions consisting of cognitive restructuring, emotional adjustment, and psychological support (number of sessions and manualization NS) by nurse	UC for 1 month	UC consisting of clinical treatment, psychological counseling, and education by nurse (regimen NS)	1	HbA1c, FBG, and SDS
86/86	50.2 ± 7.6	General	NS	Hospital (NS)	Individual CCT[a] and individual education for 3 months	Non-directive counseling sessions with an emphasis on improvement of self-esteem (number of sessions, therapist, and manualization NS)	UC for 3 months	Usual medication (regimen and therapist NS)	3	FBG, SAS, and SDS
80/71	60.4 ± 9.9	General	5.7 ± 3.1	Community health	Individual MI for 6 months	MI sessions by nurse (number of sessions and manualization NS)	UC and family education/ glucose monitoring for 6 months	Usual nursing care and one family session every 1–3 months consisting of glucose monitoring and education by nurse	6	HbA1c

95/95	56.8 ± 12.5	General	NS	Hospital (I)	Group CBT and individual education for 2 weeks	5 group CBT sessions consisting of relaxation training (therapist NS), and individual psychological support and education (number of sessions, therapist, and manualization NS)	UC for 2 weeks	UC (regimen and therapist NS)	0.5	FBG and DSQoL
200/200	52.4 ± 11.2	Depression	6.3 ± 4.2	Hospital (I and O)	Individual CBT for 1 month	8 CBT sessions consisting of behavior modification, relaxation training, psychological support, and exercise therapy (therapist and manualization NS)	UC for 1 month	Usual medication (regimen and therapist NS)	1	FBG and SDS
184/175	48.0 ± 8.0	General	4.0 ± 1.0	Hospital (O)	Individual and group CBT (duration NS)	20 CBT sessions – individual and group (therapist and manualization NS)	UC and education (duration NS)	UC and education (regimen and therapist NS)	NS	FBG and GQoLI-74
120/113	52.0 ± 12.0	General	NS (2–13)	Hospital (I)	Individual CBT[a] for 2 months	8 CBT sessions consisting of *Morita* therapy and relaxation training by psychologist (number of sessions and manualization NS)	UC for 2 months	Usual nutrition and medication (regimen and therapist NS)	2	FBG, SAS, and SDS
100/100	44.2 ± 6.8	General	4.6 ± 2.5	Hospital (I)	Individual CCT[a] and family therapy for 1 month	Non-directive counseling sessions with an emphasis on improvement of self-esteem and positive thinking (number of sessions, therapist, and manualization NS), and family therapy (number of sessions and therapist NS)	UC for 1 month	Usual nutrition and medication (regimen and therapist NS)	1	HbA1c, FBG, SAS, and SDS
150/150	32.4 ± 12.0	General	5.3 ± 2.0	Hospital (I)	Individual CCT[a], individual education, and family therapy for 3–4 weeks	Non-directive counseling sessions with an emphasis on improvement of self-esteem and positive thinking (number of sessions and manualization NS), and family therapy (number of sessions NS); all by doctor and nurse	UC for 3–4 weeks	Usual nutrition, exercise, and medication (regimen and therapist NS)	0.75–1	HbA1c and FBG

120/120	NS (36–88)	General	NS	Hospital (I)	Individual MI for 3 sessions (duration NS)	3 MI sessions (therapist and manualization NS)	Usual education (duration NS)	Usual education consisting of group seminars and individual education focusing on nutrition, medication, exercise, and blood glucose monitoring (regimen and therapist NS)	NS	HbA1c and FBG
60/60	63 (50–75)	General	NS	Hospital (I)	Individual and group CBT[a] for 1 month	8 CBT sessions consisting of relaxation training, music relaxation therapy, and emotional adjustment by doctor and nurse trained in psychology (manualization NS)	UC for 1 month	Usual nutrition, exercise, and medication by doctor and nurse (regimen NS)	1	FBG
120/106	55.9 (30–60)	General	5.5 (2–11)	Hospital (I and O)	Individual CBT[a] and individual education for 6 months	Biofeedback-assisted relaxation training (number of sessions NS), education (number of sessions NS), and 24 CBT sessions consisting of emotional adjustment and psychological support; all by psychologist (manualization NS)	UC for 6 months	Usual nutrition and medication (regimen and therapist NS)	6	HbA1c, FBG, and GQoLI-74
60/60	54.1 ± 11.9	General	NS (0.5–16)	NS	Individual CBT[a] and medication for 1 month	8 CBT sessions consisting of cognitive restructuring, emotional adjustment, relaxation training, music relaxation therapy, and psychological support (medication regimen, therapist, and manualization NS)	Medication for 1 month	Medication (regimen and therapist NS)	1	FBG, SAS, and SDS

80/75	66.9 ± 5.5	General	9.6 ± 4.7	Hospital (I)	Individual MI for 6 months	22 MI sessions by nurse (manualization NS)	Education for 6 months	6 group education sessions consisting of basic DM knowledge, nutrition, medication, exercise, glucose monitoring, and management of negative emotions (therapist NS)	6	HbA1c
128/87	Interv ention: 53.96 ± 9.63; control: 56.88 ± 8.87	General	Interv ention: 4.8 ± 5.2; control: 4.3 ± 4.2	Hospital (I)	Individual CBT[a] for 1 month	8 sessions of biofeedback-assisted relaxation training and music relaxation therapy (therapist and manualization NS)	UC for 1 month	UC (regimen and therapist NS)	8 months (1998 cohort) to 2 years (1996 cohort)	HbA1c and FBG
67/56	54.0 ± 10.0	General	NS (0.5–16)	Hospital (I)	Individual CBT[a] for 1 month	8 sessions of biofeedback-assisted relaxation training and music relaxation therapy (therapist and manualization NS)	UC for 1 month	UC (regimen and therapist NS)	1	HbA1c and FBG
59/59	57.1 ± 9.6	General	4.8 ± 5.5	Hospital (I)	Individual CBT[a] for 1 month	8–12 sessions of biofeedback-assisted relaxation training and music relaxation therapy (therapist and manualization NS)	UC for 1 month	UC (regimen and therapist NS)	1	–

Summary of meta-analyses for psychological interventions vs. control condition.

Outcomes	*K*	*N*	Effect Estimate			Heterogeneity		
			SMD	95% CI	*Z* (*P*)	χ^2	*P*	I^2 (%)
CBT vs. Control								
Glycated hemoglobin	20	2900	−0.97	−1.37 to −0.57	4.72 (<0.0001)	430.87	<0.0001	96
Depression	27	3084	−1.22	−1.51 to −0.94	8.39 (<0.0001)	331.61	<0.0001	92
Anxiety	21	2479	−1.03	−1.26 to −0.80	8.91 (<0.0001)	130.53	<0.0001	85
Blood glucose concentration	28	3802	−0.98	−1.25 to −0.72	7.20 (<0.0001)	373.18	<0.0001	93
Quality of life	5	722	−0.65	−1.35 to 0.06	1.80 (*P* = 0.07)	71.84	<0.0001	94
MI vs. Control								
Glycated hemoglobin	3	251	−0.71	−1.00 to −0.43	4.88 (<0.0001)	2.43	0.30	18
CCT vs. Control								
Glycated hemoglobin	4	451	−0.96	−1.97 to 0.05	1.86 (*P* = 0.06)	74.07	<0.0001	96
Depression	3	282	−0.86	−1.11 to −0.62	6.90 (<0.0001)	1.16	0.56	0
Blood glucose concentration	5	537	−1.31	−2.42 to −0.20	2.31 (*P* = 0.02)	130.69	<0.0001	97

Source: Chapman, A., Liu, S., Merkouris, S., Enticott, J. C., Yang, H., Browning, C. J., & Thomas, S. A. (2015). Psychological interventions for the management of glycemic and psychological outcomes of type 2 diabetes mellitus in China: A systematic review and meta-analyses of randomized controlled trials. *Frontiers in Public Health*, *3*, 252. https://doi.org/10.3389/fpubh.2015.00252 (accessed on 29th May 2025).

Yang et al. (2020) analyzed the effects of CBT on diabetes patients in RCTs published in English and Chinese between 2007 and April 2019. Analyses of 23 RCTs with 2619 patients showed improved glycemic control and depressive symptoms. The researchers recommended the incorporation of multiple aspects of CBT as per the requirement/population (Table 5.20).

Table 5.20. Effect of CBT on Glycemic Control and Other Factors in the Analyses of 23 RCTs

Study (Year)	Participants and Ethnicity (No. of C/I; Baseline % DO)	Design and Location	Age (C/I) Mean (SD)	Sex M/F (C/I)	Duration of Treatment	Intervention Aim	Methods and Delivery (C/I)	Key Intervention Outcomes (Within Groups)	Quality of Studies Assessed by PEDro Tool
Alanzi et al. (2011)	T2DM patients, Saudi Arabia (10/10) (0%/10%)	UB, Saudi Arabia	C: 52.6 (12.6); I: 50.3 (10.5)	C: 7/3; I: 8/2	6 months	Evaluate CBT-based SANAD program on glycemic control, awareness, and self-efficacy in T2DM	C: usual care; I: CBT (SANAD system via smartphone, social networking services)	−0.60 mean change in HbA1c; 2.44 in diabetes knowledge; 0.994 in self-efficacy	5, Moderate
Amsberg et al. (2009)	T1DM patients, Swedish (39/40) (2.7%/10%)	UB, Sweden	C: 41.4 (12.9); I: 41.1 (11.7)	C: 16/22; I: 20/16	48 weeks	Assess CBT impact on HbA1c, self-care, and psychosocial factors	C: usual care incl. CGM; I: same + CBT-based intervention	−0.78 in HbA1c; −1.63 in anxiety; −0.99 in depression	7, Moderate
De Greef et al. (2010)	T2DM patients, Belgian (21/20) (19%/20%)	UB, Belgium	C: 62.29; I: 61.5 (35–75 range)	C: 15/6; I: 13/7	12 weeks	Assess pedometer + group CBT effects on physical activity and health	C: usual care + single education; I: group CBT for lifestyle	−0.2 HbA1c; −2.2 SBP; −3.5 DBP; −1.7 TC; +0.4 weight; −0.1 BMI	6, Moderate
Guan et al. (2015)	T2DM patients, Chinese (45/48) (0%/0%)	UB, China	C: 53.6 (7.8); I: 54.4 (8.3)	C: 22/23; I: 25/23	6 months	Evaluate group CBT for psychological symptoms and glycemic outcomes	C: usual care + education; I: same + group CBT	−0.24 HbA1c; −0.39 fasting glucose	6, Moderate
Gregg et al. (2007)	T2DM patients, English-speaking (38/43) (13%/7%)	UB, Canada	C: 49.8 NR; I: 51.9 NR	C: 16/22; I: 22/21	3 months	Assess ACT + education on glucose control and self-management	C: education; I: education + ACT (CBT-based)	−0.72 HbA1c; +5.83 self-management	8, High
Huang et al. (2016)	T2DM w/ depression, Taiwanese (30/31) (0%/0%)	UB, Taiwan	C: 57.83 (10.38); I: 55.06 (10.44)	C: 13/17; I: 16/15	3 months	Evaluate CBT + motivational enhancement on depression and glucose	C: usual care; I: same + CBT	−3.21 HbA1c; −2.35 fasting glucose; −1.21 BMI; −5.07 depression	6, Moderate
Inouye et al. (2015)	T2DM, Asians and Pacific Islanders (103/104) (6.8%/17.3%)	SB, US	C: 57.8 (10.8); I: 57.0 (11.1)	C: 54/49; I: 59/45	6 weeks	Assess CBT on QoL, depression, and glycemia	C: education; I: same + CBT	−0.29 HbA1c; +0.4 BMI; +5.3 SBP; +0.1 DBP; −5.5 TC; −2.4 HDL-C; −6.7 LDL-C; −16.4 TG; +4.5 weight; −2.45 depression	9, Moderate

Li et al. (2018)	T2DM patients, Chinese (20/20) (10%/15%)	UB, China	C: 57.5 (11.32); I: 60.9 (7.87)	C: 10/10; I: 11/9	6 weeks	Group CBT for emotion and glucose in T2DM	C: usual care + education; I: same + group CBT	−0.46 HbA1c; −0.24 fasting glucose; −2.7 2hPG	6, Moderate
Menting et al. (2017)	T1DM patients, Dutch (60/60) (0%/1.7%)	UB, Netherlands	C: 42.9 (12.5); I: 44.4 (12.1)	C/I: 23/37	5 months	Effectiveness of CBT on fatigue and glucose in T1DM	C: waitlist; I: CBT (face-to-face + web-based)	−0.1 HbA1c; −0.4 glucose variability; −19.4 fatigue	7, High
Penckofer et al. (2012)	T2DM + depression, multiple race (36/38) (5.5%/31%)	UB, US	C: 54.0 (8.4); I: 54.8 (8.8)	All women (n = 84)	6 months	Group CBT for depression and glucose in women with T2DM	C: usual care; I: group CBT	−0.4 HbA1c; −13.8 fasting glucose; −15.1 depression; −10.1 anxiety	4, Moderate
Petrak et al. (2015)	T1DM and T2DM + depression, German (125/126) (18.4%/27%)	SB, Germany	C: 47.9 (12.8); I: 49.0 (10.6)	C: 48/77; I: 47/79	3 months	Diabetes-specific CBT group for depression + glucose	C: usual care + sertraline; I: same + CBT	−0.25 HbA1c; −12.64 depression	8, High
Piette et al. (2011)	T2DM + depression, multiracial (167/172) (12.57%/15.7%)	UB, US	C: 56.0 (10.9); I: 55.1 (9.4)	C: 77.8% F; I: 64.9% F	12 months	Telephone CBT for depression, physical activity, and diabetes	C: usual care; I: CBT by phone	+0.2 HbA1c; −5.2 SBP; −3.4 DBP; −12.5 depression	7, Moderate
Ridge et al. (2012)	T1DM patients, multiracial (117/106) (23.9%/30%)	UB, UK	C: 54.1 (10.4); I: 56.3 (10.3)	Full sample: 36 (28.1–43.8)	12 months	Assess MEF plus CBT on glycemic control in T1DM	C: motivational enhancement (4 sessions); I: same + CBT	−0.578 mean change in HbA1c	5, Moderate
Safren et al. (2014)	T2DM + depression, multiracial (42/45) (28.6%/20%)	SB, US	C: 58.31 (7.41); I: 55.44 (8.72)	C: 22/20; I: 22/23	4 months	Evaluate CBT for adherence and depression in T2DM	C: usual care; I: same + CBT	−0.95 HbA1c; −11.38 depression; −1.98 CGI	8, High
Sharif et al. (2014)	T2DM + depression, Iranian (29/29) (3.3%/3.3%)	UB, Iran	C: 55 (10.5); I: 56 (11.2)	C: 3/26; I: 8/21	2 months	Evaluate group CBT for depression and glucose in T2DM	C: usual care; I: group CBT	−1.09 HbA1c; −5.81 depression	6, Moderate
Shayeghian et al. (2016)	T2DM patients, Iranian (53/53) (3.56%/1.18%)	UB, Iran	C: 55.70 (8.98); I: 55.18 (8.26)	C: 26/27; I: 20/33	3 months	Evaluate group ACT on self-management and glucose in T2DM	C: usual care + education; I: same + group-based ACT (CBT-based)	−0.36 HbA1c; +6.98 self-care; +8.93 Acceptance and Action Diabetes	4, Moderate
Snoek et al. (2008)	T1DM patients, Dutch (41/45) (8%/27%)	UB, Netherlands	C: 37.4 (11.1); I: 38.1 (9.7)	C: 14/27; I: 18/23	12 months	Evaluate group CBT in T1DM	C: diabetes awareness; I: group CBT	No change HbA1c; −0.3 depression	5, Moderate

Sun et al. (2015)	T2DM patients, Chinese (45/45) (0%/0%)	UB, China	C: 53.6 (9.7); I: 56.6 (9.7)	C: 27/18; I: 26/19	6 months	Evaluate GCBT on health outcomes in T2DM	C: usual care; I: same + group CBT	−0.24 HbA1c; −1.48 2hPG; +1.41 FINS; −3.53 anxiety; −5.12 depression	5, Moderate
van Son et al. (2014)	T1DM and T2DM, Dutch (69/70) (10%/18.84%)	UB, Netherlands	C: 57 (13); I: 56 (13)	C: 37/32; I: 33/37	3 months	Evaluate MBCT on emotion and glucose in diabetes	C: usual care; I: CBT (MBCT)	−0.1 HbA1c; −5.1 perceived stress; −1.9 anxiety; −2.6 depression	6, Moderate
Weinger et al. (2011)	T1DM and T2DM patients, non-Hispanic White (75/74) (8%/4%)	UB, US	C: 54.7 (25.0–75.1); I: 51.8 (23.7–74.2)	C: 39/36; I: 40/34	3 months	Evaluate CBT-based structured intervention for poorly controlled diabetes	C: attention control (goal-setting); I: same + CBT	−0.82 HbA1c; −0.5 BMI; −2.5 LDL-C; −1.8 HDL-C; +686 steps (pedometer)	7, Moderate
Welschen et al. (2013)	T2DM patients, Caucasian (78/76) (2.56%/5.26%)	UB, Netherlands	C: 61.2 (8.8); I: 60.5 (9.4)	C: 50/28; I: 45/32	6 months	Assess CBT for reducing CHD risk in T2DM	C: usual care; I: same + CBT	−0.1 HbA1c; −0.1 fasting glucose; −0.3 TC; +0.9 weight; +0.2 BMI; −1.2 SBP; −2.4 DBP; −1.2 depression	7, Moderate
Whitehead et al. (2017)	T2DM patients, NZ European and Māori (34/39) (26.5%/7.6%)	DB, Australia	C: 53.76 (8.68); I: 56.1 (6.91)	C: 20/14; I: 17/22	6 months	Compare nurse-led education vs. education + ACT	C: education; I: same + ACT (CBT-based)	−0.04 HbA1c; −0.04 anxiety; −0.54 depression	8, High
Wroe et al. (2018)	T2DM + depression or anxiety, NR (52/63) (0%/0%)	DB, UK	C: 63.63 (10.71); I: 63.48 (11.04)	C: 25/27; I: 28/35	6 weeks	CBT-based intervention for depression and anxiety in T2DM	C: usual care; I: CBT-based intervention	−0.03 HbA1c; −3.4 depression; −2.86 anxiety	7, Moderate

Source: Yang, X., Li, Z., & Sun, J. (2020). Effects of cognitive behavioral therapy-based intervention on improving glycemic, psychological, and physiological outcomes in adult patients with diabetes mellitus: A meta-analysis of randomized controlled trials. *Frontiers in Psychiatry*, *11*, 711. https://doi.org/10.3389/fpsyt.2020.00711 (accessed on 29th May 2025).

5.4. Exercise and Other Recommendations

"If you don't make time for exercise, you'll probably have to make time for illness."

—Robin Sharma

Pereira et al. (2023) translated and presented the Brazilian Society of Diabetes (SBD) Guidelines 2021–2022 backed by science to guide exercises for type 1 and 2 diabetes patients. The authors reaffirmed the importance of exercise (with an emphasis on aerobics and resistance) in facilitating glycemic control and lowering cardiovascular disease (CVD) risk. A point was suggested to monitor the glucose levels precisely during these exercises to circumvent hypoglycemia (Figures 5.7 and 5.8).

Aodel of exercise guidance for individuals with diabetes

1. Increase the level of physical activity in your daily life (use stairs, walk the with tl log, take care of the garden) and reduce sedentary time (limit TV/computer TV/computer time t 10 more than two hours a day)

2. Start with aerobic exercise: ideally ---- minutes, times a week. The ideal target is 15 ninutes a week, but you can start with a few minutes a day and progressively increase by fiv ninutes each week.

3. Start a resistance exercise** 2 times a week

4. Continue with aerobic exercise* 5 days a week for at least 30 minutes per session

5. Continue with resistance exercise** 3 or more times a week

Aerobic exercise, such as walking, cycling, swimming and running, is continuous or intermitter xercise that accelerates heart rate and breathing.

* Resistance exercise involves rapid repetition exercises with live weights (or bottles with wat r sand), weight machines, elastic bands or your own body. The large muscle groups should b vorked (arms, shoulders, back, abdomen, and legs). The ideal is eight to ten different exercises, i eries with repetitions each. [1]

Figure 5.7. Orientation exercises for diabetic individuals (Sports Medicine Outpatient Clinic of the Federal University of São Paulo [UNIFESP]).

Source: Pereira, W. V. C., Vancea, D. M. M., de Andrade Oliveira, R., Silva, E. P., de Castro, J. B. P., & Lima, R. M., et al. (2023). Position of Brazilian Diabetes Society on exercise recommendations for people with type 1 and type 2 diabetes. *Diabetology & Metabolic Syndrome*, *15*, 2. https://doi.org/10.1186/s13098-022-00900-6 (accessed on 29th May 2025).

Glicemia (mg/dL)	Arrow Tendecy	Low intensity	High Intensity
>250	↑↗	Ketone Check Consider 50% of bolus correction	Avoid exercise Consider 50% of bolus correction
	→		
	↓↘	OK to begin	
181-250	↑↗	Consider 50% of bolus correction	
	→		
	↓↘	OK to begin	
126-180	↑↗	Consider 50% of bolus correction	
	→		
	↓↘	5g-10g of carbohydrates	
90-125	↑↗	5g of carbohydrates. OK to begin	
	→	5g-10g of carbohydrates. OK to begin	
	↘	10g-15g of carbohydrates. OK to begin	
	↓	20g of carbohydrates	
<90	Elevated risk for hypoglicemia		

Figure 5.8. Glucose management for diabetics during exercises.

Source: Pereira, W. V. C., Vancea, D. M. M., de Andrade Oliveira, R., Silveira, M. F., Lemos, T. V., de Castro, J. B. P., & Lima, R. M. (2023). Position of Brazilian Diabetes Society on exercise recommendations for people with type 1 and type 2 diabetes. *Diabetology & Metabolic Syndrome*, *15*, 2. https://doi.org/10.1186/s13098-022-00900-6 (accessed on 29th May 2025).

5.5. The Promise of Yoga: Research Findings

"Yoga teaches us to cure what need not be endured and endure what cannot be cured."

—B. K. S. Iyengar

A systematic review of clinical trials of 44 clinical trials of 3168 participants in the International Journal of Cardiology by Cramer et al. (2014) assessed the effect of yoga "for predefined cardiovascular risk factors in healthy participants, non-diabetic participants with high risk for CVD, or participants with T2DM." They reported that "yoga can be considered as an ancillary intervention for the general population and for patients with increased risk of CVD" (Cramer et al., 2014).

"Yoga is much more than a system of physical exercises–it is a profound path of self-transformation that encompasses a range of teachings, practices, and sacred texts that can help us cultivate wisdom, balance, and inner freedom, as well as physical health."

—Georg Feuerstein

Boston: Shambhala (2003)

The Deeper Dimensions of Yoga: Theory and Practice.

Chattopadhyay et al. (2020) developed a yoga-based approach for preventing type-2 diabetes. They initially performed a review of articles on yoga techniques that lower blood glucose (PROSPERO registration number CRD42018097216). The studies are reported in Table 5.21.

Table 5.21. List of Studies Selected to Develop a Yoga Program for Type-2 Diabetes Prevention (Yoga-DP)#

Author and Year	In Systematic Review and Year	Location	Population	Sample Size	Intervention	Comparator	Improvement in Blood Glucose Levels in the Yoga Group (from Baseline to Follow-Up)	Adverse Events
Agrawal (2003)	Aljasir (2010); Cramer (2014); Eun (2017); Innes (2016); Kumar (2016); Thind (2017); Vizcaino (2016)	Bikaner, India	T2DM, both sexes	200 (I = 100, C = 100)	Standard medical management + yoga	Standard medical management + exercise	FBG (from 183.9 ± 39.3 to 150.7 ± 34.2 mg/dl), HbA1c (from 9.4 ± 1.0 to 8.6 ± 1.0%)	Yes*

Nagarathna (2012)	Cramer (2014); Cui (2017); Innes (2016); Jayawardena (2018); Kumar (2016); Thind (2017); Vizcaino (2016)	Bangalore, India	T2DM, both sexes, above 25 years	277 (I = 141, C = 136)	Standard medical management + yoga	Standard medical management + exercise and walking	HbA1c (from 8.5 ± 1.7 to 7.3 ± 3.0%)	Yes*
Vaishali (2011, 2012)	Bhurji (2016); Chu (2016); Cramer (2014); Cui (2017); Innes (2016); Jayawardena (2018); Kumar (2016); Pai (2016); Thind (2017); Vizcaino (2016)	Mang alore, India	T2DM with cardiom etabolic risk factors, both sexes, above 60 years	60 (I = 30, C = 30)	Standard medical management + yoga	Standard medical management	FBG (from 163.5 ± 14.8 to 115.6 ± 13.7 mg/dl), HbA1c (from 10.3 ± 0.9 to 9.1 ± 0.6%)	Yes*
Yadav (2013)	Kumar (2016)	Gwalior, India	T2DM, male, 30–55 years	30 (I = 15, C = 15)	Yoga	NS	FBG (from 234.5 ± 46.9 to 127.7 ± 15.2 mg/dl)	NS
Kumar (2014)	Thind (2017); Vizcaino (2016)	Salem, India	T2DM, male, 35–60 years	30 (I = 15, C = 15)	Standard medical management + yoga	Standard medical management	FBG (from 309.5 ± 19.3 to 287.9 ± 19.9 mg/dl)	NS
Kumpatla (2015)	Thind (2017)	Chennai, India	T2DM, both sexes, 25–60 years	303 (I = 154, C = 149)	Standard medical management + yoga	Standard medical management	HbA1c (from 10.6 ± 2.5 to 7.2 ± 1.4%)	None
Sharma (2015)	Thind (2017); Vizcaino (2016)	Jaipur, India	T2DM, both sexes, 35–55 years	80 (I = 40, C = 40)	Standard medical management + yoga	Standard medical management	FBG (from 139.2 ± 16.6 to 99.8 ± 15.9 mg/dl), PPBG (from 174.1 ± 7.9 to 141.7 ± 8.4 mg/dl), HbA1c (from 9.3 ± 1.0 to 7.1 ± 0.7%)	NS
Singh (2015)	Vizcaino (2016)	Gangtok, India	T2DM, both sexes, above 20 years	337 (I–yoga = 112, I–music therapy = 110, C = 115)	Standard medical management + yoga, Standard medical management + music therapy	Standard medical management	FBG (from 166.9 ± 6.1 to 140.0 ± 3.2 mg/dl), PPBG (from 214.1 ± 7.6 to 173.3 ± 5.9 mg/dl), HbA1c (from 8.6 ± 0.6 to 7.6 ± 0.6%)	Yes*
Keerthi (2017)	–	Pudu cherry, India	Prediabetes and T2DM with normal BP, both sexes, 18–45 years	310 (He althy with normal BP: C = 62; Pred iabetes with normal BP: I = 62, C = 62; T2DM with normal BP: I = 62, C = 62)	Prediabetes and T2DM with normal BP: standard medical management + yoga	Healthy with normal BP: no change in lifestyle; Prediabetes and T2DM with normal BP: standard medical management + walking	Prediabetes with normal BP – FBG (from 112.2 ± 7.6 to 83.4 ± 12.9 mg/dl); Diabetes with normal BP – FBG (from 195.4 ± 49.9 to 152.3 ± 31.3 mg/dl)	NS

The references listed can be accessed in the chapter.

Source: Chattopadhyay, K., Mishra, P., Manjunath, N. K., Harris, T., Hamer, M., Greenfield, S. M., Wang, H., Singh, K., Lewis, S. A., Tandon, N., Kinra, S., & Prabhakaran, D. (2020). Development of a Yoga Program for Type-2 Diabetes Prevention (Yoga-DP) among high-risk people in India. *Frontiers in Public Health*, *8*, 548674. https://doi.org/10.3389/fpubh.2020.548674 (accessed on 29th May 2025).

Based on these *asanas*, the researchers developed a booklet and video for patients and a manual for instructors that were then approved by experts and tested on experts and individuals with no yoga experience. Table 5.22 lists the identified yogic techniques.

Table 5.22. The Identified Yogic Techniques in a Yoga Program for Type-2 Diabetes Prevention (Yoga-DP)

Yogic Practices	CVR	Additional Reason for Exclusion	Included in the Intervention?
Shithilikarana Vyayama	0.71	–	Yes
Surya Namaskar	0.80	–	Yes
Ardhachakrasana	0.61	–	Yes
Katichakrasana	0.90	–	Yes
Padahastasana	0.51	Part of *Surya Namaskar*	No
Prarambhasana	–0.56	–	No
Tadasana	0.37	–	Yes
Konasana	0.90	–	Yes
Paravakonasana	0.37	–	Yes
Trikonasana	0.56	–	Yes
Parivrittatrikonasana	0.27	–	No
Ardhmatsyendrasana	0.95	–	Yes
Janusirvasana	0.51	–	Yes
Kukutkasana	–0.95	–	No
Mandukasana	0.90	–	Yes
Padmasana	–0.02	–	No
Baddhapadmasana	–0.37	–	No
Paschimottanasana	0.66	–	Yes

Sukhasana	0.22	–	Yes
Ustrasana	0.66	–	Yes
Vajrasana	0.56	–	Yes
Vakrasana	1.00	–	Yes
Yoga Mudrasana 1 (Padmasana)	0.07	–	No
Yoga Mudrasana 2 (Vajrasana)	0.27	–	No
Yoga Mudrasana 3 (Sukhasana)	0.12	–	No
Bhujangasana	0.95	Part of *Surya Namaskar*	No
Poornabhujangasana	−0.71	–	No
Dhanurasana	0.80	–	Yes
Hamsasana	−0.51	–	No
Makarasana	0.66	–	Yes
Mayurasana	−0.51	–	No
Shalabhasana/ Poornashalabhasana	0.32	–	Yes
Ardhashalabhasana	0.51	–	Yes
Halasana	0.12	–	No
Ardha Halasana	0.61	–	Yes
Matsyasana	0.17	–	No
Saalmatsyasana	0.37	–	Yes
Naukasana	0.66	–	Yes
Pavanamuktasana	0.95	–	Yes
Suptavajrasana	−0.22	–	No
Sarvangasana	0.07	–	No
Uttanapadasana	0.61	–	Yes
Shavasana	0.90	Similar to *Yoga Nidra*	No
Anulom Vilom Pranayama	0.80	Similar to *Nadishodhana Pranayama*	No
Nadishodhana Pranayama	0.85	–	Yes
Chandranadi Pranayama	−0.02	–	No
Bhastrika Pranayama	0.37	–	Yes
Kapalbhati Pranayama	0.56	–	Yes

Bhramari Pranayama	0.80	–	Yes
Sheetali Pranayama	−0.17	–	No
Shitkari Pranayama	−0.27	–	No
Ujjayi Pranayama	−0.17	–	No
Vibhagiya Pranayama	0.51	–	Yes
Nadanusandhana (A Kara, U Kara, M Kara, and *AUM* chanting)	0.76	*AUM* chanting removed on religious grounds	Partially
AUM chanting	0.46	On religious grounds	No
Kayotsarga	0.80	Part of *Yoga Nidra*	No
Preksha meditation including *Anupreksha*	0.32	Part of *Yoga Nidra*	No
Yoga Nidra	0.76	–	Yes

- *Source:* Chattopadhyay, K., Mishra, P., Manjunath, N. K., Harris, T., Hamer, M., Greenfield, S. M., Wang, H., Singh, K., Lewis, S. A., Tandon, N., Kinra, S., & Prabhakaran, D. (2020). Development of a Yoga Program for Type-2 Diabetes Prevention (Yoga-DP) among high-risk people in India. *Frontiers in Public Health, 8*, 548674. https://doi.org/10.3389/fpubh.2020.548674 (accessed on 29th May 2025).

The structure of the developed program (24 weeks has been illustrated in Tables 5.23 and 5.24).

Table 5.23. Yoga-DP

Week	Group Yoga Sessions Delivered by Yoga-DP Instructors	Self-Practice of Yoga at Home Using Yoga-DP Booklet and a Video	Extra Features
1–4 (month 1)	At least two sessions of 45 min per week. An attendance register is kept.	–	At the first session, the instructor gives participants part one of the program booklet. This provides information about being at high risk of T2DM and how to prevent T2DM (i.e., by being more physically active, keeping a healthy weight, eating less fat [especially saturated fat], and eating more fiber).

5–12 (month 2–3)	At least two sessions of 75 min per week. An attendance register is kept.	–	At the last session, the instructor gives participants part two of the program booklet and a video. These provide information on Yoga practice to prevent T2DM. Also, a Yoga diary and a non-slippery Yoga mat are provided for self-practice of Yoga at home.
13–24 (month 4–6)	At least one session of 75 min every 4 weeks. An attendance register is kept.	At least two sessions of 75 min per week. Participants are given the Yoga diary to record their Yoga practice (types and minutes).	The instructor phones participants every week to offer support and help and to troubleshoot any problems.
25+ (month 7+)	–	At least two sessions of 75 min per week. Participants are given the Yoga diary to record their Yoga practice (types and minutes).	–

Source: Chattopadhyay, K., Mishra, P., Manjunath, N. K., Harris, T., Hamer, M., Greenfield, S. M., Wang, H., Singh, K., Lewis, S. A., Tandon, N., Kinra, S., & Prabhakaran, D. (2020). Development of a Yoga Program for Type-2 Diabetes Prevention (YOGA-DP) among high-risk people in India. *Frontiers in Public Health*, *8*, 548674. https://doi.org/10.3389/fpubh.2020.548674 (accessed on 29th May 2025).

Table 5.24. Yoga-DP Sessions

Yogic Practices	Week 1–4 (Each session should last for 45 min with the time split as follows)	Week 5+ (Each session should last for 75 min with the time split as follows)	Details
Shithilikarana Vyayama	Around 5 min	Around 5 min	1. Neck rotation 30 s 2. Shoulder rotation 30 s 3. Elbow flexion and extension 30 s 4. Wrist rotation 30 s 5. Finger movement 30 s
			6. Waist rotation 30 s 7. Knee flexion and extension 1 min 8. Ankle rotation 1 min 9. Toe movement 30 s
Surya Namaskar	–	Around 15 min	The below mentioned 12 steps constitute one set of *Surya Namaskar*. To complete one round of *Surya Namaskar*, participants need to repeat these 12 steps on the other side of their body (i.e., by extending their left leg behind in step number 4 and bringing their left leg forward in step number 9). Initially, they should practice *Surya Namaskar* at a slower pace. Only with practice over some time, they may try to do 12 rounds of it at a faster pace for around 15 min (i.e., a couple of seconds per step). 1. *Pranamasana* (prayer pose) 2. *Hastauttanasana* (raised arms pose) 3. *Padahastasana* (hands to feet pose) 4. *Ashwa Sanchalanasana* (equestrian pose) 5. *Dandasana* (stick pose) 6. *Ashtanga Namaskara Asana* (salute with eight parts) 7. *Bhujangasana* (cobra pose) 8. *Parvatasana* (mountain pose) 9. *Ashwa Sanchalanasana* (equestrian pose) 10. *Padahastasana* (hands to feet pose) 11. *Hastauttanasana* (raised arms pose) 12. *Pranamasana* (prayer pose)

Asana	Around 15 min	Around 30 min	Two-sided poses (right and left) are to be practiced for about 3 min (1.5 min on each side) and central-positioned poses are to be practiced for about 1.5 min. In each session, the Yogic poses are selected from the list below to prevent boredom from the similarity of routine. Advanced Yogic poses are introduced from week 5 onwards, for example, *Konasana* (angle pose), *Trikonasana* (triangle pose), *Parvakonasana* (lateral angle pose), *Ardhaustrasana* (half camel pose), *Ustrasana* (camel pose), *Dhanurasana* (bow pose), and *Naukasana* (boat pose). **(A) Standing Poses:** 1. *Tadasana* (palm tree pose) 1.5 min 2. *Ardhachakrasana* (half wheel pose) 1.5 min 3. *Katichakrasana* (waist wheel pose) 3 min 4. *Konasana* (angle pose) or *Trikonasana* (triangle pose) or *Parvakonasana* (lateral angle pose); alternatively 3 min **(B) Sitting Poses:** 1. *Vajrasana* (adamant pose) 1.5 min 2. *Mandukasana* (frog pose) 1.5 min 3. *Ardhaustrasana* (half camel pose) or *Ustrasana* (camel pose); alternatively 1.5 min 4. *Vakrasana* (twisted pose) or *Ardha Matsyendrasana* (half spinal twist pose); alternatively 3 min 5. *Paschimottanasana* (seated forward bend pose) or *Janusirsasana* (head to knee pose); alternatively 1.5 or 3 min, respectively **(C) Lying Poses– Front/Prone:** 1. *Ardha Shalabhasana* (half locust pose) or *Poornashalabhasana* (full locust pose); alternatively 3 or 1.5 min, respectively 2. *Dhanurasana* (bow pose) 1.5 min 3. *Makarasana* (crocodile pose) 1.5 min **(D) Lying Poses– Back/Supine:** 1. *Uttanapadasana* (raised legs pose) or *Ardhahalasana* (half plow pose); alternatively 1.5 min 2. *Pavanamuktasana* (wind relieving pose) 1.5 min 3. *Naukasana* (boat pose) 1.5 min 4. *Sarlamatsyasana* (easy fish pose) 1.5 min
Pranayama	Around 13 min	Around 13 min	1. *Vibhagiya Pranayama* (sectional breathing) 4 min 2. *Nadishodhana Pranayama* (alternate nostril breathing) 3 min 3. *Kapalbhati Pranayama* (skull shining breathing) or *Bhastrika Pranayama* (bellows breathing); alternatively 3 min 4. *Bhramari Pranayama* (bee breathing) 3 min

Dhyana and relaxation practices	Around 12 min	Around 12 min	In each session, the following *Dhyana* and relaxation practices are to be done in a darker room. 1. *A Kara* chanting, *U Kara* chanting, and *M Kara* chanting 3 min 2. *Yoga Nidra* (Yogic sleep) 9 min

Source: Chattopadhyay, K., Mishra, P., Manjunath, N. K., Harris, T., Hamer, M., Greenfield, S. M., Wang, H., Singh, K., Lewis, S. A., Tandon, N., Kinra, S., & Prabhakaran, D. (2020). Development of a Yoga Program for Type-2 Diabetes Prevention (YOGA-DP) among high-risk people in India. *Frontiers in Public Health*, *8*, 548674. https://doi.org/10.3389/fpubh.2020.548674 (accessed on 29th May 2025).

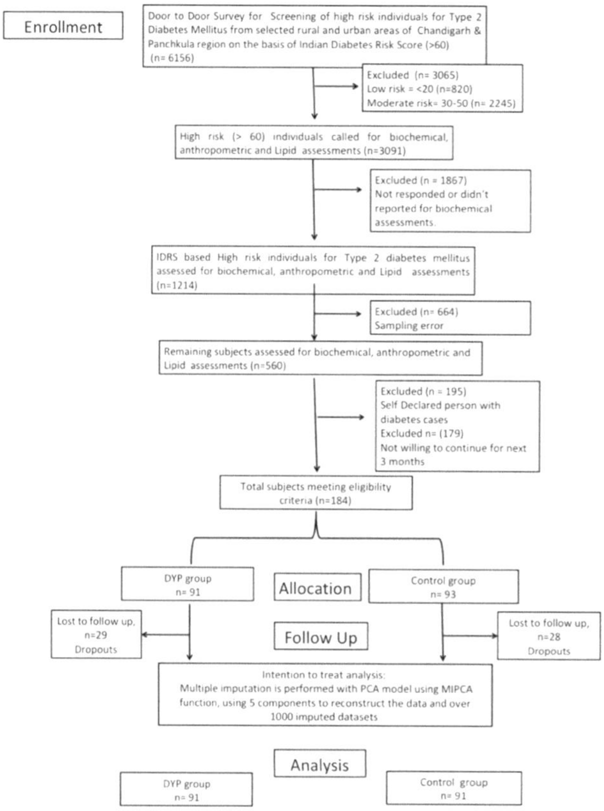

Figure 5.9. The study by Kaur et al. (2021).

Source: Kaur, N., Majumdar, V., Nagarathna, R., Patil, S. S., Badgaiyan, S., Singh, A., Sharma, R., Sharma, M., Telles, S., & Anand, A. (2021). Diabetic yoga protocol improves glycemic, anthropometric, and lipid levels in high-risk individuals for diabetes: A randomized controlled trial from Northern India. *Diabetology & Metabolic Syndrome*, *13*, 149. https://doi.org/10.1186/s13098-021-00761-1 (accessed on 29th May 2025).

An intent-to treat principal analysis as a sub-study of the Pan India trial *Niyantrita Madhumeha Bharath (NMB)* was published by Kaur et al. (2021). The patient cohort included a high-risk cohort from Chandigarh, one of the most affluent Union Territories of India with the highest reported prevalence of diabetes. The two-armed RCT conducted entailed door-to-door screening and finalized 184 individuals who were randomized into the intervention group (n = 91) and control group (n = 93). Figure 5.9 shows the approach by the authors:

The authors developed a diabetic yoga protocol (DYP) approved by the Ministry of AYUSH and Quality Council of India described as "the first protocol to be made specifically for the prediabetics and diabetics." The yoga classes were conducted for three months (one-hour sessions), and the study outcomes were analyses of glycemic and lipid profiles. Table 5.25 shows the protocol adopted as reported by the researchers.

Table 5.25. The Diabetic Yoga Protocol (DYP) of Kaur et al. (2021)

SL. No.	Name of Practice	Duration (min)
1.	Starting prayer: *Asatoma Sat Gamaya*	2
2.	Preparatory *Sukshma Vyayamas* and *Shithililarna* Practices 1. *Urdhvahastashvasana* (Hand stretching breathing – 3 rounds at 90°, 135°, and 180° each) 2. *Kati-Shakti Vikasaka* (3 rounds) a. Forward and backward bending b. Twisting 3. *Sarvangapushti* (3 rounds clockwise, 3 rounds anticlockwise)	6
3.	*Surya Namaskara* (SN) 10-step fast *Surya Namaskara* – 6 rounds 12-step slow *Surya Namaskara* – 1 round Modified version – Chair SN – 7 rounds	9

4.	*Asanas* (1 min per *asana*) 1. Standing Position *Trikonasana, Parvritta Trikonasana, Prasarita Padhastasana* 2. Supine Position *Jatara Parivartanasana, Pawanmuktasana, Viparitakarani* 3. Prone Position *Bhujangasana, Dhanurasana* followed by *Pawanmuktasana* 4. Sitting Position *Mandukasana, Vakrasana/Ardhamatsyendrasana, Paschimatanasana, Ardha Ushtrasana* At the end, relaxation with abdominal breathing in supine position (*vishranti*), 10–15 rounds (2 min)	15
5.	*Kriya* a. *Agnisara* – 1 min b. *Kapalabhati* (@60 breaths per minute for 1 min followed by rest for 1 min)	3
6.	*Pranayama* *Nadishuddhi* (for 6 min, with *antarkumbhak* and *jalandhar bandh* for 2 s) *Bhramari* – 3 min	9
7.	Meditation (for stress, deep relaxation, and silencing of mind) Cyclic meditation	15
8.	Resolve (*I am Completely Healthy*)	1
9.	Closing prayer: *Sarvebhavantu Sukhina*...	1
	Total Duration	**60**

Analyses of the glycemic (HbA1c, OGTT, and FBS), lipid (Total cholesterol, triglycerides (TGs), HDL-c, LDL-c, and VLDL-c, CDL/HDL, LDL/HDL), and body mass index (BMI) after three months revealed a significant reduction in the waist circumference (1.94 cm), lowered deterioration of post-prandial glucose levels (relative change = –2.81%, $P < 0.05$) and clinically significant improvements of LDL-C levels by 0.16 units. The findings have been summarized in Table 5.26 and 5.27.

Table 5.26. Baseline Characteristics of Subjects (Kaur et al., CTRI/2018/03/012804)

Characteristics	DYP Group $N = 91$	Control Group $N = 93$	*P* Value
Gender			
Male, *n* (%)	19 (20.88)	30 (32.26)	0.096
Age (years)	47.77 (9.59)	49.24 (10.53)	0.323
Weight, kg	70.93 (10.90)	70.80 (12.44)	0.936
Waist circumference, cm	99.34 (9.05)	99.72 (9.05)	0.794
BMI, kg/m^2	28.59 (5.75)	28.53 (5.01)	0.949
IDRS	74.07 (10.43)	75.27 (9.95)	0.425
Biochemical Variables			
FBG, mg/dL	96.89 (9.95)	97.36 (12.20)	0.776
PPBG, mg/dL	102.88 (21.91)	113.78 (33.47)	0.012*
HbA1c (%)	5.61 (0.38)	5.66 (0.38)	0.400
Total cholesterol, mg/dL	186.88 (37.64)	179.98 (34.98)	0.199
Triglycerides, mg/dL	131.93 (68.59)	138.44 (68.89)	0.522
HDL-c, mg/dL	47.76 (9.16)	48.33 (17.43)	0.780
LDL-c, mg/dL	112.75 (31.02)	104.38 (31.70)	0.072
VLDL, mg/dL	26.39 (13.72)	28.00 (13.50)	0.423

*Continuous variables are represented as mean (SD) and compared using independent t-test. Categorical variables are represented as number (percentages) and compared using chi-square test. *P* value < 0.05 were considered significant. *FBS* fasting blood sugar, *PPBG* postprandial blood glucose, *HbA1c* glycated hemoglobin, *HDL-c* high density lipid-cholesterol, *LDL-c* low density lipid-cholesterol, *VLDL* very low density lipid-cholesterol, *IDRS* Indian diabetes risk score (IDRS).

Table 5.27. Effect of the DYP on Subjects (Kaur et al., CTRI/2018/03/012804)

Variables	Baseline Mean (SD)	After 3 Months Mean (SD)	Absolute Change	Relative Change	*P* Value	Partial η^2
Waist Circumference (cm)						
DYP	99.34 (9.05)	98.14 (6.88)	–1.93	–1.94	0.032	0.029
Control	99.72 (9.05)	100.25 (7.72)	–	–	–	–
BMI, kg/m^2						
DYP	28.59 (5.75)	28.00 (6.84)	–0.40	–1.40	0.622	0.002
Control	28.53 (5.01)	28.34 (4.98)	–	–	–	–
Weight, kg						

DYP	70.93 (10.90)	69.04 (9.13)	−1.04	−1.47	0.397	0.005
Control	70.80 (12.44)	69.95 (10.44)	–	–	–	–
Postprandial Blood Glucose, mg/dL						
DYP	102.88 (21.91)	118.32 (29.89)	−1.51	−1.47	0.006	0.046
Control	113.78 (33.47)	130.73 (36.98)	–	–	–	–
Fasting Blood Glucose, mg/dL						
DYP	96.89 (9.95)	99.82 (9.49)	1.44	1.49	0.287	0.007
Control	97.36 (12.20)	98.85 (9.26)	–	–	–	–
HbA1c (%)						
DYP	5.61 (0.38)	5.61 (0.39)	−0.02	−0.36	0.077	0.020
Control	5.66 (0.38)	5.68 (0.38)	–	–	–	–
Total Cholesterol, mg/dL						
DYP	186.88 (37.64)	189.01 (25.64)	−0.40	−0.21	0.130	0.014
Control	179.98 (34.98)	182.51 (20.82)	–	–	–	–
Triglycerides (TG), mg/dL						
DYP	131.93 (68.59)	148.14 (54.92)	−13.98	−10.60	0.138	0.014
Control	138.44 (68.89)	168.63 (75.06)	–	–	–	–
HDL-C, mg/dL						
DYP	47.76 (9.16)	47.01 (9.16)	2.20	4.61	0.097	0.017
Control	48.33 (17.43)	45.38 (12.57)	–	–	–	–
LDL-C, mg/dL						
DYP	112.75 (31.02)	103.39 (21.44)	−17.56	−15.57	0.044*	0.025
Control	104.38 (31.70)	112.58 (21.99)	–	–	–	–
VLDL, mg/dL						
DYP	26.39 (13.72)	28.85 (10.47)	−1.23	−4.66	0.229	0.009
Control	28.00 (13.50)	31.69 (10.57)	–	–	–	–

*Absolute change = [(intervention group follow-up) – (intervention group baseline)] – [(control group follow-up) – (control group baseline)]. Relative change = (absolute change/intervention group baseline) × 100%; *P* value for difference between the intervention and the control groups by MANCOVA adjusting for age, gender, status of diabetes/prediabetes/normoglycemia baseline values of glycemic and lipid variables, length of time having had prior exposure of yoga.

A 2024-published study scrutinized the effect of yoga on health outcomes/parameters of CVD, including high blood pressure (BP). While the promise of yoga on improved parameters cannot be denied, the application of larger sample sizes and randomized studies were suggested to fortify the findings (Angusubalakshmi et al., 2024). The results compiled by the authors are presented in Tables 5.28 and 5.29.

Table 5.28. Summary of Results as Compiled by Angusubalakshmi et al. (2024)*

Authors	Year	Title	Key Findings	Limitations
Sharma et al.	2015	Effect of yoga and health education on stress and cardiovascular risk factors among police personnel	Yoga and health education significantly reduced stress and improved cardiovascular risk factors	Small sample size; short duration of intervention
Singh et al.	2016	Cardiovascular benefits of yoga: a review of studies in Indian police personnel	Yoga was associated with improved cardiovascular health markers, including reduced BP and cholesterol levels	Lack of control groups
Patel et al.	2017	Impact of yoga on cardiovascular health in Indian police personnel	Significant improvements in cardiovascular health parameters, including lower incidence of hypertension	High dropout rate; varied adherence to yoga practice
Kumar et al.	2018	Health education and yoga interventions for cardiovascular health: evidence from police personnel	Combined interventions led to a notable reduction in cardiovascular risk factors among police personnel	Short follow-up period; self-reported data
Joshi et al.	2019	Yoga and cardiovascular health in police personnel	Yoga practice resulted in better cardiovascular outcomes compared to standard health education alone	Limited generalizability; regional differences
Reddy et al.	2020	Effectiveness of yoga-based stress management on cardiovascular health among police personnel	Yoga-based stress management effectively reduced stress and improved cardiovascular health indicators	Small sample size; lack of long-term follow-up
Gupta et al.	2021	Integration of yoga and health education for cardiovascular health in police personnel	Yoga combined with health education showed improvements in cardiovascular health and overall well-being	Variability in intervention protocols
Bhatia et al.	2022	Long-term effects of yoga and health education on cardiovascular health among police personnel in India	Long-term yoga practice led to sustained improvements in cardiovascular health and reduced risk factors	Potential biases due to selection

*The reference listed here can be accessed in the chapter.

Source: R, A., Mary Vaishali, P., & Parasuraman, G. (2024). Beyond the badge: A scoping review among police personnel in South India exploring the impact of yoga and health education on cardiovascular health. *Cureus, 16*(9), e68370. https://doi.org/10.7759/cureus.68370 (accessed on 29th May 2025). PMID: 39355455; PMCID: PMC11443585.

Table 5.29. The Effects of Yoga [LDL: Low-Density Lipoprotein; and HDL: High-Density Lipoprotein]

Authors	Year	Parameters Checked	Parameters Increased	Parameters Decreased	Reason for Changes Among Body Parameters
Sharma et al.	2015	BP, cholesterol levels, heart rate variability	Heart rate variability	BP, cholesterol levels	Regular yoga practice improved autonomic function.
Singh et al.	2016	BP, cholesterol levels, LDL, triglycerides	N/A	BP, cholesterol levels, LDL, triglycerides	Yoga's emphasis on relaxation and stress reduction led to lower BP and lipid levels.
Patel et al.	2017	BP, fasting blood glucose, LDL cholesterol, HDL cholesterol	HDL cholesterol	BP, fasting blood glucose, LDL cholesterol	Regular yoga improved lipid profiles by increasing HDL cholesterol and decreasing LDL and blood glucose due to enhanced metabolic function.
Kumar et al.	2018	BMI, waist-to-hip ratio, BP, physical fitness level	Physical fitness level	BMI, waist-to-hip ratio, BP	Combined interventions of yoga and health education promoted physical activity and dietary changes, leading to improved BMI and cardiovascular health.
Joshi et al.	2019	BP, cholesterol levels, exercise tolerance	Exercise tolerance	BP, cholesterol levels	Yoga increased exercise tolerance by improving cardiovascular efficiency and reducing stress, leading to decreased BP and cholesterol.
Reddy et al.	2020	Resting heart rate, BP, stress resilience	Stress resilience	Resting heart rate, BP	Yoga-based stress management enhanced stress resilience, leading to lower resting heart rate and BP.
Gupta et al.	2021	BP, fasting glucose, waist circumference, quality of life	Quality of life	BP, fasting glucose, waist circumference	Integrating yoga with health education improved overall well-being, reducing stress-related parameters like BP and waist circumference.
Bhati et al.	2022	BP, cholesterol levels, long-term health compliance	Long-term health compliance	BP, cholesterol levels	Sustained yoga practice fostered long-term adherence to healthy behaviors, resulting in ongoing reductions in cardiovascular risk factors.

Source: R, A., Mary Vaishali, P., & Parasuraman, G. (2024). Beyond the badge: A scoping review among police personnel in South India exploring the impact of yoga and health education on cardiovascular health. *Cureus*, *16*(9), e68370. https://doi.org/10.7759/cureus.68370 (accessed on 29th May 2025). PMID: 39355455; PMCID: PMC11443585.

5.5.1. Clinical Studies

A systematic review published in the Journal of Diabetes Research of results from 25 controlled trials (13 nonrandomized, 12 randomized) (N = 2170 participants) highlighted the promise of yoga in managing glucose levels (glycemic control), lipid profiles, sleep quality, and also lower the usage of medications (Innes et al., 2016) (Table 5.30).

Table 5.30. A Summary of Yoga on Glycemic Control and Other Parameters Presented by Innes et al. (2016)*

First Author, Year, and Location	Tx Dura tion	Study Population	N Enrolled/ Completed (per Group) [% Retention]	Yoga Intervention	Comparison Condition	Assessment Times	Major Findings	
Nonrandomized Controlled Trials (NRCTs)								
Dash, 2014, India	40 days	Adults 40–60 yo w/DM2 for 0–10 y; Excl: BMI > 25; DM1; DM2 w/nephropathy, CAD, retinopathy, alcoholism; practicing any yoga; 37% F	60 (30Y, 30C) [100%]#	Yoga (AS, PR, SH, and M): 30–40 min/d; + prescribed diet, oral meds	Prescribed diet, oral meds	Before and after: FBG, PPBG, A1c, TC, TG, LDL, HDL, and VLDL	Yoga: sig ↓ in FBG, PPBG, A1c, TC, TG, LDL, VLDL; sig ↑ HDL; C: sig ↓ in FBG, PPBG, VLDL; Y vs. C: sig ↓ in FBG, PPBG, A1c, TC, TG, LDL; sig ↑ HDL	4
Popli, 2014, India [43]	6 mos	Adults 30–60 yo w/DM2, no previous yoga experience; Excl: pts already on oral hypoglycemic meds or insulin, w/alcoholism, BG > 300 mg/dL, or end-organ damage (e.g., retinal detachment, nephropathy, and peripheral neuropathy)	130 (80Y, 50C)	Yoga (AS, PR): 1 hr with yoga trainer, 5 d/wk for 1st month, then continuing practice at home for remaining 5 mos	No treatment	Monthly: FBG; 3×/mo: PPBG, A1c	Yoga: sig ↓ in FBG, PPBG, A1c; C: NS	1
Bindra, 2013, India	Up to 90 days	Adults 35–65 yo w/DM2 for ≤10 y and no complications; Excl: those w/RA, cancer, TB, MI and not willing to do yoga	100 (50Y, 50C) [100%]#	Yoga (not described) + oral DM meds	Oral DM meds only	Before and after: FBG, A1c, TC, LDL, HDL, TG	Baseline yoga vs. C: NS differences between the groups; After 90 days, yoga vs. C: signif differences in FBG, A1c, TC, LDL, HDL	5
Balaji, 2011, India	3 mos	Uncomplicated DM2 pts 40–55 yo w/DM duration 1–10 y	44 (22Y, 22C) [100%]#	Yoga (AS, PR, SH): daily for 1 hr; Subgroup T1 (n = 16): + oral drugs; Subgroup T2 (n = 6): + oral drugs and insulin	22 controls	Before and after: FBG, PPBG, A1c, TC, TG, LDL, HDL, insulin/d (T2), wt, BMI, W:H	Yoga T1: sig ↓ in FBG, A1c, TG, LDL, wt, BMI, W:H; Yoga T2: sig ↓ in FBG, PPBG, A1c, TG, LDL, wt, BMI, W:H, insulin/d; C: NS	2

Hegde, 2011, India	3 mos	DM clinic pts w/DM2; age: 40–75 y; Excl: smoking, alcoholism	123/120 (60Y, 63C); strat'd by complications [98%]***	Yoga (AS, PR, and SH): at least 3 d/wk; + standard care	Standard care (given general oral and written information about diet and exercise)	Before and after: FBG, PPBG, A1c, oxidative stress (MDA, glutathione, SOD, Vit. C, and Vit. E), BMI, waist circumference, W:H, and BP	Y vs. C: sig ↓ in FBG, PPBG, A1c, BMI, MDA; sig ↑ glutathione, Vit. C	4
Kyizom, 2010, India	45 days; groups matched for age and sex	DM clinic pts, 35–60 yo, w/ uncomplicated DM2 from 2–10 y	60 (30Y, 30C) [100%]#	Yoga (AS, PR, and SH): daily for 45 min/d; + standard care	Standard care	Before and after: FBG, PPBG, event-related evoked potentials at frontal (Fz), vertex (Cz), and parietal (Pz) areas, peak latencies, and baseline to peak amplitudes of N2 and P3	Yoga: sig ↓ in FBG, PPBG; sig ↓ in latency of N2 at Cz and P300 at all montages (Fz, Cz, and Pz); sig ↑ in amplitude of wave N2 at Cz and P300 at Pz montage; C: NS	2
Malhotra, 2010, India	40 days; controls matched on age and DM severity	Pts from endocrine metabolic clinic w/DM2 for 0–10 y, 30–60 yo, on recommended diet and oral DM meds; Excl: CAD, nephropathy, and proliferative retinopathy	106 (56Y, 50C)/64 (26Y, 38C) [60%]	Yoga (AS, PR, and SH): 40–60 min/d; + diet and DM meds	Standard care: meds, diet, and light exercises (walking)	Before and after: FBG, PPBG, TC, TG, HDL, LDL, VLDL, MDA, insulin; wt, W:H, BMI, LBM, and BSA; SBP, DBP, HR, and QT interval; SVC, FEV1, FVC, FEV1:FVC ratio, PEFR, and MVV; median nerve conduction velocity (m/sec), amplitude (mV), and latency (msec) measured proximally (at elbow) and distally (at wrist)	Yoga: sig ↓ in FBG, TC, TG, MDA, SBP, DBP, HR, W:H; sig ↑ in pulmonary and CV fxn; sig ↑ in left hand nerve conduction velocity and amplitude (distal); C: sig ↓ in LBM (worsening), nerve conduction amplitude (right proximal), sig ↑ in TG (worsening), insulin (in 4 pts), HR, PEFR; Y vs. C: not analyzed	2
Mahapure, 2008, India	6 wks	Pts 40–58 yo, w/DM2 on regular diet and antidiabetic drug regimen	40 (30Y, 10C) [100%]#	Yoga (AS, PR, SH): 1 hr/d, every day except Sundays; + standard care	Standard care: diet and meds	Before and after: FBG, A1c, and SOD	Yoga: sig ↓ in FBG, A1c; sig ↑ SOD; C: NS; Y vs. C: sig ↓ in FBG, A1c; sig ↑ SOD	3
Singh, 2008, India	45 days	Pts 35–60 yo, w/ uncomplicated DM2 for 1–10 y	60 (30Y, 30C) [100%]#	Yoga (AS, PR, and SH): daily for 45 min/d; + standard care	Standard care (conventional meds)	Before and after: FBG, PPBG, A1c, TC, TG, LDL, VLDL, HDL, insulin, wt, and BMI	Yoga: sig ↓ in wt, FBG, PPBG, insulin, TC, TG, VLDL, LDL; sig ↑ in HDL; C: sig ↑ wt; Y vs. C: not given	2
Agte, 2004, India	4 mos	Previously diagnosed DM2 pts 45–65 yo; having stabilized glucose levels and taking conventional prescribed medications; BMI: 25.4 (Y), 25.6 (C); 53% F	87 (57Y, 30C)/65 (35Y, 30C) [75%]	SKY + PR, AS, and M; interactive discussions on stress-free living; nutritional counseling with emphasis on eating fresh fruits and vegetables; 6 d course	Without SKY training	Before and after: FBG, PPBG, A1c, TC, TG, HDL, and MDA	Yoga: sig ↓ in FBG, PPBG, TC, TG, MDA; C: NS; Y vs. C: not presented	1

Agrawal, 2003, India	3 mos	Pts randomly selected from diabetes clinic (type of DM not specified, but background implies that study targeted DM2); Excl: pts with liver disease, alcoholism, malnutrition, thyrotoxicosis, TB, or who were noncooperative	200/154 (82Y, 72C) [77%]	Yogic lifestyle program: health rejuvenation exercises (5 min), AS (18 min), abdominal exercises (7 min), and R/M/PR (30 min); at least 5 d/wk + diet	Standard medical tx or standard home exercise program	Before and after: FBG, A1c, TC, HDL, LDL, VLDL, BP, BMI, W:H, QOL (satisfaction, impact, and worry), psychological assessment, self-evaluation, doses of metformin, glipizide, and insulin, BP, and renal function	Y vs. C: sig ↓ in FBG, A1c, BMI, W:H, TC, LDL, VLDL, SBP, DBP; metformin, glipizide, and insulin doses; QOL satisfaction, impact, and worry scores, psychological assessment, and self-evaluation; sig ↑ HDL	3
Malhotra, 2002, India	40 days; controls matched on age, sex, SES, and DM severity	DM2 for 0–10 y; 30–60 yo; Excl: cardiac, renal, and proliferative retinal complications	40 (20Y, 20C) [100%]	Supervised yoga (AS, PR, and SH): daily for 30–40 min/d; + medication, diet	Medication, diet, and light exercise (walking)	Before and after 40-day treatment: median nerve conduction velocity (m/sec), amplitude (mV), and latency (msec) measured proximally (at elbow) and distally (at wrist)	Yoga: sig ↑ conduction velocity in left hand; C: sig ↓ in amplitude at right elbow (proximal)	4
Khare, 1999, India	3 mos; non-DM controls matched for age, sex	60 DM2 pts (DM for 1–2 y) from DM clinics (in yoga/diet groups), 20 non-DM matched on age, sex; 40–70 y on vegetarian diet	80 (20, 20, 20, 20) [100%][#]	(1) Yoga: AS (3 poses, 2–5 min each) and SH (20 min) only; (2) Yoga + strict diet; Yoga: 2×/d	(1) No intervention (non-DM adults); (2) Strict diet alone (20 DM adults)	Baseline and 1, 2, and 3 mos: BG, serum fructosamine, TC, and wt	Yoga (3 mos): sig ↓ in BG, Fruc, TC, and wt; Yoga + diet: sig ↓ in BG, Fruc, TC, and wt; Diet: sig ↓ in TC and wt; Non-DM, no tx: NS	1
Randomized Controlled Trials (RCTs)								
Habibi, 2013, Iran	12 wks	Women w/DM2, 45–60 yo, not taking insulin; without DM complications or hx of CVD	26 (16Y, 10C) [100%][#]	Yoga: 75 min, 3 d/wk	Standard care	Before and after: BP, FBG, fasting insulin, TC, HDL, LDL, leptin, wt, and BMI	Y vs. C: sig ↓ in FBG, insulin, TG	4[†]
Jyotsna, 2012, India	6 mos	Adults w/DM2 + lifestyle modification, A1c of 6–9%, and oral hypoglycemic agents for past 6 mos; Excl: pts w/retinopathy, glaucoma, uncontrolled HTN, CAD, overt complications of diabetes, and nephropathy; mean age (y): 49.92 ± 11.46 (Y), 47.25 ± 10.80 (C)	120 (64Y, 56C) [100%][#]	*Sudarshan Kriya Yoga* (SKY: a rhythmic cyclical breathing, preceded by PR); 3 d group training program followed by classes 1×/wk (long *kriya*) and daily home practice (short *kriya*) + standard care	Standard care (oral antidiabetic drugs and diet and exercise advice)	Before and 6 mos after tx: CAFTs, FBG, PPBG, and A1c; Before and 3 and 6 mos after tx: QOL (domains: (1) physical health; (2) psychological well-being; (3) social relationships; (4) environment)	Yoga: sig ↑ sympathetic fxn; C: NS; Y vs. C: sig ↑ overall cardiac autonomic fxn; sig ↓ PPBG; sig ↑ QOL: at 3 mos—domains 1 and 2 and total QOL; at 6 mos—domains 2 and 4 and total QOL	4[†]; 4; 5[†]

Naga rathna, 2012, India	9 mos	Pts >25 yo w/DM2 >1 y (FBG >120 mg% at dx), stable dose of oral hypoglycemic agents or insulin for ≥3 wks, no prior yoga, no major complications; mean age: 52.4 y; 31% F	277 (141Y, 136C)/173 (88Y, 85C) [62%]	Yoga (AS, PR, M, devotional sessions, and lectures): 1 hr/d, 5 d/wk for 12 wks [cleansing techniques (*kriyas*) 1×/wk]; 1 2-hr class/wk and 1-hr daily home practice for 9 mos	Exercises and walking to match intensity, nonyogic breathing, supine rest, and lectures: 1 hr/d, 5 d/wk for 12 wks; 1 2-hr class/wk and 1-hr daily home practice for 9 mos	Before and after: TC, TG, HDL, LDL, VLDL, FBG, PPBG, A1c, and oral hypoglycemic medication requirement	Yoga: sig ↓ meds, FBG, PPBG, A1c, TG, TC, LDL, VLDL; sig ↑ HDL; C: sig ↓ PPBG, A1c, TG, TC, VLDL; Y vs. C: sig ↓ meds, LDL; sig ↑ HDL	6
Shanta kumari, 2012, India	3 mos	Pts w/DM2 + HTN and dyslipidemia, 35–55 yo; Excl: those w/known retinopathy, nephropathy, CAD, and cerebrovascular diseases; avg DM duration: 5–10 y; 48% F	100 (50Y, 50C) [100%][#]	Yoga: 1 hr daily; AS (30–35 min), PR (10 min), and M (15 min); + standard care	Standard care (oral hypoglycemic drugs, no yoga)	Before and after: FBG, PPBG, TC, HDL, LDL, TG, wt, W:H, BMI, SBP, and DBP	Yoga: sig ↓ wt, W:H, TG, TC, LDL; C: sig ↑ wt	6[†]; 5[†]
Subram aniyan, 2012, India	15 days	Males ≥18 yo w/DM2 on standard care and medically eligible for walking/yoga per physician; age: 55% were 31–40 yo	20 [100%][#]	Yoga: 60 min (6–7 a.m.) daily; AS (~30 min), sun salutation (~6 min), SH (~25 min) + routine meds	Brisk walking: 60 min (6–7 a.m.) daily + routine meds	Before and after: FBG	Yoga: sig ↓ in FBG; Walking: sig ↓ in FBG	4
Vaishali, 2011, India	12 wks	Diabetic clinic pts >60 yo w/ DM2 >15 y and ≥1 metabolic risk factor (high FBG, pre-HTN, overweight/obese, high TC), on antidiabetic meds >10 y; Excl: uncontrolled HTN, severe neuropathy, hx of foot lesions, unstable proliferative retinopathy, and nephropathy	60/57 [95%]	Yoga (individualized AS, PR, and SH): 45–60 min under supervision, 6 d/wk	Educational group (general healthy lifestyle and exercise): 1×/ mo	Before and after: FBG, A1c, TC, TG, LDL, and HDL	Yoga: sig ↓ FBG, A1c, TC, TG, LDL; sig ↑ HDL; C: NS; Y vs. C: sig ↓ A1c, FBG, TC, TG, LDL; sig ↑ HDL	6[†]; 6
Pardasany, 2010, India	12 wks	Adults w/DM2, 40–60 yo; Excl: hx of renal disease, arthritis, HBP, intermittent claudication, foot injury or ulcers, breathlessness, and cardiac disease; 38% F	45 (15, 15, 15) [100%][#]	*Hatha Yoga* (12 AS and 6–7 PR): 3×/wk; oral hypoglycemic meds	(1) Yang-style tai chi (TC, 24 forms): 3×/wk + oral hypoglycemic meds; (2) Oral hypoglycemic meds only (C)	Before and after: FBG, PPBG, A1c, TC, and LDL	Yoga: sig ↓ FBG, PPBG, A1c, TC, LDL; TC: sig ↓ FBG, PPBG, A1c, TC, LDL; C: NS; Y vs. C: sig ↓ FBG, PPBG, TC, LDL; TC vs. C: sig ↓ FBG, PPBG, A1c, TC; Tai chi vs. Y: NS	4[†]

Amita, 2009, India	Up to 90 days	Middle-aged (35–65 yo) DM2 pts on oral hypoglycemics; Excl: >200 mg/dL FBG, >300 mg/dL PPBG; hx of DM complications or other systemic conditions; 29% F	41 (20Y, 21C) [100%][#]	*Yoga Nidra* (deep relaxation): 45 min, daily	Standard care (no yoga)	Every 30 days: FBG, PPBG, and symptoms related to DM (e.g., insomnia, palpitations, sweating, distress, headache, and anxiety)	Yoga: sig ↓ FBG (60 and 90 d), PPBG (90 d), total symptoms (insomnia, distress, etc., after 3 mos); C: not given	1[†]
Skoro-Kondza, 2009, UK (London)	12 wks	Adults (>18 yo) w/DM2, not on insulin; most well-controlled (A1c x = 6.9); mean DM2 duration: 30 ± 5 y; mean age: 60 ± 10 y; nonwhite: 55% at one site, 40% at the other; 61% F	59 [100%][#]*	Yoga (PR, AS, and SH): 90 min class, 3×/wk	Wait list (both groups received healthy lifestyle leaflets and were encouraged to exercise)	Before, after, and 6 mos later: A1c, wt, waist circumference, W:H, BMI, TC, LDL, TG, HDL, SBP, and DBP (used to calculate cardiovascular risk score); diabetes-related QOL and self-efficacy	Yoga: NS; C: NS; Y vs. C: NS; Note: Quantitative data provided only for A1c	4[†]
Gordon, 2008, Cuba	24 wks; age- and sex-matched controls	Pts 40–70 yo w/DM2 (1–10 y) with ≥3 mos of DM education, exercise, diet, and medication (per IDF); no severe complications; nonsmoker; nonalcoholic	231 (77 pts: 62 females, 15 males per group) [100%][#***]	Yoga: PR (20 min), warm-up exercises (25 min), AS (60 min), and SH (15 min); 1 class/wk for 24 wks + home yoga exercises (per IDF criteria)	(1) PT: warm-up (15 min), aerobic walking (30 min), flexibility (20 min), aerobic dance (20 min), games (25 min), warm-down (10 min); 1 class/wk for 24 wks + home exercise 3–4×/wk; (2) Control: tx plan as per their doctors, no active exercise tx	Baseline, 3 mos, and 6 mos: FBG, A1c, insulin, TC, TG, HDL, LDL, VLDL, BMI, MDA, PLA2 activity, POX, SOD, catalase activity; microalbuminuria, creatinine, cortisol, TSH, T3, T4	Yoga: 3 mos: sig ↓ FBG, TC; 6 mos: sig ↓ FBG, A1c, TC, VLDL, microalbuminuria, MDA; sig ↑ SOD; PT: 3 mos: sig ↓ FBG, TC; 6 mos: sig ↓ FBG, TC, VLDL, microalbuminuria, MDA; sig ↑ SOD; C: NS at 3 and 6 mos; Y vs. C: 3 mos: sig ↓ FBG, A1c, TC; 6 mos: sig ↓ FBG, A1c, TC, MDA, BMI, microalbuminuria; sig ↑ % insulin receptor binding; PT vs. C: 3 mos: sig ↓ FBG, A1c, TC; 6 mos: sig ↓ FBG, A1c, TC, MDA, BMI, microalbuminuria; sig ↑ % insulin receptor binding	6[†]; 4[†]

Céspedes, 2002, Cuba	12 mos	DM2 patients, 50–70 y, DM duration 2–5 y, without malnutrition or severe complications, in good mental health	40 (22Y, 18C) [100%][#]	Moderate intensity yoga (PR, AS): 60 min class, 3×/wk + lifestyle advice, soybean-rich diet	Moderate intensity aerobic exercise: 60 min class, 3×/wk + lifestyle advice, soybean-rich diet	Before and after: BG, TC, HDL, LDL, TG, and creatinine	Yoga: sig ↓ TC, LDL, TG, creatinine; sig ↑ HDL; PT: sig ↓ TC, LDL, TG, creatinine; sig ↑ HDL; Y vs. C: sig ↓ TC, LDL, TG, creatinine; sig ↑ HDL	5
Monro, 1992, UK	12 wks	DM2 controlled with meds (N = 13; yoga group = 8) or diet (N = 8); Excl: end-stage liver or kidney disease or congestive cardiac failure; age: 45–67 y	21 (11Y, 10C) [100%]**	Yoga (PR, AS, and R) + standard care: 90 min, classes offered 5×/wk (most attended 1–2×/wk and practiced at home 1–2×/wk)	Standard care (continuing on medication, diet)	Before and after: FBG and A1c	Y vs. C: sig ↓ in A1c, FBG	5[†]

*Summary of study characteristics and major findings.

[#]Assumed (retention not specifically reported), [*]adherence very low, [**]adherence moderate, [***]adherence excellent, and [†]score from PEDro database.

A1c: glycosylated hemoglobin A1c, AHA: American Heart Association, AS: yoga asanas or postures, avg: average, BF: biofeedback, BP: blood pressure, BSA: body surface area, C: control, CAD: coronary artery disease, CAFT: cardiac autonomic function tests, cal: calorie, Clin: clinical, comp: composition, CVD: cardiovascular disease, d: day, DM: diabetes mellitus, Excl: excluded, F: female, FBG: fasting blood glucose, FEV1: forced expiratory value in first second, FVC: forced vital capacity, h: hour, HDL: high density lipoprotein, HR: heart rate, HTN: hypertension, hx: history, IFNγ: interferon gamma, a cytokine critical for innate and adaptive immunity against viral and intracellular bacterial infections and for tumor control, IR: insulin resistance (markers of), KR: kriyas or cleansing exercises, LBM: lean body mass, LDL: low density lipoprotein, M: meditation, MDA: malondialdehyde, MI: myocardial infarction, mo: month, MVV: maximal voluntary ventilation, PEFR: peak expiratory flow rate, PLA2: phospholipase A2, PMR: progressive muscle relaxation, POX: protein oxidation, PPBG: postprandial blood glucose, PR: pranayama or yogic breathing exercises, QOL: quality of life, R: relaxation poses (nonspecified), RA: rheumatoid arthritis, Resid: residential, SH: shavasana or corpse pose, a traditional yoga relaxation pose, Sig: significant, SNS/PNS: markers of sympathetic/parasympathetic activation, including heart rate and catecholamine levels, SOD: superoxide dismutase, SVC: slow vital capacity, TB: tuberculosis, TC: total cholesterol, Tg: triglycerides, veg: vegetarian, VLDL: very low density lipoprotein, W : H: waist-hip ratio, wk: week, wt: weight, y: years, and yo: years old.

Source: Innes, K. E., & Selfe, T. K. (2016). Yoga for adults with type 2 diabetes: A systematic review of controlled trials. *Journal of Diabetes Research*, *2016*, 6979370, 23 pages. https://doi.org/10.1155/2016/6979370 (accessed on 29th May 2025).

A few of these studies analyzed showed that there were reductions in glycemic indicators, such as glycosylated HbA1c, insulin, and fasting blood glucose. While the potential of yoga cannot be ruled out, further studies are warranted to address pending gaps, including participant heterogeneity and study design (Table 5.31).

Table 5.31. The Effect of Yoga on Metabolic Parameters in Diabetes Reviewed by Innes et al. (2016)

Findings, by Clinical Measure	**Study Design**			
	Nonrandomized Controlled Trials (NRCTs)		**Randomized Controlled Trials (RCTs)**	
	Yoga vs. Baseline	**Yoga vs. Controls**	**Yoga vs. Baseline**	**Yoga vs. Controls**
Measures of Insulin Resistance				
Fasting glucose	14.33–33.23%	9.87–29.75%	7.21–27.53%	13.46–36.2%
Postprandial glucose	5.92–38.65%	11.61–35.5%	7.03–18.89%	11.17–14.22%
Fasting glycosylated hemoglobin (HbA1c)	1.55–21.23%	1.03–7.44%	0.31–14.17%	7.77–17.78%
Blood Lipid Profiles				
Total cholesterol	5.97–14.61%	4.11–8.63%	1.37–37.01%	4.74–18.3%
Triglycerides	3.97–16.35%	3.53%	14.33–38.0%	1.06–10.96%
Low-density lipoprotein (LDL)	2.18–14.88%	1.38–15.05%	8.33–48.45%	3.39–11.42%
High-density lipoprotein (HDL)	8.28–15.21%	5.01–24.96%	6.99–101.59%	9.1–54.92%
Very low-density lipoprotein (VLDL)	15.17–16.06%	13.28%	7.23–22.66%	–
Anthropometric Measures				
BMI	7.52–10.34%	2.72–3.56%	–	4.32%
Body weight	3.48–6.95%	–	–	4.18%
Waist-hip circumference ratio	5.38–8.99%	3.17%	–	5.32%
Blood Pressure (BP)				
Systolic blood pressure (SBP)	11.27%	5.03%	–	–
Diastolic blood pressure (DBP)	12.92%	3.46%	–	–

Summary: Meta-analyses of the effects of yoga on risk indices relevant to T2DM (the references cited here can be accessed in the chapter)

Measure	First Author, Year	Population	Included Studies			Comparator	Mean Difference (95% CI)	P
			Design	Number	Total Pts			
Glucose Tolerance								
Fasting blood glucose (mg/dL)	Cramer, 2014	DM2	RCTs	7	525	Usual care	−25.56 (−39.60, −11.53)	<0.01
	Chu, 2014	DM or MS	RCTs	6	315	All	−8.77 (−26.77, 9.23)	0.34
HbA1c	Cramer, 2014	DM2	RCTs	7	550	Usual care	−0.49 (−1.03, 0.05)	0.07
Lipid Profiles								
Total cholesterol	Cramer, 2014	DM2	RCTs	5	516	Usual care	−13.09 (−19.60, −6.59)	<0.01
	Cramer, 2014	DM2	RCTs	2	317	Exercise	−8.08 (−19.20, 3.03)	0.21
	Chu, 2014	DM or MS	RCTs	5	365	All	−20.98 (−33.23, −8.72)	0.0008
	Chu, 2014	CVD risk factors	RCTs	2	109	All	−18.85 (−37.24, −0.46)	0.04
HDL	Cramer, 2014	DM2	RCTs	5	516	Usual care	5.51 (3.56, 7.47)	<0.01
	Cramer, 2014	DM2	RCTs	2	317	Exercise	4.24 (1.75, 6.72)	0.01
	Chu, 2014	DM or MS	RCTs	5	365	All	2.45 (−0.33, 5.24)	0.08
	Chu, 2014	CVD risk factors	RCTs	2	109	All	3.95 (1.69, 6.21)	0.0006
LDL	Cramer, 2014	DM2	RCTs	5	515	Usual care	−10.26 (−20.85, 0.32)	0.06

	Cramer, 2014	DM2	RCTs	2	317	Exercise	−9.24 (−16.55, −1.93)	0.01
	Chu, 2014	DM or MS	RCTs	5	365	All	−21.27 (−32.93, −9.62)	<0.00001
	Chu, 2014	CVD risk factors	RCTs	2	109	All	−14.42 (−20.47, −8.36)	0.0003
VLDL	Cramer, 2014	DM2	RCTs	2	308	Usual care	−4.81 (−6.67, −2.96)	<0.01
Triglycerides	Cramer, 2014	DM2	RCTs	5	509	Usual care	−23.60 (−36.78, −10.43)	<0.01
	Cramer, 2014	DM2	RCTs	2	317	Exercise	−22.98 (−60.97, 15.00)	0.24
	Chu, 2014	DM or MS	RCTs	5	365	All	−18.61 (−32.61, −4.60)	0.009
	Chu, 2014	CVD risk factors	RCTs	2	109	All	−27.47 (−60.09, 5.15)	0.10
Body Composition								
Waist-hip ratio	Cramer, 2014	DM2	RCTs	3	311	Usual care	−0.02 (−0.03, −0.00)	<0.01
BMI	Chu, 2014	DM or MS	RCTs	3	155	All	−1.63 (−2.25, −1.01)	<0.00001
	Chu, 2014	CVD risk factors	RCTs	2	77	All	−0.99 (−2.38, 0.40)	0.16
Weight (kg)	Chu, 2014	DM or MS	RCTs	3	151	All	−3.27 (−4.99, −1.54)	0.0002
	Chu, 2014	CVD risk factors	RCTs	6	273	All	−1.95 (−5.25, 1.35)	0.25
Blood Pressure (BP) (mmHg)								
Systolic BP	Cramer, 2014	DM2	RCTs	3	237	Usual care	−6.87 (−14.68, 0.94)	0.08

	Cramer, 2014	Non-DM high risk	RCTs	8	347	Usual care	−10.00 (−16.42, −3.59)	<0.01
	Cramer, 2014	HT	RCTs	6	278	Usual care	−9.65 (−17.66, −2.06)	0.01
	Hagins, 2013	HT (all)	RCTs, NRCTs	11	431	Usual care	−7.96 (−10.65, −5.27)	0.0002
	Hagins, 2013	HT (Y incl M, PR, AS)	RCTs, NRCTs	13	656	All	−8.17 (−12.45, −3.89)	NR
	Hagins, 2013	HT (Y > 58.9 h)	RCTs, NRCTs	6	215	All	−9.73 (−17.66, −1.79)	NR
	Chu, 2014	DM or MS	RCTs	3	80	All	−9.39 (−15.14, −3.63)	0.001
	Chu, 2014	CVD risk factors	RCTs	10	461	All	−7.36 (−13.39, −1.33)	0.001
Diastolic BP	Cramer, 2014	DM2	RCTs	2	210	Usual care	−0.79 (−5.22, 3.65)	0.73
	Cramer, 2014	Non-DM high risk	RCTs	8	347	Usual care	−7.45 (−12.70, −2.21)	<0.01
	Cramer, 2014	HT	RCTs	6	278	Usual care	−7.22 (−12.83, −1.62)	0.01
	Hagins, 2013	HT (all)	RCTs, NRCTs	11	431	Usual care	−6.14 (−9.39, −2.89)	NR
	Hagins, 2013	HT (Y incl M, PR, AS)	RCTs, NRCTs	13	656	All	−5.52 (−7.92, −3.11)	NR
	Chu, 2014	DM or MS	RCTs	3	80	All	−5.41 (−8.82, −2.01)	0.002
	Chu, 2014	CVD risk factors	RCTs	10	461	All	−6.97 (−11.80, −2.13)	0.005
Autonomic fxn								
Heart rate	Cramer, 2014	Non-DM high risk	RCTs	3	133	Usual care	−10.89 (−22.83, 1.04)	0.07

Abbreviations: AS: *Asana*; CAD: Coronary artery disease; CI: Confidence interval; CVD: Cardiovascular disease; fxn: Function; HT: Hypertension; M: *Meditation*; MS: Metabolic syndrome; NR: Not reported; NRCT: Nonrandomized controlled trial; PR: *Pranayama*; Pts: Participants; Y: *Yoga*.

Source: Innes, K. E., & Selfe, T. K. (2016). Yoga for adults with type 2 diabetes: A systematic review of controlled trials. *Journal of Diabetes Research, 2016*, 6979370, 23 pages. https://doi.org/10.1155/2016/6979370 (accessed on 29th May 2025).

"The yoga mat is a good place to turn when talk therapy and antidepressants aren't enough"

—Amy Weintraub

5.6. Case Study: The NNMB-Trial

The potential of a yoga-based lifestyle modification protocol (YLP) in preventing diabetes in high-risk individuals was reported in the Niyantrita Madhmeha Bharata Abhiyaan (NMB-trial).

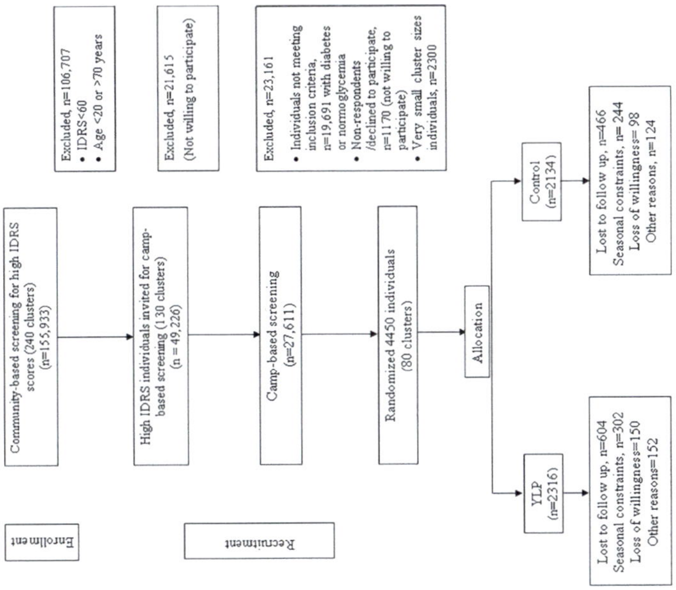

Figure 5.10. The NMB trial.

Source: Raghuram, N., Ram, V., Majumdar, V., SK, R., Singh, A., Patil, S., Anand, A., Judu, I., Bhaskara, S., Basa, J. R., & Nagendra, H. R. (2021). Effectiveness of a yoga-based lifestyle protocol (YLP) in preventing diabetes in a high-risk Indian cohort: A multicenter cluster-randomized controlled trial (NMB-Trial). *Frontiers in Endocrinology, 12*, 664657. https://doi.org/10.3389/fendo.2021.664657 (accessed on 29th May 2025).

The study: Clinical Trials Registry–India (CTRI) Trial Registration Number: CTRI/2018/03/012804) was a multicenter cluster-randomized trial conducted on Indian participants (20–70 years) with prediabetes (blood glycosylated HbA1c values in the range of 5.7–6.4%) and Indian IDRS ≥ 60. The control group was advised home care guidelines and the yoga group received YLP training for 9 days (done daily and supervised weekly for 3 months) (Raghuram et al., 2021). The approach is shown in Figure 5.10; Tables 5.32 and 5.33.

Table 5.32. The Yoga Regimen in the NMB Trial (Practiced All Days of the Week)

SL. No.	Name of the Practice	Duration
1.	Starting prayer	2 mins
2.	Preparatory *Sukshma Vyayamas* and *Shithililarana* Practices (loosening practices) · *Urdhvahastashvasana* (Hand stretch and breathing, 3 rounds at 90°, 135°, and 180° each) · *Kati-Shakti Vikasaka* (Trunk twisting pose, 3 rounds each) · *Sarvangapushti* (3 rounds clockwise, 3 rounds anti-clockwise)	6 mins
3.	*Surya Namaskara* (Sun salutation) · 10-step fast *Surya Namaskara* – 6 rounds · 12-step slow *Surya Namaskara* – 1 round	9 mins
4.	Standing postures: · *Trikonasana* (triangle pose), *Parvritta Trikonasana* (revolved triangle pose), *Prasarita Padhastasana* (intense leg stretch) Supine postures: · *Jatara Parivartanasana* (abdominal twist pose), *Pavanamuktasana* (wind-relieving pose), *Viparitakarani* (inverted lake pose) Prone postures: · *Bhujangasana* (cobra pose), *Dhanurasana* (bow pose) followed by *Pavanamuktasana* Sitting postures: · *Mandukasana* (frog pose), *Vakrasana/Ardhamatsyendrasana* (spine twisting posture), *Paschimatanasana* (seated forward bending), *Ardha Ushtrasana* (half camel pose) At the end: relaxation with abdominal breathing in supine position (*vishranti*), 10–15 rounds (2 mins)	15 mins

5.	*Kriya* (cleansing techniques) · *Agnisara* – 1 min · *Kapalabhati* – 60 breaths per minute for 1 min followed by 1 min rest	3 mins
6.	*Pranayama* · *Nadishuddhi* (alternate nostril breathing – 6 mins) · *Bhramari* – 3 mins	9 mins
7.	Meditation	15 mins
8.	Resolve	½ min
9.	Closing prayer: *Sarvebhavantu Sukhinaha...*	⅓ min
	Total	**60 mins**

Category	ADA Recommendation	Yoga Lifestyle
Diet	Rich in whole grains, fruits, vegetables, legumes, and nuts; low in refined grains, red or processed meats; without sugar and sweetened beverages	*Satvic* diet Wholesome lacto-vegetarian diet
Physical activity	Minimum 2.5 hrs of moderate to vigorous intensity physical activity per week (e.g., brisk walking, water aerobics, swimming, or jogging)	Daily loosening practices – 6 mins *Surya Namaskara* – 9 mins *Asanas* and *Kriyas* – 18 mins × 7 days = 126 mins **Total:** ~231 minutes (~3.85 hrs) of mild to moderate physical activity

Source: Raghuram, N., Ram, V., Majumdar, V., SK, R., Singh, A., Patil, S., Anand, A., Judu, I., Bhaskara, S., Basa, J. R., & Nagendra, H. R. (2021). Effectiveness of a yoga-based lifestyle protocol (YLP) in preventing diabetes in a high-risk Indian cohort: A multicenter cluster-randomized controlled trial (NMB-Trial). *Frontiers in Endocrinology, 12*, 664657. https://doi.org/10.3389/fendo.2021.664657 (accessed on 29th May 2025).

Table 5.33. The Diet (Healthy Choices) Advised in the NMB Trial

Dietary Constituents	Baseline			Post-Intervention		
	Yoga	Control	*P* Value	Yoga	Control	*P* Value
Cereals (Staple Food)						
Intake of Dairy Items						
Usually/often	864 (32.0%)	435 (31.0%)	0.794	801 (29.7%)	412 (29.4%)	<0.001
Sometimes	1251 (46.4%)	657 (46.9%)		998 (37.0%)	491 (35.0%)	
Never/rarely	582 (21.6%)	310 (22.1%)		877 (32.5%)	498 (35.5%)	
Intake of Meat						
Usually/often	371 (14.1%)	205 (14.9%)	0.425	388 (14.8%)	178 (13.0%)	<0.001
Sometimes	1234 (47.0%)	616 (44.9%)		1005 (38.3%)	524 (38.2%)	
Never/rarely	1018 (38.8%)	551 (40.2%)		1194 (45.5%)	669 (48.7%)	
Intake of Fatty Foods						
Usually/often	361 (13.6%)	204 (14.8%)	0.599	299 (11.3%)	155 (11.2%)	<0.001
Sometimes	1353 (50.9%)	693 (50.1%)		1086 (40.9%)	526 (38.0%)	
Never/rarely	942 (35.5%)	486 (35.1%)		1234 (46.4%)	701 (50.6%)	
Intake of Salty Foods						
Usually/often	354 (13.4%)	187 (13.6%)	0.928	313 (11.9%)	112 (8.1%)	<0.001
Sometimes	1202 (45.7%)	621 (45.0%)		874 (33.2%)	535 (38.8%)	
Never/rarely	1076 (40.9%)	571 (41.4%)		1412 (53.6%)	730 (53%)	
Intake of Sweets						
Usually/often	301 (11.4%)	152 (11.0%)	0.939	318 (12.0%)	127 (9.2%)	<0.001
Sometimes	1202 (45.5%)	629 (45.6%)		881 (33.4%)	527 (38.2%)	
Never/rarely	1137 (43.1%)	597 (43.3%)		1407 (53.2%)	719 (52.1%)	
Intake of Aerated Beverages						
Usually/often	382 (13.4%)	162 (11.7%)	0.307	359 (13.7%)	130 (9.4%)	<0.001
Sometimes	1055 (40.2%)	561 (40.6%)		854 (32.5%)	485 (35.1%)	
Rarely/never	1220 (46.4%)	660 (47.7%)		1384 (52.6%)	763 (55.1%)	
Eating Behavior (Skipping Breakfast)						
Usually/often	923 (34.2%)	488 (34.3%)	0.148	852 (31.6%)	432 (30.4%)	–
Sometimes	836 (31.0%)	477 (33.5%)		647 (24.0%)	364 (25.6%)	–
Rarely/never	940 (34.8%)	458 (32.2%)		1174 (43.4%)	625 (44%)	–

Source: Raghuram, N., Ram, V., Majumdar, V., SK, R., Singh, A., Patil, S., Anand, A., Judu, I., Bhaskara, S., Basa, J. R., & Nagendra, H. R. (2021). Effectiveness of a Yoga-Based Lifestyle Protocol (YLP) in preventing diabetes in a high-risk Indian cohort: A multicenter cluster-randomized controlled trial (NMB-Trial). *Frontiers in Endocrinology, 12*, 664657. https://doi.org/10.3389/fendo.2021.664657 (accessed on 29th May 2025).

Diabetes developed in 726 (21.44%) participants; of these, the YLP group had lower occurrence (n = 192, 11.21%) than the control group (n = 534, 32.01%). The relative risk (RR) of conversion from prediabetes to type 2 diabetes was also lower in the YLP group vs. the control. These results are documented in Table 5.34. Further, no adverse effects were reported apart from mild lumbar/dorsal region that was addressed by relevant yoga poses.

Table 5.34. Follow-Up Results in the NMB Trial

	Imputed data-based analyses						
Subgroups	**Conversion from prediabetes to diabetes, number of events, n (%)**		**Test statistic (χ^2)**	**Unadjusted RRR (95% CI)**	**RRR-adjusted for covariates (95% CI)**	**Cluster-adjusted RRR (95% CI)**	**$P_{interaction}$**
	YLP (n = 2316)	**Control (n = 2134)**					
Overall, n = 4450	266 (11.48)	669 (32.01)	264.09	63.36 (58.31–67.81)	64.19 (57.22–64.19)	63.81 (56.55–69.85)	
					#64.24 (58.09–69.49)	# 63.95 (56.96–69.81)	
≤40 years	58 (9.45)	143 (26.48)	57.97	64.33 (52.69–73.10)	64.47 (56.01–71.30)	64.76 (50.70–74.82)	0.99
>40years	208 (12.22)	526 (32.99)	205.29	62.97 (57.17–67.97)	62.92 (44.13–75.39)	64.64 (57.71–70.44)	
Gender							
Male	87 (9.64)	260 (29.61)	113.03	58.92 (41.94–70.94)	59.99 (46.03–70.33)	61.10 (49.35–70.12)	0.80
Female	208 (14.71)	526 (41.88)	153.46	64.59 (53.85–72.84)	66.01 (57.46–72.84)	62.40 (46.19–73.73)	
Location							
Rural	108 (10.66)	301 (33.33)	146.16	69.29 (60.49–76.13)	68.40 (60.06–75.00)	62.04 (36.73–77.22)	0.62
Urban	158 (12.13)	368 (29.90)	121.50	41.03 (11.10–60.88)	54.78 (39.03–66.46)	55.71 (42.65–65.80)	
BMI, kg/m²							
≤23	198 (11.40)	505 (30.93)	194.38	63.19 (57.18–68.27)	64.47 (56.01–71.30)	59.08 (40.58–71.82)	0.72
>23	68 (11.74)	164 (32.73)	70.16	64.12 (53.65–72.53)	63.21 (73.48–48.97)	63.53 (49.95–73.43)	
Physical activity							
No	95 (12.45)	246 (31.91)	83.70	64.49 (49.40–75.08)	66.47 (53.98–75.57)	66.66 (56.56–74.41)	
Mild	70 (11.38)	161 (29.98)	62.49	69.02 (55.88–78.24)	66.55 (49.73–77.75)	64.58 (51.45–74.16)	0.73
Moderate	46 (9.81)	137 (33.41)	74.43	53.02 (27.90–69.40)	53.66 (30.05–69.31)	45.22 (4.02–71.16)	0.89
Vigorous	55 (11.85)	125 (30.12)	45.10	60.73 (47.61–70.56)	66.55 (49.73–77.75)	46.66 (33.85–78.07)	0.99

	Complete case records analyses						
Subgroups	**Conversion from prediabetes to diabetes, number of events, n (%)**		**Test statistic (χ^2)**	**Unadjusted RRR (95% CI)**	**RRR-adjusted for covariates (95% CI)**	**Cluster-adjusted RRR (95% CI)**	**$P_{interaction}$**
	YLP (n = 1712)	**Control (n = 1668)**					
Overall, n = 3380	192 (11.21)	534 (32.01)	216.65	64.97 (59.28–64.97)	63.03 (54.45–69.99)	63.20 (54.79–70.04)	
					62.98 (54.38–69.96)	#63.16 (54.74–70.02)	
Age, years				64.62 (57.70-70.42)			
≤40 years	40 (8.26)	120 (26.67)	55.63	69.01 (56.72–69.01)	64.78 (44.57–77.62)	66.79 (48.81–78.46)	0.90
>40 years	152 (12.38)	414 (33.99)	160.59	63.58 (56.92–63.58)	62.13 (51.97–70.15)	62.31 (52.22–70.26)	
Gender							
Male	68 (10.00)	210 (30.30)	86.82	66.86 (57.35–66.86)	58.92 (41.94–70.94)	59.75 (43.28–71.44)	0.90
Female	124 (12.01)	324 (33.33)	131.05	63.95 (56.52–63.95)	64.59 (53.85–72.84)	64.89 (54.39–72.97)	
Location							
Rural	40 (8.06)	282 (33.73)	146.16	75.98 (67.18–75.98)	69.29 (60.49–76.13)	69.48 (60.78–76.24)	0.36
Urban	152 (12.50)	252 (30.0)	121.50	58.93 (50.79–58.93)	52.38 (46.42–57.68)	44.30 (17.19–62.53)	
BMI, kg/m²							
≤23	109 (.27)	410 (31.67)	130.16	64.40 (56.77–64.40)	62.59 (49.83–72.11)	63.07 (53.12–70.90)	0.90
>23	35 (11.59)	124 (33.24)	43.46	65.14 (50.87–65.14)	64.00 (44.00–76.86)	64.35 (45.37–76.74)	
Physical activity							
No	62 (11.78)	228 (32.29)	70.43	63.50 (52.80–63.50)	64.49 (49.40–75.08)	64.82 (50.04–75.23)	
Mild	63 (11.75)`	157 (30.13)	54.16	61.00 (49.10–61.00)	69.02 (55.88–78.24)	69.14 (56.11–78.31)	0.89
Moderate	39 (10.10)	127 (34.14)	64.00	70.41 (58.86–70.41)	53.02 (27.90–69.40)	54.04 (29.73–69.94)	0.85
Vigorous	28 (10.61)	22 (31.88)	19.41	66.74 (45.62–66.74)	46.95 (23.50–77.21)	49.61 (17.19–78.33)	0.86

The Chi-Square test was used to calculate χ^2 values, and t-values were derived from independent samples t-test result. Relative risk reduction (RRR) was calculated by mixed-effects logistic regression models. Models were adjusted for all the covariates age, gender, location, baseline BMI levels, and physical activity levels except for the categorizing variables. Clusters were entered as random effects and the RRRs were separately presented under sensitivity analyses. Interaction between YLP and subgroups was calculated as per the statistical notes reported by Altman and Bland, 2003, results are mentioned in terms of $P_{interaction}$ Assessments were also done on the imputed datasets generated by conducting 50 iterations under intention-to-treat basis. #RRRs were additionally adjusted for post-BMI levels.

Source: Raghuram, N., Ram, V., Majumdar, V., SK, R., Singh, A., Patil, S., Anand, A., Judu, I., Bhaskara, S., Basa, J. R., & Nagendra, H. R. (2021). Effectiveness of a Yoga-Based Lifestyle Protocol (YLP) in preventing diabetes in a high-risk Indian cohort: A multicenter cluster-randomized controlled trial (NMB-Trial). *Frontiers in Endocrinology*, *12*, 664657. https://doi.org/10.3389/fendo.2021.664657 (accessed on 29th May 2025).

Additionally, analyses revealed that YLP facilitated regression to normoglycemia (adjusted odds ratio [adjOR] = 1.20 [95% CI, 1.02–1.43]), particularly in younger participants (≤40 years). Overall, the authors highlighted the "proof" of the potential of yoga in handling yoga (Table 5.35).

Table 5.35. Statistical Analyses (NMB Trial) Highlighting the Potential of Yoga

	Conversion to normoglycemia			Logistic regression		$P_{interaction}$
	YLP	Control	Test statistic (χ^2)	Adjusted Odd's Ratio (95% CI)	p-value	
Overall, n (%)	904 (55.55)	630 (59.47)	4.09*	1.20 (1.02–1.43) #1.21 (1.02–1.44)	0.030 0.029	
Age						
Age ≤ 40 years, n (%)	264 (54.54)	138 (30.67)	23.60*	2.17 (1.53–3.07)	<0.001	<0.001
Age>40 years, n (%)	640 (52.11)	492 (40.39)	0.56	1.04 (0.84–1.29)	0.69	
Gender						
Females, n (%)	520 (57.27)	342 (52.78)	3.09*	1.32 (1.05–1.67)	0.018	0.319
Males, n (%)	384 (62.74)	288 (59.26)	1.39	1.13 (0.85–1.51)	0.386	
Area						
Rural, n (%)	228 (50.00)	360 (64.52)	21.70**	1.57 (1.19–2.07)	<0.001	0.063
Urban, n (%)	676 (63.52)	270 (46.87)	42.49**	2.08 (1.65–2.62)	<0.001	
BMI						
≤23 kg/m², n (%)	510 (59.44)	505 (57.06)	1.03	1.14 (0.93–1.40)	0.196	0.251
>23 kg/m², n (%)	158 (59.18)	125 (50.20)	4.19*	1.72 (1.17–2.53)	0.002	
Physical activity						
No (n = 942)	904 (59.47)	630 (55.55)	0.70	1.13 (0.85–1.50)	0.410	
Mild (n = 837)	285 (60.25)	206 (56.59)	1.14	1.19 (0.88–1.61)	0.256	0.95
Moderate (n = 592)	206 (59.36)	138 (56.32)	0.54	1.32 (0.93–1.89)	0.123	0.86
Vigorous (n = 283)	150 (63.56)	28 (59.57)	0.27	1.20 (0.16–9.04)	0.859	0.99

*Pearson's chi-square test, *p < 0.05, **p < 0.001 Odd's ratio calculated by logistic regression, Models used clusters as random effects and were adjusted for all the covariates age, gender, location, baseline BMI levels and physical activity levels except for the categorizing variables. $P_{interaction}$ values were calculated as per the statistical notes reported by Altman and Bland, 2003; #additionally adjusted for post BMI levels.*

Source: Raghuram, N., Ram, V., Majumdar, V., SK, R., Singh, A., Patil, S., Anand, A., Judu, I., Bhaskara, S., Basa, J. R., & Nagendra, H. R. (2021). Effectiveness of a Yoga-Based Lifestyle Protocol (YLP) in preventing diabetes in a high-risk Indian cohort: A multicenter cluster-randomized controlled trial (NMB-Trial). *Frontiers in Endocrinology, 12*, 664657. https://doi.org/10.3389/fendo.2021.664657 (accessed on 29th May 2025).

These findings have shown the potential of yoga in managing diabetes. However, it should be noted that a complex condition like diabetes needs a multipronged approach encompassing optimal treatment modules backed by strong research.

"We are not going to change the whole world, but we can change ourselves and feel free as birds. We can be serene even in the midst of calamities and, by our serenity, make others more tranquil. Serenity is contagious. If we smile at someone, he or she will smile back. And a smile costs nothing. We should plague everyone with joy. If we are to die in a minute, why not die happily, laughing? (136–137)"

—Sri S. Satchidananda, The Yoga Sutras of Patanjali

References

1. Angusubalakshmi, R., Mary Vaishali, P., & Parasuraman, G. (2024). Beyond the badge: A scoping review among police personnel in South India exploring the impact of yoga and health education on cardiovascular health. *Cureus, 16*(9), e68370. https://doi.org/10.7759/cureus.68370.
2. Bablis, P., Day, R. R., & Pollard, H. (2024). Treatment of type 2 diabetes and stress using neuro-emotional technique: Case report. *Frontiers in Endocrinology, 15*, 1382757. https://doi.org/10.3389/fendo.2024.1382757.
3. Baharvand-Ahmadi, B., Bahmani, M., Tajeddini, P., Naghdi, N., & Rafieian-Kopaei, M. (2016). An ethno-medicinal study of medicinal plants used for the treatment of diabetes. *Journal of Nephropathologist, 5*(1), 44–50. https://doi.org/10.15171/jnp.2016.08.
4. Chapman, A., Liu, S., Merkouris, S., Enticott, J. C., Yang, H., Browning, C. J., & Thomas, S. A. (2015). Psychological interventions for the management of glycemic and psychological outcomes of type 2 diabetes mellitus in China: A systematic review and meta-analyses of randomized controlled trials. *Frontiers in Public Health, 3*, 252. https://doi.org/10.3389/fpubh.2015.00252.
5. Chattopadhyay, K., Mishra, P., Manjunath, N. K., Harris, T., Hamer, M., Greenfield, S. M., Wang, H., Singh, K., Lewis, S. A., Tandon, N., Kinra, S., & Prabhakaran, D. (2020). Development of a Yoga Program for Type-2 Diabetes Prevention (YOGA-DP) among high-risk people in India. *Frontiers in Public Health, 8*, 548674. https://doi.org/10.3389/fpubh.2020.548674.
6. Chattopadhyay, K., Wang, H., Kaur, J., Nalbant, G., Almaqhawi, A., Kundakci, B., Panniyammakal, J., Heinrich, M., Lewis, S. A., Greenfield, S. M., Tandon, N., Biswas, T. K., Kinra, S., & Leonardi-Bee, J. (2022). Effectiveness and safety of Ayurvedic medicines in type 2 diabetes mellitus management: A systematic review and meta-analysis. *Frontiers in Pharmacology, 13*, 821810. https://doi.org/10.3389/fphar.2022.821810.
7. Cho, E., & Kim, W. (2021). Effect of acupuncture on diabetic neuropathy: A narrative review. *International Journal of Molecular Sciences, 22*(16), 8575. https://doi.org/10.3390/ijms22168575.
8. Cramer, H., Lauche, R., Haller, H., Steckhan, N., Michalsen, A., & Dobos, G. (2014). Effects of yoga on cardiovascular disease risk factors: A systematic review and meta-analysis. *International Journal of Cardiology, 173*(2), 170–183. https://doi.org/10.1016/j.ijcard.2014.02.017.
9. Dening, J., Islam, S., George, E., & Maddison, R. (2020). Web-based interventions for dietary behavior in adults with type 2 diabetes: Systematic review of randomized controlled trials. *Journal of Medical Internet Research, 22*(8), e16437. https://doi.org/10.2196/16437.
10. Elmi, G. R., Anum, K., Saleem, K., Fareed, R., Noreen, S., Wei, H., Chen, Y., Chakraborty, A., Rehman, M. U., Liyuan, S., Abbas, M., & Duan, Y. (2023). Evaluation of clinical trials of ethnomedicine used for the treatment of diabetes: A systematic review. *Frontiers in Pharmacology, 14*, 1176618. https://doi.org/10.3389/fphar.2023.1176618.
11. Healy, S. J., Black, D., Harris, C., Lorenz, A., & Dungan, K. M. (2013). Inpatient diabetes education is associated with less frequent hospital readmission among patients with poor glycemic control. *Diabetes Care, 36*(10), 2960–2967. https://doi.org/10.2337/dc13-0108.

12. Innes, K. E., & Selfe, T. K. (2016). Yoga for adults with type 2 diabetes: A systematic review of controlled trials. *Journal of Diabetes Research, 2016*, 6979370. https://doi.org/10.1155/2016/6979370.
13. Islam, S. M. S., Mishra, V., Siddiqui, M. U., Moses, J. C., Adibi, S., Nguyen, L., & Wickramasinghe, N. (2022). Smartphone apps for diabetes medication adherence: Systematic review. *JMIR Diabetes, 7*(2), e33264. https://doi.org/10.2196/33264.
14. Istepanian, R. S. H. (2022). Mobile health (m-Health) in retrospect: The known unknowns. *International Journal of Environmental Research and Public Health, 19*(7), 3747. https://doi.org/10.3390/ijerph19073747.
15. Kaur, N., Majumdar, V., Nagarathna, R., Anand, A., Sharma, K., Patil, S. S., & Raghuram, N. (2021). Diabetic yoga protocol improves glycemic, anthropometric and lipid levels in high-risk individuals for diabetes: A randomized controlled trial from Northern India. *Diabetology & Metabolic Syndrome, 13*, 149. https://doi.org/10.1186/s13098-021-00761-1.
16. Kirwan, M., Vandelanotte, C., Fenning, A., & Duncan, M. (2013). Diabetes self-management smartphone application for adults with type 1 diabetes: Randomized controlled trial. *Journal of Medical Internet Research, 15*(11), e235. https://doi.org/10.2196/jmir.2588.
17. Modak, M., Dixit, P., Londhe, J., Ghaskadbi, S., & Devasagayam, T. P. (2007). Indian herbs and herbal drugs used for the treatment of diabetes. *Journal of Clinical Biochemistry and Nutrition, 40*(3), 163–173. https://doi.org/10.3164/jcbn.40.163.
18. Murudkar, P. H., Tambe, M. S., Chandrasekar, S. B., Boddeda, B., & Pawar, A. T. (2022). Common Ayurvedic, Chinese traditional and Unani antidiabetic formulations–A review. *Frontiers in Pharmacology, 13*, 991083. https://doi.org/10.3389/fphar.2022.991083.
19. National Institutes of Health Office of Dietary Supplements. (2011). *Botanical Dietary Supplements: Background Information*. http://ods.od.nih.gov/factsheets/botanicalbackground.asp (accessed on 21 May 2025).
20. Pereira, W. V. C., Vancea, D. M. M., de Andrade Oliveira, R., et al. (2023). Position of Brazilian Diabetes Society on exercise recommendations for people with type 1 and type 2 diabetes. *Diabetology & Metabolic Syndrome, 15*, 2. https://doi.org/10.1186/s13098-022-00945-3.
21. Raghuram, N., Ram, V., Majumdar, V., S. K., R., Singh, A., Patil, S., Anand, A., Judu, I., Bhaskara, S., Basa, J. R., & Nagendra, H. R. (2021). Effectiveness of a Yoga-Based Lifestyle Protocol (YLP) in preventing diabetes in a high-risk Indian cohort: A multicenter cluster-randomized controlled trial (NMB-trial). *Frontiers in Endocrinology, 12*, 664657. https://doi.org/10.3389/fendo.2021.664657.
22. Rashrash, M., Schommer, J. C., & Brown, L. M. (2017). Prevalence and predictors of herbal medicine use among adults in the United States. *Journal of Patient Experience, 4*(3), 108–113. https://doi.org/10.1177/2374373517706612.
23. Roca, S., Lozano, M. L., García, J., & Alesanco, Á. (2021). Validation of a virtual assistant for improving medication adherence in patients with comorbid type 2 diabetes mellitus and depressive disorder. *International Journal of Environmental Research and Public Health, 18*(22), 12056. https://doi.org/10.3390/ijerph182212056.
24. Rodríguez, I. A., Serafini, M., Alves, I. A., Lang, K. L., Silva, F. R. M. B., & Aragón, D. M. (2023). Natural products as outstanding alternatives in diabetes mellitus: A patent review. *Pharmaceutics, 15*(1), 85. https://doi.org/10.3390/pharmaceutics15010085.

INDEX